Novak's
Gynecology

Jonathan S. Berek, editor

Self-Assessment and Review

Novak's
Gynecology

Jonathan S. Berek, editor

Self-Assessment and Review

David L. Olive, MD

Professor and Chief
Reproductive Endocrinology and Infertility
Department of Obstetrics and Gynecology
Yale University School of Medicine
New Haven, Connecticut

Jonathan S. Berek, MD, MMSc

Professor and Vice Chair
Chief of Gynecology and Gynecologic Oncology
Department of Obstetrics and Gynecology
UCLA School of Medicine
Director, UCLA Women's Gynecologic Oncology Center
Jonsson Comprehensive Cancer Center
Los Angeles, California

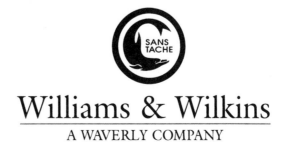

Williams & Wilkins
A WAVERLY COMPANY

BALTIMORE • PHILADELPHIA • LONDON • PARIS • BANGKOK
BUENOS AIRES • HONG KONG • MUNICH • SYDNEY • TOKYO • WROCLAW

Editor: Charles W. Mitchell
Managing Editor: Marjorie Kidd Keating
Marketing Manager: Peter Darcy
Project Editor: Robert D. Magee
Designer: Tim Hengst

Library of Congress Cataloging-in-Publication Data

Novak's gynecology : self-assessment and review / [edited by] David L. Olive,
    Jonathan S. Berek.
        p.   cm.
    Includes bibliographical references.
    ISBN 0-683-00589-8
        1. Gynecology—Examinations, questions, etc.   2. Gynecology—Outlines, syllabi, etc.
    I. Olive, David L.   II. Berek, Jonathan S.   III. Novak, Emil, 1883–1957.
        [DNLM: 1. Genital Diseases, Female examination questions.
    2. Pregnancy Complications examination questions.   3. Gynecology—methods examination
    questions.   WP 18.2 N935 1998]
    RG111.N68   1998
    618.1'0076—dc21
    DNLM/DLC   97-50305
    for Library of Congress   CIP

Dedication
We dedicate this book to our spouses, Katie and Deborah
and to our children, Zachary, Matthew, and Alex, and
Jonathan, James, and Jessica

Preface

Novak's Gynecology has established a proud tradition, and the Twelfth Edition has been well received. Our colleagues and students suggested that we develop a study guide to complement the book. The purpose of this guide is to facilitate the review of the text and to help the reader retain concepts presented in the longer format. We have chosen the same design as *Novak's Gynecology, 12th Edition,* with selected figures and tables to enhance the reader's understanding of the book. Several appendices summarize frequently used information.

Each chapter contains several questions, along with brief explanations of their answers and references to the source material in *Novak's Gynecology, 12th Edition.* We encourage our readers to use the questions to prompt a more careful study of the material and a more thorough understanding of the subject.

David L. Olive
Jonathan S. Berek

Acknowledgment

We wish to acknowledge the support we have received from the publishers, especially Charley Mitchell and Margie Keating; the excellent manuscript processing of Annabelle Perez and Leslie Radcliffe; Tim Hengst for his superb illustrations; and all of our colleagues who contributed their time and effort to assist in the completion of this study guide.

Contents

Contributors

David A. Baram, MD

Associate Professor Department of Obstetrics, Gynecology, and Psychiatry
University of Rochester School of Medicine and Dentistry
Rochester, New York

Ross S. Berkowitz, MD

William H. Baker Professor of Gynecology
Harvard Medical School
Director of Gynecology and Gynecologic Oncology
Co-Director of New England Trophoblastic Disease Center
Brigham and Women's Hospital
and Dana Farber Cancer Institute
Boston, Massachusetts

Robert E. Bristow, MD

Gynecologic Oncology Fellow
Department of Obstetrics and Gynecology
UCLA School of Medicine
Los Angeles, California

Lee-may Chen, MD

Gynecologic Oncology Fellow
Department of Obstetrics and Gynecology
UCLA School of Medicine
Los Angeles, California

Daniel L. Clarke-Pearson, MD

James M. Ingram Professor and Director
Division of Gynecologic Oncology
Department of Obstetrics and Gynecology
Duke University Medical Center
Durham, North Carolina

Daniel W. Cramer, MD, ScD

Associate Professor
Department of Obstetrics, Gynecology and Reproductive Biology
Brigham and Women's Hospital
Harvard Medical Center
Boston, Massachusetts

Oliver Dorigo, MD

Resident
Obstetrics and Gynecology
Department of Obstetrics and Gynecology
UCLA School of Medicine
Los Angeles, California

Joseph C. Gambone, DO

Associate Professor
Department of Obstetrics and Gynecology
UCLA School of Medicine
Los Angeles, California

Armando E. Giuliano, MD

Clinical Professor of Surgery
Department of Surgery
UCLA School of Medicine
Los Angeles, California
Director, Joyce Eisenberg Keefer Breast Center
John Wayne Cancer Institute
Saint John's Hospital and Health Center
Santa Monica, California

Donald P. Goldstein, MD

Associate Professor of Obstetrics, Gynecology,
and Reproductive Biology
Harvard Medical School
Director, New England's Trophoblastic
Disease Center
Brigham and Women's Hospital
Boston, Massachusetts

Joseph A. Hill, MD

Director of Reproductive Medicine
Department of Obstetrics, Gynecology,
and Reproductive Biology
Harvard Medical School
Brigham and Women's Hospital
Boston, Massachusetts

Paula A. Hillard, MD

Associate Professor
Department of Obstetrics and Gynecology
Department of Pediatrics
University of Cincinnati College of Medicine
Cincinnati, Ohio

William W. Hurd, MD

Associate Professor and Director
Division of Reproductive Endocrinology
Department of Obstetrics and Gynecology
University of Indiana Medical Center
Indianapolis, Indiana

John R. Lurain, MD

John and Ruth Brewer Professor of
Gynecology and Cancer Research
Section Head, Gynecologic Oncology
Department of Obstetrics and Gynecology
Northwestern University Medical School
Chicago, Illinois

Howard D. McClamrock, MD

Associate Professor
Department of Obstetrics and Gynecology
Division of Reproductive Endocrinology
University of Maryland School of Medicine
Baltimore, Maryland

Malcolm G. Munro, MD

Associate Professor of
Clinical Obstetrics and Gynecology
Olive View/UCLA Medical Center
UCLA School of Medicine
Los Angeles, California

Robert W. Rebar, MD

Professor and Director
Department of Obstetrics and Gynecology
College of Medicine
University of Cincinnati
Cincinnati, Ohio

Wendy J. Scherzer, MD

Assistant Professor
Department of Obstetrics and Gynecology
Temple University Hospital
Philadelphia, Pennsylvania

Anne P. Shapter, MD

Gynecologic Oncology
Lahey Hitchock Medical Center
Burlington, Massachussetts

Nada L. Stotland, MD

Associate Professor
Departments of Psychiatry and Obstetrics and Gynecology
The University of Chicago
Medical Coordinator
Division of Mental Health
Illinois Department of Mental Health and Developmental Disabilities
Chicago, Illinois

Phillip G. Stubblefield, MD

Professor and Chair
Department of Obstetrics and Gynecology
Boston University School of Medicine
Boston, Massachusetts

Gillian M. Thomas, MD

Head, Department of Radiation Oncology
Toronto-Sunnybrook Regional Cancer Centre
North York, Ontario, Canada
Associate Professor
Departments of Radiation Oncology, and Obstetrics and Gynecology
University of Toronto
Toronto, Ontario, Canada

Felipe L.G. Videla, MD

Instructor
Department of Obstetrics and Gynecology
Louisiana State University Medical Center
New Orleans, Louisiana

L. Lewis Wall, MD, DPhil

Associate Professor
Department of Obstetrics and Gynecology
Louisiana State University Medical Center
New Orleans, Louisiana

Robert C. Young, MD

President
Fox Chase Cancer Center
Philadelphia, Pennsylvania

PRINCIPLES
OF PRACTICE

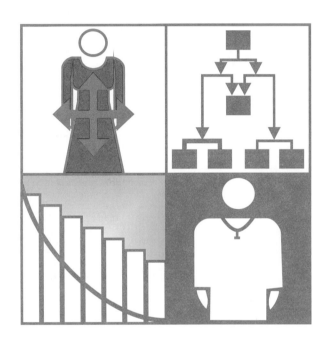

1

Initial Assessment and Communication

Paula A. Hillard
Jonathan S. Berek

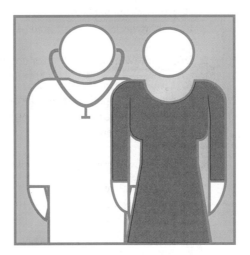

Learning Objectives

1. Be aware of the importance of communication in physician/patient interactions.

2. Recognize the value of open-ended questions in interviewing.

3. Be aware of the extent to which the patient's psychological reaction to her illness affects her responses.

4. Be able to describe and document the female genital examination for the medical record.

5. Be able to recognize and choose an appropriately sized vaginal speculum for individual patients.

Questions

1. A 30-year-old married woman comes to the office with the stated symptom of a vaginal discharge. During the interview, she appears anxious. She describes a yellow, malodorous discharge. Each of the following techniques would be helpful in determining the cause of her distress **except:**

    A. Asking her what she fears may be the cause of her symptoms
    B. Allowing her to describe her symptoms without interruption
    C. Direct questioning about the possibility of STDs
    D. Confronting her with suspicions about her sexual practices
    E. Asking her about associated psychological symptoms

2. Of the following techniques for communication with a patient, the physician should:

    A. Listen more and talk less
    B. Interrupt the patient when she comes to the essential point in her history
    C. Provide a lecture to the patient on her disease
    D. Avoid open-ended questions

3. Of the following, which portion of the physical examination should be performed last:

    A. Uterine palpation
    B. Vulvar inspection
    C. Rectal examination
    D. Cervical inspection
    E. Abdominal palpation

4. A 42-year-old woman presents to the office with pelvic and abdominal pain, bloating, painful but regular menses, and weight loss. Each of the following is indicated during the physical examination **except:**

    A. Pap smear
    B. Bimanual examination
    C. Rectovaginal examination
    D. Examination of stool for occult blood
    E. Endometrial biopsy

5. A 16-year-old young woman presents to the emergency department with severe abdominal and pelvic pain. Her last menstrual period was six weeks before, and a urine pregnancy test is positive. She states that she has been sexually active, and that condoms were used inconsistently. She states that she has never before had a pelvic examination. The most appropriate vaginal speculum for this patient would be:

    A. Grave's extra-long
    B. Grave's regular
    C. Pederson extra-long
    D. Pederson regular
    E. Pediatric short speculum

Answers

1. **D**

    The art and techniques of obtaining a medical history vary with the patient, the type of problem with which she presents, and the physician's own style. Techniques not conducive to appropriate communication between the physician and the patient, and which are generally best avoided, include behavior that is confrontational, combative, condescending, overbearing, or judgmental. Open-ended questions that allow the patient to

talk about her chief complaint are appropriate. After allowing her to describe the symptoms most bothersome to her, additional information can be obtained by direct questioning. This allows the clinician to formulate hypotheses that can be tested using additional questioning to formulate a differential diagnosis. A review of symptoms also may be helpful if the diagnosis does not seem obvious. The clinician should be aware of the influence of the patient's emotional state on her reaction to disease. Psychological factors or a psychiatric diagnosis may be complicating the presentation of illness. In addition, the patient may well have a different understanding, interpretation, or concern about her symptoms. It is often helpful to elicit that information.
Reference: Pages 3–9

2. A

In general, the physician needs to be a good listener. The physician needs to give the patient maximum opportunity to speak freely, avoiding interruptions, lectures, and soliloquies. It is advisable to ask open-ended questions to encourage maximum responses. The following are techniques to help achieve rapport with patients:

- Use positive language, e.g., agreement, approval, and humor.
- Build a partnership, e.g., acknowledge understanding, ask for opinions, paraphrase and interpret the patient's words.
- Ask rephrased questions.
- Give complete responses to the patient's questions.

Some general guidelines that help to improve communication follow:

- Listen more and talk less.
- Encourage the pursuit of topics introduced by and important to the patient.
- Minimize controlling speech habits such as interrupting, issuing commands, and lecturing.
- Seek out questions and provide full and understandable answers.
- Become aware of discomfort in an interview, recognize when it originates in an attempt by the physician to take control, and redirect that attempt.
- Assure patients that they have the opportunity to fully discuss their problem.
- Recognize when patients may be seeking empathy and validation of their feelings rather than a solution. Sometimes all that is necessary is to be a compassionate human being.

An interview that permits maximum transmission of information to the physician is best achieved by the following approach:

- Begin with an "open" question.
- As the patient begins to speak, pay attention not only to her answers but also to her emotions and general body language.
- Extend a second question or comment, encouraging the patient to talk.
- Allow the patient to respond without interrupting, perhaps by using silence, nods, or small facilitative comments to encourage the patient to talk while the physician is listening.
- Summarize and express empathy and understanding at the completion of the interview.

Attentiveness, rapport, and collaboration characterize good medical interviewing techniques. Open-ended questions are generally desirable, particularly when coupled with good listening skills.
Reference: Pages 6–9

3. C

Typically, the abdominal examination should be done prior to the pelvic examination. The rectal examination should be performed after the direct examination and should be

performed in premenopausal women as needed to assist the examiner in the assessment of the pelvic structures; when there is a suspicion of colorectal pathology (e.g., when appendicitis has been excluded, or the patient complains of passing blood per rectum); and routinely in postmenopausal women.
Reference: Pages 12–18

4. E

The patient described could have a number of gynecologic problems, including ovarian or cervical cancer. The possibility of rectal disease or a gastrointestinal malignancy should also be kept in mind. The examination is designed to evaluate these possible causes of her symptoms. Screening for cervical cancer with a Pap smear and for colon cancer using a test for occult blood in the stool are both appropriate tests. A rectovaginal examination or a rectal exam alone is indicated given these symptoms. An endometrial biopsy is not indicated, given that the patient describes only dysmenorrhea, without menstrual abnormalities.
Reference: Pages 13–18

5. D (see Fig. 1.2)

The choice of an appropriate vaginal speculum can make the difference between an examination that is painful for the patient and thus relatively unrevealing, and an exam that is uncomfortable, yet tolerable, which allows valuable information to be gained. In general, the smallest speculum necessary to produce adequate visualization should be used. The speculum should be warmed (on a heating pad or with warm water) prior to insertion. The most appropriate speculum for *most* individuals during a routine examination is the Pederson speculum. Sexually active adult women may require a Grave's speculum if the vagina is particularly redundant or cervical procedures are indicated. A long speculum is rarely required, but may be indicated if the woman's buttocks preclude sufficient depth of insertion. The first pelvic examination for an adolescent is typically an anxiety-provoking experience. Most young women, even those who have not been sexually active, can tolerate an examination with the Pederson speculum. Some young women who are virginal may require a Huffman speculum (also called the narrow or virginal speculum) if the hymenal ring is tight. The so-called "pediatric" speculum, a short speculum, is almost never indicated in prepubertal girls for an exam in the office, but may occasionally be required for an examination under anesthesia. Its short length is inadequate to allow visualization of the cervix in menarchal women, and thus should not be used.
Reference: Pages 15–16

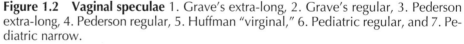

Figure 1.2 Vaginal speculae 1. Grave's extra-long, 2. Grave's regular, 3. Pederson extra-long, 4. Pederson regular, 5. Huffman "virginal," 6. Pediatric regular, and 7. Pediatric narrow.

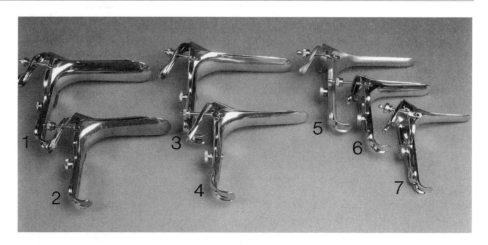

2 Principles of Patient Care

David L. Olive

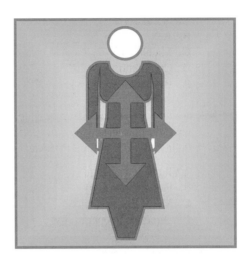

Learning Objectives

1. Know the principles and concepts for ethical decision-making.

2. Understand the purpose of confidentiality and informed consent.

3. Be able to identify and deal with conflicts of interest.

4. Understand the concept of justice in the provision of health care.

Questions

1. A patient presents to her physician's office for HIV testing, but is concerned that the information resulting from the test could be damaging to her career. The ethical principle that prohibits the phyician from revealing such information to a third party without consent of the patient is:

   A. Autonomy
   B. Justice
   C. Maleficence
   D. Confidentiality
   E. Beneficence

2. An interactive discussion in which one participant has greater knowledge about medical information and the other participant has greater knowledge about that individual's value system and circumstances affected by the information is termed:

   A. Informed consent
   B. Patient autonomy
   C. Mutual expressivity
   D. Directive cooperativity

3. A patient with severe pelvic pain presents to your office after seven prior surgeries in the previous two years. You assess her situation, review her records, examine her, and conclude that her best option is to begin medical therapy and that surgery has no role in her future care. She refuses and demands surgery immediately. Your ethical obligation is to:

   A. Operate on the patient
   B. Insist upon medical therapy
   C. Do not institute medical therapy, but refuse to operate
   D. Have the situation arbitrated by a third party

4. The effect of therapy on the patient's experience of living, based on her perspective, is called:

   A. Experiential care
   B. Quality of life
   C. Patient-based outcome assessment
   D. Efficacy

5. A local physician owns partial interest in a magnetic resonance imaging scanner down the road. He sees a patient with multiple leiomyomata desiring conservative surgery. He believes that to perform optimal surgery, MRI assessment of the exact size and location of the tumors is required prior to the procedure. There is no state law that addresses the appropriate actions of the physician in this setting. His most appropriate course of action is:

   A. Avoid the MRI and proceed directly to surgery
   B. Perform the MRI at the local scanner, but inform the patient of the financial conflict of interest
   C. Perform an alternative imaging study
   D. Send the patient to the MRI scanner in the next county

6. The fair and equitable distribution of the burdens and benefits of health care delivery is termed:

   A. Justice
   B. Maleficence
   C. Covenant
   D. Beneficence

Answers

The practice of gynecology, as true for all aspects of medicine, is based on ethical principles that guide patient care. These principles and concepts create a framework for ethical decision-making that applies to all aspects of practice:

- Autonomy: A person's right to self-rule, to establish personal norms of conduct, and to choose a course of action based on a set of personal values and principles derived from them.
- Beneficence: The obligation to promote the well-being of others.
- Confidentiality: A person's right to decide how and to whom personal medical information will be communicated.
- Covenant: A binding agreement between two or more parties for the performance of some action.
- Fiduciary Relationship: A relationship founded on faith and trust.
- Informed Consent: The patient's acceptance of a medical intervention after adequate disclosure of the nature of the procedure, its risks and benefits, and alternatives.
- Justice: The right of individuals to claim what is due them based on certain personal properties or characteristics.
- Maleficence: The act of committing harm (nonmaleficence obliges one to avoid doing harm).

1. D

Confidentiality is an expression of the trust or covenantal relationship between physician and patient. The patient seeking assistance from a health professional has the right to be assured that the information exchanged during the interaction is private. The right to privacy prohibits a physician from revealing information regarding the patient unless the patient waives that privilege. The only exceptions to this principle are when this right impinges on the legal and ethical rights of institutions and society at large, or if so declared by legislation.
Reference: Pages 22–23

2. A

Informed consent is a process that involves an exchange of information directed toward reaching mutual understanding and informed decision-making. Ideally, informed consent should be the practical manifestation of respect for patient preferences (autonomy). In essence, informed consent is a conversation between physician and patient that teaches the patient about the medical condition, explores her values, and informs her about the reasonable medical alternatives.
Reference: Page 23

3. C

Autonomy, the patient's right to choose to receive or refuse medical care, is an important ethical principle. However, it is not respect for a patient's wishes against good medical judgment. The physician's ethical obligation is to seek the best for the patient's care (beneficence) and avoid harm (maleficence) of surgery, even if that is what the patient wants. Physicians are not obligated to offer treatment they believe to be of no benefit to the patient. The patient does, however, have the right to refuse treatment if it does not conform with her values. Thus, the patient can refuse medical therapy, but she has no right to demand any treatment she wishes.
Reference: Pages 23–24

4. B

Quality of life (QOL) is a much used but often unclear term. Basically, it refers to assessing the results of treatment intervention from the patient's perspective, not that of the physician, family members, or other interested parties. It is perilous and wholly speculative to assume that physicians know what QOL represents for a particular patient. Often, the patient may bring a host of modifying feelings, attitudes, and desires to any decision-making or evaluative process—factors known or understood only by the patient herself.

Controversy exists regarding whether currently available QOL measurement systems will provide information to help patients make decisions. Informing patients of others' experiences with alternative treatments may help in their decision-making, but this is never a substitute for individual patient decision-making.
Reference: Page 25

5. B

The reality of care in the 1990s is that health care givers make many decisions under the pressure of multiple conflicts of interest. Physicians are continually caught between self-interest and professional integrity. Focusing clearly on meeting the patient's best interest and responsibly rejecting choices that compromise the patient's needs are ethical requirements. Frequently, state law will address physician behavior in these situations. However, in the absence of such directive, it is still ethically necessary for financial conflicts of interest to be revealed to patients.
Reference: Pages 26–27

6. A

Justice is the right of individuals to claim what is due them based on certain personal properties or characteristics. However, distributing benefits in an equitable manner is a matter of great debate. There are various methods of proposed distribution:

- Equal shares (everyone has the same number of health care dollars per year).
- Need (only those people who need health care get the dollars).
- Queuing (the first in line for a transplant gets it).
- Merit (those with more serious illnesses receive special benefits).
- Contribution (those who have paid more into their health care fund get more health care).

Each may be just in some situations, but each will effect an individual patient in a different way. The principle of justice applies when a resource is desired or beneficial and to some extent scarce. With scarce resources, the overall benefits for all patients are considered in conjunction with the individual benefits for one patient. These decisions are frequently among the most difficult in health care delivery.
Reference: Page 28

3 Quality Assessment and Improvement

Joseph C. Gambone

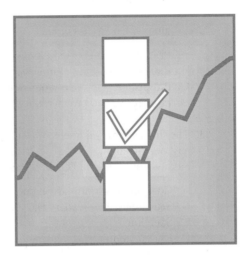

Learning Objectives

1. Understand the concept of quality assurance.

2. Be able to enumerate the principles of quality assessment.

3. Understand the principles of outcomes assessment, including quality-of-life measurement.

4. Be aware of the mechanisms for quality improvement.

Questions

1. The U.S. health care expenditure of 14% of gross domestic product (GDP) in 1996 was:

    A. About the same as other industrialized countries
    B. Less than other countries because of decreased access to care in the United States
    C. Higher than most but with much better outcomes
    D. Higher than any other country with lower overall outcomes

2. Traditional Quality Assurance (QA) compared to Quality Improvement (QI) is:

    A. Prospective and periodic rather than retrospective and continuous
    B. Retrospective and periodic rather than prospective and continuous
    C. Prospective and continuous rather than retrospective and periodic
    D. Prospective and preventative rather than retrospective and self-imposed

3. The first essential element or step to establish a quality improvement (QI) process in any organization, whether it is called continuous quality improvement (CQI), total quality management (TQM), or performance improvement (PI) is:

    A. Controlling variation by using scientific methods
    B. Selecting strong leaders and putting them totally in charge
    C. Spending a great deal of money
    D. Understanding the customer(s) and incorporating this knowledge into the system

4. The terms efficacy, effectiveness, and efficiency are similar but differ importantly in the following way:

    A. Working under ideal conditions versus working under ordinary practice conditions versus representing the best value
    B. Working under ordinary practice conditions versus the best value versus working under ideal conditions
    C. The best value versus working under ideal conditions versus working under ordinary practice conditions
    D. Best practice versus best outcomes versus best value

5. Optimally effective health care is most closely related to:

    A. Effectiveness
    B. Value
    C. Efficiency
    D. Efficacy

6. Improvement in health-related quality of life is primarily determined by:

    A. The process of care, or how the care is delivered
    B. The structure of care, or the quality of the people and equipment
    C. The outcomes of care, or how the patient actually is helped
    D. All of the above

7. Variation or differences in the way that medical or surgical care is delivered:

    A. Should be totally eliminated
    B. Is always appropriate and represents the "art of medicine"
    C. Should be controlled in a way that allows for desirable variation due to patient differences
    D. Is due to financial considerations

8. Studying the variation in resources used (procedures and tests) in women's health care can help improve health care services by:

   A. Identifying overutilization and waste
   B. Identifying underutilization and lack of access to care
   C. Identifying uncertainty and the need for outcomes research
   D. All of the above

9. The PDCA cycle is a quality improvement tool that is used to test small-scale change. The acronym stands for:

   A. Plan, Do, Control, and Advance
   B. Process, Do, Check, and Adjust
   C. Plan, Do, Check, and Act
   D. Process, Direct, Control, and Adjust

10. The basic "essential" element(s) of adequate informed consent are:

    A. Risks and benefits
    B. Risks and alternatives
    C. Rationale, risks, benefits, and alternatives
    D. A thorough discussion of risks and complications

Answers

1. **D**
   Overall health care spending in the United States was estimated to be 14% of gross domestic product (GDP) in 1996. This percent of gross domestic spending has been rising since health care spending statistics were first calculated in the early 1960s, when only 6% of gross domestic product was spent for health care goods and services. Figure 3.1 shows the dramatic drop in out-of-pocket expenditures as compared to those monies that are spent by governments, including federal, state, and local, and by insurance companies. No other country in the world spends as much of their GDP on health care. Despite this, the United States has overall health outcomes, such as longevity, perinatal, and neonatal mortality rates, that are less than other industrialized countries including the United Kingdom, Japan, and Canada where health care spending is significantly less.
   Reference: Pages 33–34

2. **B**
   The traditional methods for assessing and improving quality in health services has tended to be self-imposed and retrospective and takes the form of peer review. Studies indicate that this methodology is not very effective at bringing about improvements in the way that health care is delivered. Health services investigators feel that this retrospective and periodic method of review, with its emphasis on finding "bad apples," is less effective than a process that is designed to be prospective and continuous. This methodology emphasizes that periodic review leads to only periodic improvement, and in order for systems such as health care services to continually improve, the process for quality review must be continuous. Figure 3.2 illustrates how QA or quality assurance is designed to deal with the small percentage of substandard care which is represented on the left side of the figure. Sanctions are used to attempt to eliminate this kind of care. Continuous quality improvement (CQI), on the other hand, attempts to shift the level of care to the right by examining in a nonpunitive fashion the processes of care. Traditional QA is retrospective and periodic rather than prospective and continuous.
   Reference: Pages 34–37

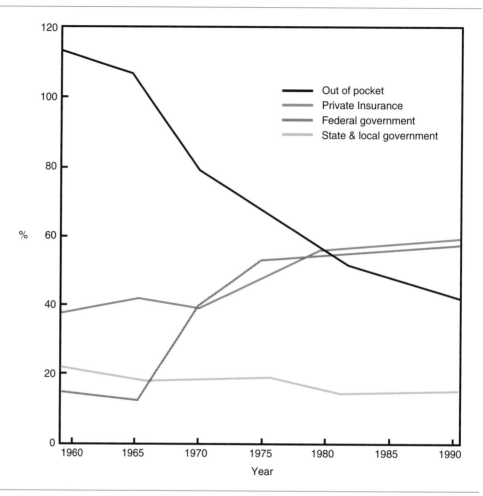

Figure 3.1 Sources of spending in U.S. health care, 1960–1990. Note that third-party payment has steadily replaced direct payment during this interval. (Data from U.S. Congressional Budget Office, 1992).

3. D

Proponents of modern quality management recognize that in order to improve the quality of goods and services, the providers of these products must have a thorough understanding of who their customers are and how these customers view the goods or services in terms of quality and value. The presence of strong leadership and controlling variation using scientific methods, however, are important as a first step.
Reference: Pages 34–37

4. A

Knowing how well health care interventions really work is an essential element for quality assessment and quality improvement. Unfortunately, measurements of the success of health care interventions have tended to be based upon more theoretical or "off line" measurements of true effectiveness. The Institute of Medicine (IOM), along with a number of other organizations and agencies, has defined theoretical effectiveness, or efficacy of a health care intervention, as how it works under ideal conditions that usually exist in traditional clinical trials. Effectiveness, on the other hand, indicates the measurement of how interventions work under ordinary every day clinical practice. A third term, efficiency, is similar to both efficacy and effectiveness; however, efficiency indicates the measurement of effectiveness with the least waste in terms of cost and complications. In other words, efficiency indicates the best value in a given health care intervention.
Reference: Pages 36–37

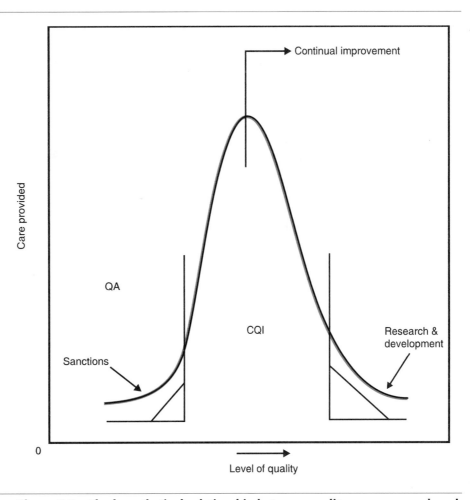

Figure 3.2   The hypothetical relationship between quality assurance and quality improvement.

5. B

Donabedian has differentiated between optimally effective additions to health care and maximally effective additions to that care. Figure 3.3 identifies a "Point A" where the additional benefits for a health care intervention begin to level off or even decrease at a time when costs continue to increase at a greater rate. In the bottom panel, considering costs along with benefits results in a curve that begins to decrease further to "Point B." Point B identifies maximal benefits, but does not consider the proportionately higher addition of costs and, therefore, does not identify the optimally effective level or the level of greatest value.
Reference: Pages 36–37

6. C

The consumers of health care services—patients and potential patients—are increasingly more concerned about health-related quality of life and how it is affected or improved by health care services. Donabedian's model for assessing the quality of health care involves evaluating the structure of care, i.e., the resources, equipment, and people who provide the care; the process of care, i.e., the method by which a health care procedure or treatment is carried out; and, finally, the outcomes of care, which include both short-term adverse events such as complications and side effects as well as the longer term outcomes of health and functional status and health-related quality of life. Improvement, therefore, in health-related quality of life and functional

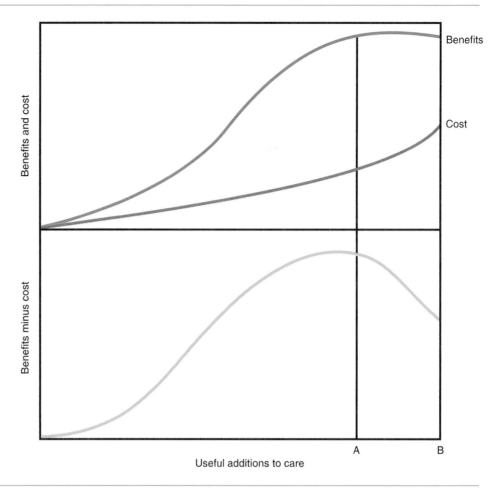

Figure 3.3 The "optimal" versus the "maximal" benefits and costs of medical treatments. *On the top panel,* the benefits to health and the costs of care are plotted. *On the bottom panel,* the cost is subtracted from the benefits, illustrating that after a certain point, additions of care may detract from the benefits. (Reproduced with permission from **Donabedian A.** The quality of care: How can it be assessed. *JAMA* 1988;260:1743–8.)

status is most related to outcomes of care or how a patient is actually helped by a procedure or treatment.
Reference: Pages 38–39

7. **C**

Variation is present in every aspect of life, including health care processes. Also, variation may be either desirable or undesirable. Examples of undesirable variation in health care would be allowing for individual provider preferences for medication, suture materials, catheters, and other equipment without scientifically based reasons for these expensive variations; or allowing for significant variation in the technique or the equipment used during a procedure, resulting in more time and expense, without evidence of improved patient outcomes. It is important to reduce undesirable variation in order to increase efficiency, while at the same time preserving desirable or intended variation that is needed to account for legitimate patient differences and preferences and to allow for innovation in health care technology.
Reference: Pages 40–43

8. D

The scientific study of variation in utilization rates allows clinicians to identify both over- and underutilization of health care services including health care procedures such as hysterectomy and cesarean delivery. Variation in utilization of health care services can be categorized as follows:

- Necessary and intended variation due to well-recognized patient differences such as severity of illness, comorbidity, and legitimate patient preferences.
- Acceptable but reducible variation because of uncertainty and lack of accurate information about outcomes.
- Unacceptable variation because of nonclinical factors such as habitual differences in practice style that are not grounded in knowledge or reason.

The identification of variation can identify over- and underutilization of health care services.
Reference: Pages 40–43

9. C

One model for scientifically testing changes in health care improvement, also used in other industries, is the PDCA cycle, which stands for Plan, Do, Check, and Act. "Do" means to implement the plan or process and collect the data. "Check" means to check the data to determine if the change to the process represents an improvement, and the "Act" means to incorporate the change into the process if it is found to be an improvement. Another cycle with a different change is initiated if an improvement was not measured in the first cycle.
Reference: Page 43

10. C

The process of informed consent evolved in the United States largely because of medical-legal liability that arose secondary to failure to properly inform patients before treatment, in particular, surgical procedures. Recent research has indicated that even the four basic or essential elements for adequate informed consent are not always covered during the informed consent process. Results from the study illustrated that rationale was covered only 43% of the time, a discussion of the benefits only 34% of the time, a discussion of the risks only 14% of the time, and alternatives, 12% of the time. Because clinical outcomes have been shown to improve with more participation of the patient in both decision-making and the delivery of care, researchers are now suggesting a process of informed collaborative choice. One model to accomplish this is the PREPARED checklist.

Procedure:	The course of action being considered
Reason:	The indication or rationale
Expectation:	The chances of benefit and failure
Preferences:	Patient-centered priorities (utilities) affecting choice
Alternatives:	Other reasonable options
Risks:	The potential for harm from procedures
Expenses:	All direct and indirect costs
Decision:	Fully informed collaborative choice

This sequenced checklist has been shown to improve health care decision-making by increasing patient satisfaction and self-efficacy and, therefore, facilitating more appropriate patient choice.
Reference: Pages 43–45

4

Epidemiology for the Gynecologist

Daniel W. Cramer
Jonathan S. Berek

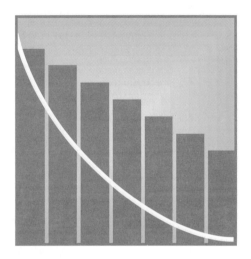

Learning Objectives

1. Be able to distinguish a descriptive study, a nonexperimental study, and an experimental analytic study.

2. Know the difference between incidence and prevalence.

3. Know the difference between a case-control and a cohort study.

4. Be able to define the measures of validity for a screening test including sensitivity and specificity.

5. Know what information is conveyed by a "P value" and a "confidence interval" and the principal types of statistical biases that may affect analytic studies.

6. Gain an appreciation of key exposures that can affect women's health.

7. Gain an appreciation of the principal cancers and other causes of death that occur in women of various age groups.

8. Gain an appreciation of the frequency of key benign gynecologic conditions such as endometriosis, fibroids, ovarian cysts, and PID.

Questions

1. The term "randomization" is most likely to be found in the context of describing:

    A. A case series
    B. A cross-sectional study
    C. A clinical trial
    D. A case-control study
    E. A community intervention trial

2. Which of the following data collections would not describe incidence?

    A. The frequency of births among California women between 1995 and 1996
    B. The frequency of new ovarian cancers among Massachusetts women between 1995 and 1996
    C. The frequency of deaths from breast cancer among New York women between 1995 and 1996
    D. The proportion of women found to have fibroids among all women coming to autopsy at a major teaching hospital during 1996
    E. All of the above describe incidence.

3. Concerning differences between case-control and cohort studies, all of the following statements are true **except:**

    A. Case-control studies are always retrospective and cohort studies are always prospective.
    B. Rare diseases may be more feasibly studied by case-control means.
    C. Rare exposures may be more feasibly studied by cohort means.
    D. Attributable risk cannot be derived from a cohort study.
    E. A case-control study is generally less costly.

4. To evaluate endometrial biopsy as a screening test, a clinician decides to biopsy all patients about to have hysterectomy. What measure is defined by the number of women who had endometrial cancer found in both their endometrial biopsy and surgical specimen divided by the total number of women who had endometrial cancer in their surgical specimen?

    A. Predictive value of positive test
    B. Sensitivity
    C. Specificity
    D. None of the above

5. Which of the following statements is true concerning the statistical validity of analytic studies?

    A. A "P value" less than 0.05 rules out chance as an explanation for a study finding.
    B. Stratification is an analytic technique to correct for selection bias.
    C. Meta-analysis is a statistical technique used to correct for confounding variables.
    D. Recall bias concerning exposure is less likely to occur in a cohort study.
    E. All of the above are true.

6. Which of the following exposures and diseases have not been linked in current epidemiologic studies?

    A. Smoking may cause cervical cancer.
    B. Tubal ligation may protect against ovarian cancer.
    C. Alcohol use may increase breast cancer risk.
    D. Smoking may cause early menopause.
    E. Oral contraceptives may protect against ovarian cancer.
    F. All of the above associations are described.

7. You are asked by your HMO to recommend programs for mortality prevention in women. Which is *least* likely to be justifiable on the basis of leading causes of death in women?

    A. A program to encourage seat belt use among all women
    B. A colon cancer screening program for women over age 55
    C. A cardiac risk modification program for women over 35
    D. A violence prevention program for women 15–34
    E. A mammographic screening program for women 15–34

8. Which is the most frequent cause of hospitalization for gynecologic disease among women 15–45?

    A. PID
    B. Endometriosis
    C. Ectopic pregnancy
    D. Uterine fibroids
    E. Cervical neoplasia

Answers

1. **C**

   Randomization is the cornerstone of an experimental clinical trial. Trials are conducted "prospectively." In cancer trials, randomized trials are usually called phase III clinical trials. Nonrandomized clinical trials are phase I and II, which are "one arm feasibility" and "response studies," respectively. Community interventional trials are also experimental trials, but they are typically nonrandomized.

   Case-series and cross-sectional studies are both "descriptive" studies and do not involve randomization. They are nonexperimental analytic studies.

   Case-control studies are also "nonexperimental" in that they are not randomized. These studies typically use historical or population-based controls and are thus "retrospective" rather than "prospective."
   Reference: Pages 51–56

2. **D**

   Incidence is defined as the rate of occurrence of a new disease or new condition over a specified time interval, whereas prevalence is defined as disease existing in a population at a particular point in time. While these two terms are frequently confused, the easy way to remember the distinction is that any disease frequency that is examined over a period of time is an incidence. The first three (A-C) are examples of incidence, whereas the proportion of women found to have fibroids at autopsy is a prevalence.
   Reference: Page 53

3. **A**

   Case-control and cohort studies are both considered to be "nonexperimental," in that neither one is randomized, and they are often retrospective. Case-control studies typically start with the identification of individuals with a disease and a suitable control population without the disease. Rare diseases may be studied more feasibly with this approach.

   A cohort study is one in which a group of individuals has a particular factor in common, e.g., a disease, that is followed over time. An example is a survival analysis in which 100% of the individuals are alive at the beginning of the study and, over time, the percentage of survival of the cohort is measured. Rare exposures may be studied more feasibly with this type of study. Both attributable risk (the difference between the occurrence measure in the exposed and the unexposed cohort) and relative risk (the occurrence in the exposed cohort divided by the occurrence in the unexposed cohort) can be obtained from a cohort study.
   Reference: Pages 54–55

4. B

Sensitivity of a test is defined as the true positive results out of all those who have the disease, while the specificity is the proportion of true negative results out of all those who do not have the disease. The predictive value of a positive test is defined as the number of true positive results out of all those screened with positive results. Conversely, the predicative value of a negative test is defined as the number of true negative results out of all those screened with negative results (see Table 4.1).
Reference: Page 57

5. D

In a cohort study, recall bias is not likely to be a problem because the study group is typically being evaluated for a particular observable finding, such as mortality. In a survival study, most studies require the actual report of an event that occurs during the study, not one that requires recall.

Table 4.1   Measures of Validity for a Screening Procedure

Status Determined by Screening	True Disease Status		Total
	Positive	Negative	
Positive	a (true positives)	b (false-positives)	a + b (all screened positive)
Negative	c (false-negatives)	d (true negatives)	c + d (all screened negative)
Total	a + c (all diseased)	b + d (all nondiseased)	N (all subjects)

Measure	Definition	Formula
Sensitivity	True positives / All diseased	$\dfrac{a}{a + c}$
Specificity	True negatives / All nondiseased	$\dfrac{d}{b + d}$
Predictive value of a positive screen	True positives / All screened positive	$\dfrac{a}{a + b}$

Reproduced from **Cramer DW.** Epidemiology and biostatistics. In: **Berek JS, Hacker NF,** eds. *Gynecologic Oncology*. 2nd ed. Baltimore: Williams & Wilkins, 1994: 193.

Table 4.4   Estimated number of annual hospitalizations among women of reproductive age in the United States

Group of Diagnosis	Hospitalizations*
Pelvic inflammatory disease	287,343
Benign cysts of the ovary	190,548
Endometriosis	188,805
Menstrual disorders	182,988
Uterine leiomyomas	177,082
Prolapse/stress incontinence	101,907
Cervical intraepithelial neoplasia	60,320

*Based on discharge diagnoses for women 15 through 45 years of age in nonmilitary hospitals averaged for the period 1988–1990.
From **Velebil P, Wingo PA, Xia A, Wilcox LS, Peterson HB.** Rate of hospitalization for gynecologic disorders among reproductive-age women in the United States. *Obstet Gynecol* 1995;86:764–9.

A low P value, especially p<0.05, indicates a low likelihood that a result occurs merely as a result of chance; however, it does not exclude the possibility.

Stratification is a technique that permits subgroups within the larger study population to be analyzed separately for a particular variable. This approach cannot, however, correct for selection bias.

The statistical technique meta-analysis combines the results of several independent studies and seeks to take an average of the results. Thus, the larger studies will contribute the greatest information. Confounding variables that exist in particular studies will still contribute to the confounding of the meta-analysis result.

Reference: Page 58

6. E

All of these associations have been described. Ovarian cancer risk is lower in women who have taken the oral contraceptive or have undergone a tubal ligation. The risk of ovarian cancer is progressively lower in women who have a longer exposure to the oral contraceptive; in women who have taken "the pill" for five years or longer, the relative risk is 0.5, i.e., the risk is cut in half. Pregnancy also decreases the risk of ovarian cancer. The hypothesis is that the fewer times a woman ovulates during her lifetime, the less disruption of the ovarian surface epithelium occurs, and therefore, the cells are less likely to undergo neoplastic transformation.

Figure 4.5 Age-specific incidence of hospitalization for various benign gynecologic conditions around 1990. (From **Velebil P, Wingo PA, Xia A, Wilcox LS, Peterson HB.** Rate of hospitalization for gynecologic disorders among reproductive-age women in the United States. *Obstet Gynecol* 1995;86:764–9.)

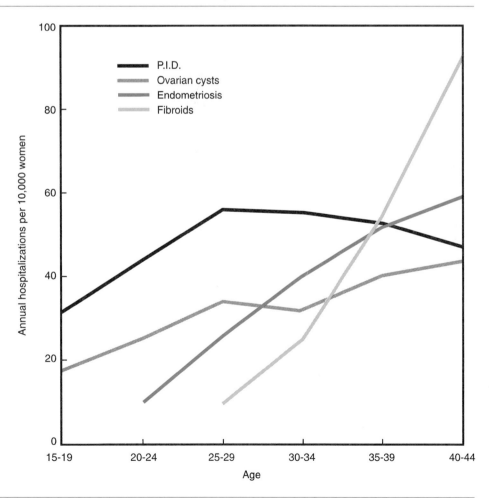

Smoking not only increases the risk of cancer of the respiratory system, especially lung cancer, but it has been associated with the higher risk of malignancies of the female reproductive tract, especially cervical cancer. It should be noted that the most common cause of death from cancer in women in the United States is now lung cancer. Smoking also tends to decrease circulating levels of estrogen, which presumably could lead to a higher risk of hypoestrogenism. This condition is associated with early menopause and a lower risk of endometrial cancer, but this is not a suitable means of cutting risk of the latter condition.

Although the effect of alcohol on the incidence of breast cancer is somewhat controversial, most studies reveal an increased risk.
Reference: Pages 59–60

7. E

Breast cancer among 15–34 year olds accounts for far fewer deaths than accidents in all women, colon cancer in women over 55, heart disease in women over 35, or homicides in women 15–34.

Indeed, the value of mammography screening in premenopausal women is controversial. There are no data that support routine mammography screening of women in the general population who are younger than 40 years. In women ages 40 to 49, there may be some benefit, perhaps a reduction in mortality as much as 17%. In addition to the relatively lower prevalence of the condition at any time in the screened population, the premenopausal breast is more difficult to assess because of its density, and therefore, there are more "false positives" requiring more breast biopsies.
Reference: Pages 60–62

8. A

The rate of hospitalization for pelvic inflammatory disease in women between the ages of 15 and 45 is greater than the other conditions listed (see Table 4.4). However, if one examines Figure 4.5, which illustrates age-specific incidence figures, the incidence of PID is clearly greater by age group up to the age of 35 years. Thereafter, the incidence of hospitalization for uterine myomata increases rapidly, equaling the figures for PID within the 35-to-39-year age group, and becoming the most common cause for hospitalization in the age group 40–45 years.
Reference: Pages 62–64

BASIC SCIENCE

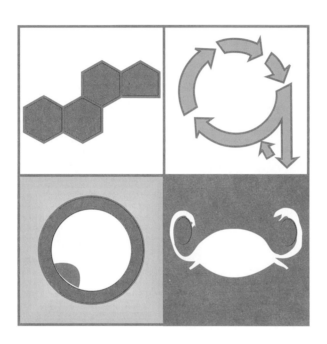

5 Anatomy and Embryology

Jonathan S. Berek

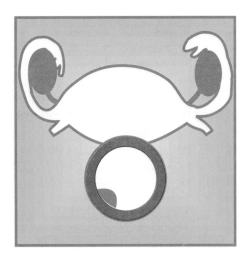

Learning Objectives

1. Be able to identify the bony structures, muscles, blood vessels, lymphatics, nerves, and viscera of the pelvis.

2. Understand the embryologic development of the pelvic viscera.

3. Know the anatomy of the anterior abdominal wall.

4. Understand the development of the urinary tract.

5. Know the anatomy of the perineum.

6. Be able to identify the structures of the retroperitoneum.

7. Know the complete course of the ureter, including its relationship to other important anatomic structures.

8. Be able to illustrate the anatomy of the pelvic floor.

Questions

1. A 72-year-old woman has developed progressive urinary stress incontinence and a decision is made to perform a retropubic cystourethropexy. One of the principal ligaments used in bladder suspensions is Cooper's ligament, which is comprised of the following ligaments:

   A. inguinal and lacunar
   B. piriformis and perineal
   C. urogenital and cardinal
   D. pectineal and iliopectineal

2. The levator ani muscle is composed of several muscles that comprise the pelvic floor and support the pelvic viscera. The muscles are:

   A. piriformis, obturator internus, and iliopsoas
   B. bulbocavernosus, deep and superficial perineal
   C. puboccoccygeus, iliococcygeus, and coccygeus
   D. superficial transverse perineal, ischiocavernosus, and gluteus maximus

3. A 28-year-old woman is undergoing a cesarean section and develops intractable postpartum hemorrhage. After most techniques of controlling the blood loss have been attempted, the surgeon decides to perform a bilateral "hypogastric artery ligation." Some of the main branches of the internal iliac (hypogastric) artery are:

   A. obturator, uterine, superior vesical
   B. inferior rectal, perineal, clitoral
   C. external pudendal, inferior epigastric, and deep circumflex
   D. sigmoid, superior hemorrhoidal, and left colic

4. The principal collateral anastamoses of the ovarian arteries are which of the following arteries:

   A. uterine
   B. superior rectal
   C. deep iliac circumflex
   D. iliolumbar

5. A woman with invasive squamous carcinoma of the cervix has a visible lesion apparently confined to the cervix (FIGO stage Ib). The surgeon performs a radical hysterectomy and is most concerned about the possibility of lymphatic dissemination. Which lymphatic channels are most likely to be the first site of early metastases from the invasive cervical cancer?

   A. common iliac
   B. obturator
   C. inguinal
   D. sacral

6. During pelvic surgery, injury to the genitofemoral nerve would result in sensory loss in which of the following locations:

   A. mons and upper labia majora
   B. anterior vulva and anterior thigh
   C. lateral perineum and labia majora
   D. buttocks and contiguous perineum

7. A 26-year-old woman with chronic pelvic pain secondary to endometriosis and associated scarring is advised to undergo a transection of the presacral nerve. The success

of the operation would depend on complete transection of the nerve. This is difficult because the presacral nerve:

A. overlies the middle sacral vessels and is usually composed of two or three incompletely fused trunks
B. is a subsidiary of the celiac plexus and is located along the inferior mesenteric artery
C. is part of the ovarian plexus, which transverses the infundubulopelvic ligament
D. is Frankenhauser's ganglion, which also innervates the uterus and vagina

8. Although genetic sex is predetermined at the time of fertilization, the early genital system is indistinguishable between the two sexes—the "indifferent stage." Clinically, gender is not apparent until approximately which week of embryonic life:

A. 8th
B. 10th
C. 12th
D. 14th

9. The development of the external genitalia in the embryo begins its differentiation around the seventh embryonic week. If the process is defective, hermaphrodites can occur. True hermaphrodism is when:

A. the genetic sex indicates one gender and the external genitalia have characteristics of the other gender
B. individuals have both ovarian and testicular tissue, most commonly ovotestes but occasionally with an ovary on one side and a testes on the other
C. the gonads remain undifferentiated and produce both male and female sex hormones
D. there are abnormal levels of müllerian-inhibiting substance, which produce a disruption of embryonic development

10. A 27-year-old woman has had two spontaneous abortions and an evaluation of the uterus suggests a uterine anomaly. On hysterosalpingography she is found to have a bicornuate uterus. Of the following, which illustrates a bicornuate uterus (as opposed to a uterine didelphus, septate, or unicornuate uterus):

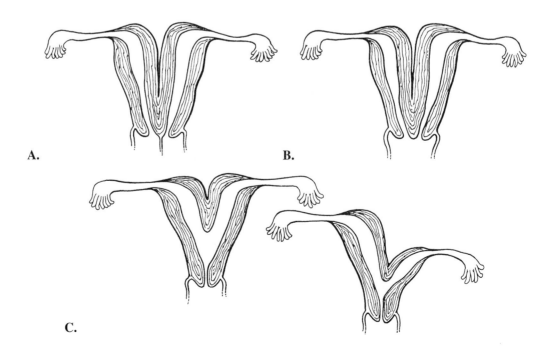

A.

B.

C.

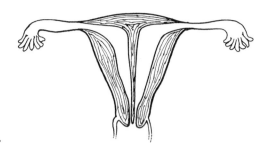
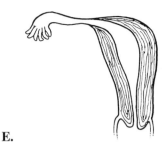

D.   **E.**

11. A 32-year-old woman is referred to you for an evaluation of an "enlarged ovarian" with an ovarian cyst. The patient has a transvaginal ultrasound which demonstrates a left ovary measuring 5 × 4 × 3 cm with a 1.1 cm single ovarian cyst. The right ovary is 4 × 3 × 3 cm. You should indicate to her that the left ovary is:

    A. abnormal because it is approximate twice the size of a normal ovary
    B. abnormal because it contains a cyst
    C. normal in size and the cyst is likely functional
    D. normal because ovaries can be twice the average anticipated size

12. In entering the abdomen to perform a hysterectomy, a transverse lower incision is used. As the incision is extended laterally, the aponeurosis of the rectus abdominus and the lateral muscles (the aponeurosis of the external and internal oblique and the transversus oblique muscles) join caudal to the arcuate line. Which blood vessel runs superiorly in the transverse fascia to reach the arcuate line where it enters the rectus sheath?

    A. inferior epigastric
    B. superior epigastric
    C. circumflex iliac
    D. external pudendal

13. Perineal trauma can result in damage to vessels in the superficial perineal compartment. The deep layer of the superficial perineal fascia, or Colles' fascia, is continuous superiorly with the deep layer of the superficial abdominal fascia, which is called the:

    A. deep transverse perineal fascia
    B. urogenital fascia
    C. Scarpa's fascia
    D. Camper's fascia

14. The subperitoneal area of the true pelvis is partitioned into potential spaces by the various organs and their respective fascial coverings, and by the selective thickenings of the endopelvic fascia into ligaments and septa. The paravesical and pararectal spaces are separated by which ligaments:

    A. vesicouterine
    B. pararectal
    C. cardinal
    D. rectal

Answers

1. D

The Cooper's ligament is used frequently in the performance of a bladder neck suspension using the retropubic approach, i.e., the Burch operation. Cooper's ligament is a strong ridge of fibrous tissue extending along the pectineal line (also known as the pectineal ligament), which merges laterally with the iliopectineal ligament and medially with the lacunar ligament.
Reference: Page 74

2. C (see Figure 5.2)

The levator ani are the supporting muscular structure for the pelvic floor. The puboccoccygeus can also be divided into the pubovaginalis, the puborectalis, and the iliococcygeus. Together they form a broad, curved sheet of muscle that stretches from the symphysis pubis anteriorly and the coccygeus posteriorly and from one side of the pelvis to another. They are perforated by the urethra, vagina, and anal canal. The levator ani assists the anterior abdominal wall in containing the abdominal and pelvic contents. This important group of muscles supports the posterior wall of the vagina, facilitates defecation, and is an important component of the mechanism of fecal continence.
Reference: Pages 74–79, 119–121

3. A (see Figure 5.4)

The internal iliac artery, otherwise known as the hypogastric artery (an interesting name as there are many arteries that are caudal to the stomach!) provides one of the principal blood supplies to the pelvic viscera. Each vessel (one on the left and one on the right) has an anterior and posterior division. The posterior division has three branches—the iliolumbar, lateral sacral, and posterior gluteal; the anterior division has ten—obturator; internal pudendal; umbilical; superior, middle, and inferior vesicals; middle rectal (hemorrhoidal); uterine; vaginal; and inferior gluteal. There is some variation in this pattern. However, the branches of the internal artery serve as the blood supply to most of the pelvic viscera, the pelvic, and lower abdominal muscles. Bilateral "hypogastric artery ligation" is an important technique for control of pelvic hemorrhage when other methods have failed, as it results in a dramatic reduction in the pulse pressure in the pelvis, which converts the blood flow characteristics from that of an arterial system to a venous system. For a list of the branches of internal iliac hypogastric artery, see Table 5.2 (partial).
Reference: Pages 75–83

4. A

The primary anastomosing arteries of the uterine vessels are the ascending vaginal and the uterine arteries. The ovarian arteries arise from the aorta and anastomose with the branches of the internal iliac arteries.
Reference: Page 82

5. B (see Figure 5.6 and Table 5.4)

The cervix and upper vagina drain laterally to the parametrial, obturator, and external iliac lymph nodes.
Reference: Pages 79, 86

6. B (see Table 5.5)

The genitofemoral nerve arises from the nerve roots L1 and L2 and follows a course through the pelvis over the psoas muscle and ultimately splits into two branches—the genital branch, which enters the inguinal canal with the round ligament and passes through the superficial inguinal ring to the anterior vulva, and the femoral branch, which intervates a portion of the skin of the anterior and medial thigh.
Reference: Pages 85–88

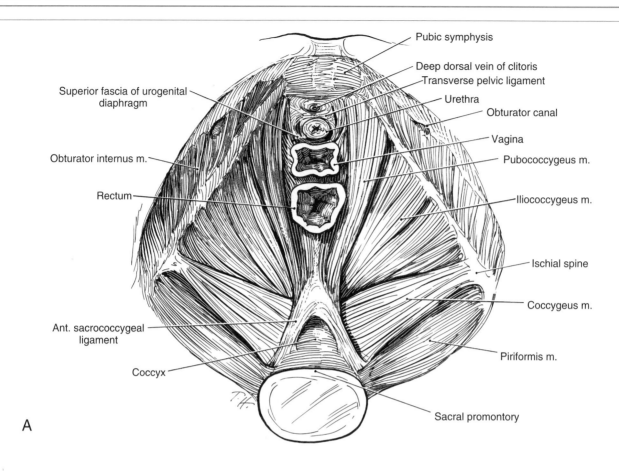

A

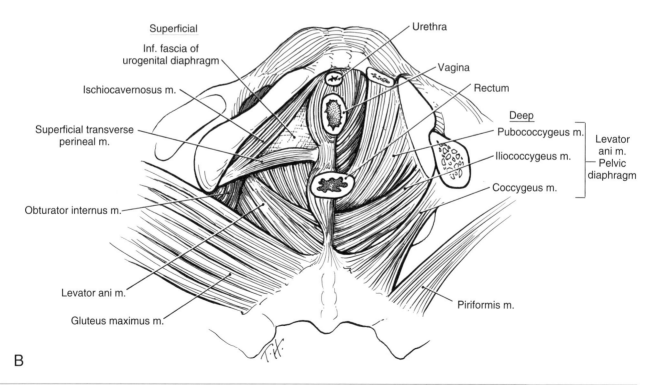

B

Figure 5.2   The pelvic diaphragm. *A,* A view into the pelvic floor that illustrates the muscles of the pelvic diaphragm and their attachments to the bony pelvis. *B,* A lateral, sagittal view of the pelvic diaphragm. *C,* A view from outside the pelvic diaphragm illustrating the divisions of the levator ani muscles.

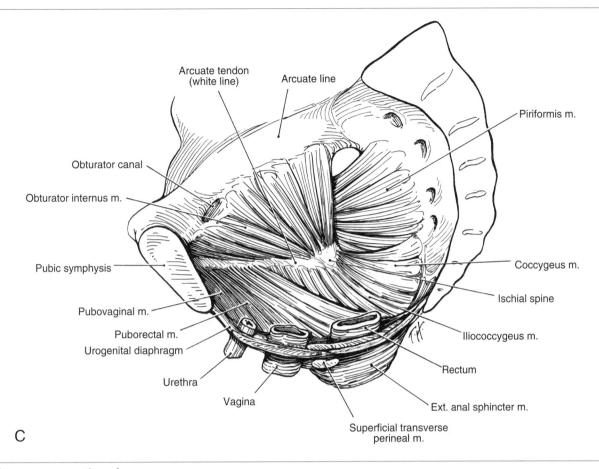

Arcuate tendon (white line)

Arcuate line

Piriformis m.

Obturator canal

Obturator internus m.

Pubic symphysis

Pubovaginal m.

Puborectal m.

Urogenital diaphragm

Urethra

Vagina

Coccygeus m.

Ischial spine

Iliococcygeus m.

Rectum

Ext. anal sphincter m.

Superficial transverse perineal m.

C

Figure 5.2—*continued*

7. A (see Figure 5.8)

The presacral neurectomy is an operation in which the superior hypogastric plexus is divided and resected in order to interrupt sensory fibers from the uterus and cervix, and has been associated with relief of dysmenorrhea secondary to endometriosis in about 50 to 75% of cases. Because there are several branches and their locations vary, and because other nerves supply these structures, the resection of these nerves does not uniformly relieve the pain.
Reference: Pages 88–90

8. C (see Table 5.6)

Approximately the 12th week of embryonic life, the differentiation of the gonads takes place. The process depends on the elaboration of testis-determining factor (TDF) and, subsequently, by androgens produced by the male gonad.
Reference: Pages 92–95

9. B

True hermaphrodism is an extremely rare condition associated with chromosomalmosaicism, mutation, or abnormal cleavage involving the X and Y chromosomes. In pseudohermaphrodism, the genetic sex indicates one gender and the external genitalia has the characteristics of the other gender.
Reference: Pages 96–97

10. C

Reference: Page 98

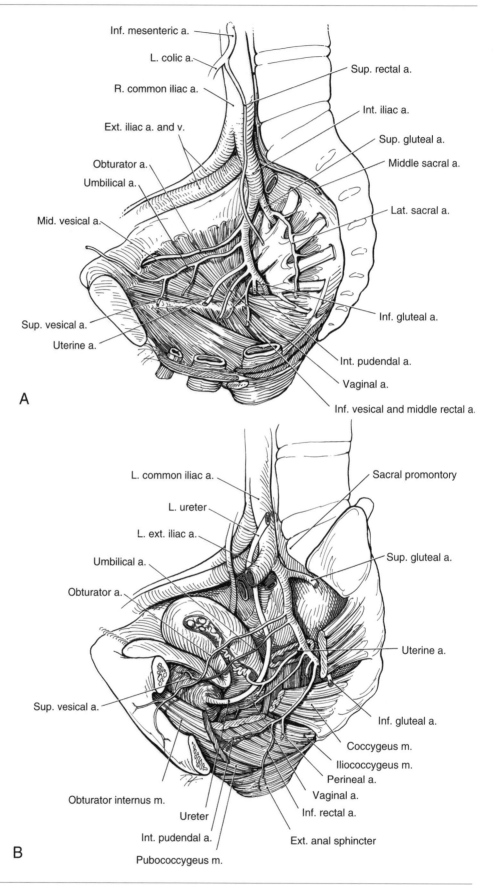

Figure 5.4   The blood supply to the pelvis. *A,* The sagittal view of the pelvis without the viscera. *B,* The blood supply to one pelvic viscera.

Table 5.2   Branches of Internal Iliac Hypogastric Artery

Branches

Posterior division:
1. *Iliolumbar*—anastomoses with lumbar and deep circumflex iliac arteries; helps supply lower abdominal wall, iliac fossa
2. *Lateral sacral*—supplies contents of sacral canal, piriformis muscle
3. *Superior gluteal*—supplies gluteal muscles

Anterior division:
1. *Obturator*—supplies iliac fossa, posterior pubis, obturator internus muscle
2. *Internal pudendal*
3. *Umbilical*—remnant of fetal umbilical artery; after giving off branches, as the medial umbilical ligament
4. *Superior, middle, inferior vesical*—supply bladder and one or more branches to the ureter
5. *Middle rectal (hemorrhoidal)*—supplies rectum, branches to mid vagina
6. *Uterine*—supplies uterine corpus and cervix, with branches to upper vagina, tube, round ligament, and ovary
7. *Vaginal*—supplies vagina
8. *Inferior gluteal*—supplies gluteal muscles, muscles of posterior thigh

---

11. C

The normal sized ovary in a reproductive aged women varies in size but is about 5 × 3 × 3 cm, and frequently contains small functional cysts.
Reference: Page 102

12. A

This vessel is vulnerable to damage with a transverse abdominal incision in which the rectus muscle is completely or partially transacted.
Reference: Pages 108–109

13. C

The deep layer of the superficial abdominal fascia is called Scarpa's fascia, which attaches from the ischiopubic rami and ischial tuberosities. The superficial perineal compartment is continuous superiorly with the superficial fascial spaces of the anterior abdominal wall. Thus, blood and infection can spread along this route.
Reference: Pages 111–112

14. C (see Figure 5.22)

Otherwise known as Mackenrodt ligament, this structure is traversed by the uterine vessels and contains lymphatic channels in the parametrium.
Reference: Page 116–117

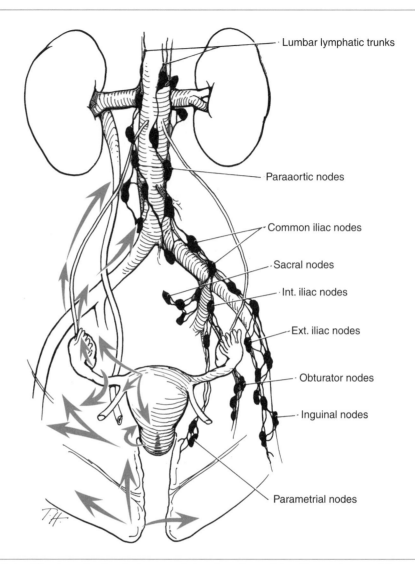

Labels (top to bottom, right side):
- Lumbar lymphatic trunks
- Paraaortic nodes
- Common iliac nodes
- Sacral nodes
- Int. iliac nodes
- Ext. iliac nodes
- Obturator nodes
- Inguinal nodes
- Parametrial nodes

Figure 5.6 The lymphatic drainage of the female pelvis. The vulva and lower vagina drain to the superficial and deep inguinal nodes, sometimes directly to the iliac nodes (along the dorsal vein of the clitoris) and to the other side. The cervix and upper vagina drain laterally to the parametrial, obturator, and external iliac nodes and posteriorly along the uterosacral ligaments to the sacral nodes. Drainage from these primary lymph node groups is upward along the infundibulopelvic ligament, similarly to drainage of the ovary and fallopian tubes to the para-aortic nodes. The lower uterine body drains in the same manner as the cervix. Rarely, drainage occurs along the round ligament to the inguinal nodes.

Table 5.4   Primary Lymph Node Groups Providing Drainage to Genital Structures

Nodes	Primary Afferent Connections
Aortic/para-aortic	Ovary, fallopian tube, uterine corpus (upper); drainage from common iliac nodes
Common iliac	Drainage from external and internal iliac nodes
External iliac	Upper vagina, cervix, uterine corpus (upper); drainage from inguinal nodes
Internal iliac Lateral sacral Superior gluteal Inferior gluteal Obturator Vesical Rectal Parauterine	Upper vagina, cervix, uterine corpus (lower)
Inguinal Superficial Deep	Vulva, lower vagina; (rare: uterus, tube, ovary)

Table 5.5   Lumbosacral Plexus

Nerve	Spinal Segment	Innervation
Iliohypogastric	T12, L1	Sensory—skin near iliac crest, just above symphysis pubis
Ilioinguinal	L1	Sensory—upper medial thigh, mons, labia majora
Lateral femoral cutaneous	L2, L3,	Sensory—lateral thigh to level of knee
Femoral	L2, L3, L4	Sensory—anterior and medial thigh, medial leg and foot, hip and knee joints Motor—iliacus, anterior thigh muscles
Genitofemoral	L1, L2	Sensory—anterior vulva (genital branch) middle/upper anterior thigh (femoral branch)
Obturator	L2, L3, L4	Sensory—medial thigh and leg, hip and knee joints Motor—adductor muscles of thigh
Superior gluteal	L4, L5, S1	Motor—gluteal muscles
Inferior gluteal	L4, L5, S1, S2	Motor—gluteal muscles
Posterior femoral cutaneous	S2, S3	Sensory—vulva, perineum
Sciatic	L4, L5, S1, S2, S3	Sensory—much of leg, foot, lower extremity joints Motor—posterior thigh muscle, leg and foot muscles
Pudendal	S2, S3, S4	Sensory—perianal skin, vulva and perineum, clitoris, urethra, vaginal vestibule Motor—external anal sphincter, perineal muscles, urogenital diaphragm

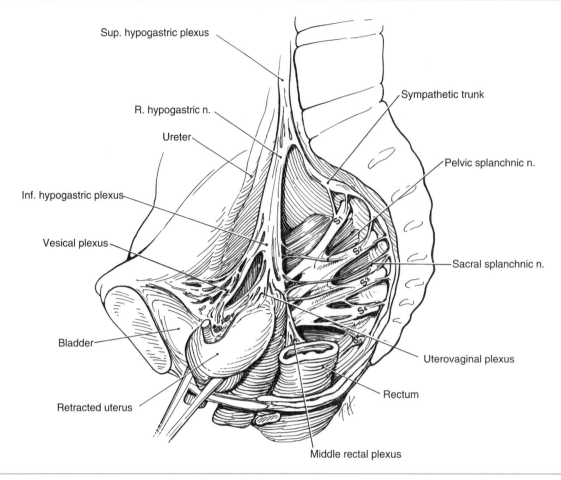

Figure 5.8   The presacral nerves.

Table 5.6   Development of Genital and Urinary Tracts by Embryologic Age

Weeks of Gestation	Genital Development	Urinary Development
4–6	Urorectal septum	Pronephros
	Formation of cloacal folds, genital tubercle	Mesonephros/mesonephric duct
		Ureteric buds, metanephros
	Genital ridges	Exstrophy of mesonephric ducts and ureters into bladder wall
6–7	End of indifferent phase of genital development	Major, minor calyces form
	Development of primitive sex cords	Kidneys begin to ascend
	Formation of paramesonephric ducts	
	Labioscrotal swellings	
8–11	Distal paramesonephric ducts begin to fuse	Kidney becomes functional
	Formation of sinuvaginal bulbs	
12	Development of clitoris and vaginal vestibule	
20	Canalization of vaginal plate	
32		Renal collecting duct system complete

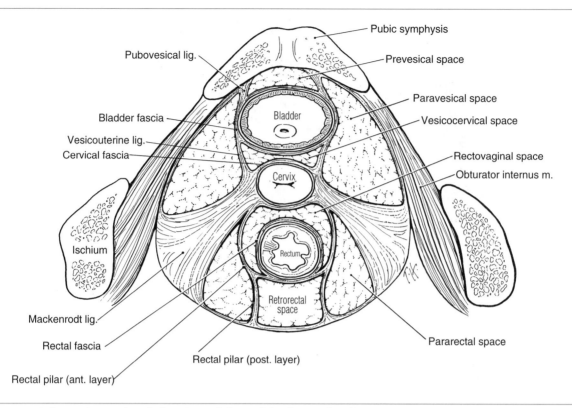

Labels in figure:

Pubovesical lig.
Bladder fascia
Vesicouterine lig.
Cervical fascia
Ischium
Mackenrodt lig.
Rectal fascia
Rectal pilar (ant. layer)
Rectal pilar (post. layer)
Pubic symphysis
Prevesical space
Paravesical space
Vesicocervical space
Rectovaginal space
Obturator internus m.
Pararectal space

Bladder
Cervix
Rectum
Retrorectal space

Figure 5.22   Schematic sectional drawing of the pelvis shows the firm connective tissue covering. The bladder, cervix, and rectum are surrounded by a connective tissue covering. The Mackenrodt ligament extends from the lateral cervix to the lateral abdominal pelvic wall. The vesicouterine ligament originating from the anterior edge of the Mackenrodt ligament leads to the covering of the bladder on the posterior side. The sagittal rectum column spreads both to the connective tissue of the rectum and the sacral vertebrae closely nestled against the back of the Mackenrodt ligament and lateral pelvic wall. Between the firm connective tissue bundles is loose connective tissue (paraspaces). (Reproduced with permission from **Von Peham H, Amreich JA.** *Gynaekologische Operationslehre.* Berlin: S Karger, 1930.)

6 Molecular Biology and Genetics

Oliver Dorigo
Jonathan S. Berek

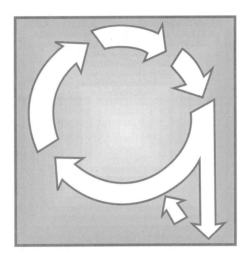

Learning Objectives

1. Be able to identify the phases of the normal cell cycle.

2. Be able to identify factors that regulate the normal cell cycle.

3. Understand the process of apoptosis.

4. Be able to identify the components of the immune system.

5. Be aware of the factors that trigger neoplasia.

Questions

1. Which of the following statements about the normal cell cycle is incorrect?

   A. Red blood cells, uterine muscle cells, and nerve cells are terminally differentiated cells and, therefore, cannot reenter the cell cycle.
   B. The G_2 phase of the cell cycle is the most variable phase.
   C. The DNA content of the cell is copied during the S phase of the cell cycle.
   D. During mitosis, the DNA content is equally distributed to each of the daughter cells to yield diploid genetic material.
   E. Proteins are synthesized during the G_2 phase of the cell cycle.

2. Which of the following effects is caused by the tumor suppressor gene p53?

   A. Cell cycle arrest at the G_2/M boundary
   B. Inhibition of microtubuli formation during mitosis
   C. Prevention of apoptosis
   D. Increased amount of cells in the G_2 phase
   E. Arrest of cells at the G_1/S boundary

3. Which of the following statements about apoptosis is incorrect?

   A. Apoptosis is a process that occurs in normal tissue to maintain a balance between cell proliferation and cell death.
   B. Apoptosis is an energy-dependent process.
   C. Apoptosis can hardly be distinguished from cell necrosis.
   D. Apoptotic cells exhibit cellular condensation and fragmentation of the nucleus.
   E. Apoptosis is an important factor in the growth of neoplasm.

4. Which of the following statements about oncogenes is correct?

   A. erbB2, c-myc, and k-ras are examples of oncogenes.
   B. erbB2 plays a role as oncogenic protein in ovarian cancer.
   C. Normal cells do not express oncogenes.
   D. Expression of oncogenes might be induced by environmental factors.
   E. The proto-oncogene fms encodes a receptor for colony stimulating factor.

5. Which of the following statements about Transforming Growth Factor Beta (TGF-β) is correct?

   A. TGF-β is exclusively produced by the embryo and theca cells.
   B. TGF-β has a mainly stimulating effect on the immune system.
   C. TGF-β activates intracytoplasmatic serine kinases.
   D. TGF-β does not play a role in gynecologic malignancies.
   E. None of the above statements is correct.

6. Which of the following statements about the effect of growth factors on intracellular signaling is incorrect?

   A. The interaction between growth factors and their receptors can result in activation of intracytoplasmatic kinases.
   B. Proteins encoded by proto-oncogenes do not participate in intracellular signal transduction.
   C. G-proteins are guanyl nucleotide-binding proteins.
   D. G-proteins display GTPase activity.
   E. Adenylate cylase molecules can be activated by G-proteins.

7. Which of the following DNA alterations play a role in gynecologic cancer?

    A. Amplification
    B. Point mutations
    C. Deletions
    D. Rearrangements
    E. All of the above

8. Which of the following gene therapy modalities has shown to be most effective in pre-clincal as well as clinical studies?

    A. Replacement of mutated p53 tumor suppressor genes with wild type p53 gene
    B. Inhibition of oncogenes and proto-oncogenes
    C. Cytokine gene modified tumor cell vaccines
    D. Suicide gene therapy
    E. None of the above

9. Which of the following tumor-associated antigens is specific for the associated gynecologic malignancy?

    A. Squamous cell carcinoma (SCC) antigen for cervical cancer
    B. CA125 for ovarian cancer
    C. Carcinoembryonic antigen (CEA) for endometrial cancer
    D. β-hCG for ovarian germ cell tumor
    E. None of the above

10. Which of the following classes of cluster determinants (CD) are present in all mature T cells?

    A. CD3
    B. CD4
    C. CD8
    D. CD20
    E. CD56

11. Which of the following statements about differences between T and B cells is incorrect?

    A. T cells are part of the cellular immune response, B cells produce a humoral immune response.
    B. B cells are able to produce antibodies specific for a certain antigen.
    C. B-cell and T-cell receptors interact with the antigen in similar ways.
    D. Both B and T cells can go into clonal expansion upon recognition of an antigen.
    E. Both T cells and B cells have been isolated from gynecologic malignancies.

12. Which one of the following cell types is considered the most important and effective in mediating lysis of tumor cells?

    A. CD4 positive helper cells
    B. CD8 positive killer cells
    C. Macrophages
    D. Natural killer cells
    E. B cells

13. Which of the following cell types is able to generate a memory response?

    A. NK cells
    B. T cells
    C. Macrophages
    D. Eosinophils
    E. Monocytes

14. Which of the following cytokines is produced in a predominantly TH1-like T-cell response?

    A. Interleukin-2
    B. Interleukin-4
    C. Interleukin-5
    D. Interleukin-10
    E. Granulocyte macrophage colony stimulating factor

15. Which of the following cytokines is primarily involved in generaton of inflammatory responses?

    A. Interleukin-1
    B. Interleukin-2
    C. Interleukin-6
    D. Interleukin-10
    E. Interleukin-12

16. Which of the following cytokines is similar to granulocyte macrophage colony stimulating factors (GM-CSF) in its biological activities?

    A. Interleukin-2
    B. Interleukin-3
    C. Interleukin-6
    D. Interleukin-12
    E. Interferon-γ

17. Which of the following cytokines have been found in large amounts in ascites from ovarian cancer patients?

    A. Interleukin-2
    B. Interleukin-8
    C. Interleukin-10
    D. Interleukin-15
    E. Interferon-α

18. Which of the following is a potentially lethal side effect of interleukin-2 therapy?

    A. Anaphylaxis
    B. Neutropenia
    C. Dehydration
    D. Vascular leak syndrome
    E. T-cell lymphoma

19. Which of the following is the single most important risk factor for the development of cancer?

    A. Smoking
    B. Radiation
    C. Advanced age
    D. Exposure to environmental carcinogens
    E. Genetic disposition

Answers

1. **B (see Figure 6.2)**

    The highest degree of variation is found in the G_1 phase of the cell cycle. Depending on the cell type, the G_1 phase can range from 8 hours to more than 100 hours. These variations account for different generation times exhibited by various cell types. This

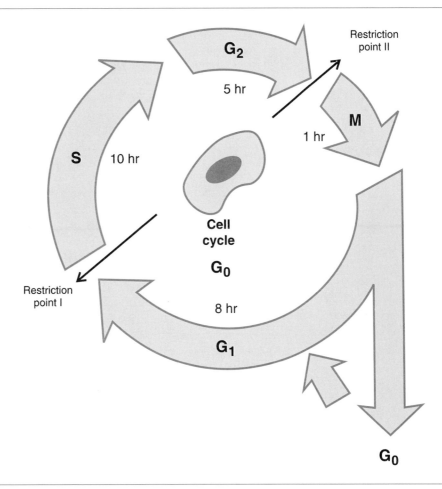

Figure 6.2   The cell cycle.

is an important biological phenomenon, since a number of antineoplastic drugs are active in the G_1 or G_1/S transition point of the cell cycle. This phase is characterized by diverse biosynthetic activity. Enzymes and regulatory proteins necessary for DNA synthesis are being produced to prepare the cell for the mitosis.

Terminally differentiated cells, such as red blood cells, uterine smooth muscle cells, and nerve cells, cannot reenter the cell cycle and must be generated from stem cells. They differ from cells in the quiescent G_0 phase. Cells in G_0 can be stimulated to enter the cell cycle following exposure to specific stimuli. The stimuli can include steroid hormones, irradiation, cytotoxic drugs, or trauma. Rapidly proliferating cells are in general more susceptible to the effect of antineoplastic drugs. These cells are mainly found in the gastrointestinal tract or the skin.

During the S phase, the DNA content of the cell is copied. After initiation of DNA synthesis, the replication of DNA proceeds as an "all-or-none" phenomenon. Cells that contain more than diploid genetic material, such as polyploid cancer cells for example, might produce either more or less than twice the amount of DNA during the S phase.

During the G_2 phase of the cell cycle, proteins are synthesized (e.g., proteins with structural and enzymatic properties). Errors of replication, which occur during DNA replication, are repaired in this phase. Failure to detect and correct genetic errors might allow genetically aberrant cells to continue through the cell cycle. These cells may ultimately avoid cell cycle control and display malignant transformation.
Reference: Pages 123–126

2. E

The p53 tumor suppressor gene elicits its main function via cell cycle control by arresting cells in the G_1/S check boundary. Errors of replication not repaired in the G_2 phase or resulting from mitosis, are repaired in the G_1 phase. The tumor suppressor gene p53 encodes for protein with diverse transcriptional activity. The induced mechanisms ultimately lead to growth arrest in the G_1/S transition point, allowing time for the cell to repair DNA damage. If DNA repair is successful, the cell will continue to cycle and undergo DNA replication during the S phase. If DNA repair fails, however, p53 is able to induce apoptosis or cell suicide via a number of different pathways. A cell with extensive DNA damage would subsequently disintegrate and die. Cells with normal or nonmutated p53 protein, therefore, possess a strong control mechanism for preventing genetically aberrant cells from continous proliferation.

The gene p53 is still the most important tumor suppressor gene in gynecologic malignancies. Overall, approximately 30% of ovarian cancers have been found to display aberrant p53 expression. The importance of mutations in the p53 gene lies in the inability of the cell to arrest in the G_1/S transition point. The cell, therefore, has less time to repair DNA defects. Furthermore, the apoptosis-inducing effect of the wild type p53 protein is missing in cells that have mutated p53 gene sequences. The resulting mutated or truncated proteins fail to induce the transcriptional mechanisms that induce cell suicide or apoptosis. Knowledge of this mechanism had lead to the development of novel therapeutic approaches in cancer gene therapy. The introduction of the wild type p53 gene into cells with mutated p53 has been shown to restore the growth arrest and apoptosis in a variety of different cancer cell lines.
Reference: Pages 126–128

3. C

Apoptosis can be distinguished from necrosis by a number of features. In apoptosis, the cell condenses with fragmentation of the nucleus. This is an energy-dependent process, which is regulated by the expression of specific genes. In contrast, cell necrosis is an energy-independent process. In necrosis, cells undergo spontaneous lysis.

Apoptosis is required to maintain a balance between proliferation and cell death in normal tissue. This mechanism, for example, accounts for the development of intestinal mucosa or palatal fusion. It is regulated by complex interactions between certain genes such as Bcl2, c-myc, and p53.

Apoptosis is also an important factor in the genesis of neoplasms. Cancer cells fail to show an adequate rate of apoptosis as found in normal tissue. Genes involved in the regulation of apoptotic pathways are frequently mutated in cancer cells. Lack of functional apoptotic pathways contribute to increased and uncontrolled proliferation of cells. The development of novel therapies for cancer uses replacement of genes in cancer cells to restore the apoptotic machinery.
Reference: Pages 127–128

4. C (see Table 6.1)

Many oncogenes are expressed at low levels in normal cells and are required for cellular functions such as cell division. Although more than 100 oncogenes have been identified, only a small minority seem to participate in the development of the majority of oncogene-associated tumors. Oncogenes exist within a cell in a latent state as a proto-oncogene and must be activated endogenously by genetic rearrangement or exogenously by environmental factors to produce the oncogenic effect.

A variety of different oncogenes have been associated with ovarian cancer, including erbB2, c-myc, jun, or k-ras. The oncogene erbB2 is a 185 kDa oncogenic protein that directly correlates with prognosis. A protein present in normal adult tissue, erbB2 is overexpressed in cancer tissue.

Table 6.1 Proto-oncogenes

Proto-oncogenes	Gene Product/Function
	Growth factors
	Fibroblast growth factor
fgf-5	
sis	Platelet-derived growth factor beta
hst, int-2	
	Transmembrane receptors
erbB	Epidermal-growth-factor (EGF) receptor
HER-2/neu	EGF-related receptor
fms	Colony-stimulating-factor (CSF) receptor
kit	Stem-cell receptor
trk	Nerve-growth-factor receptor
	Inner-membrane receptor
bcl-2	
Ha-ras, N-ras, N-ras	
fgr, lck, src, yes	
	Cytoplasmic messengers
crk	
cot, plm-1, mos, raf/mil	
	Nuclear DNA binding proteins
erbB-1	
jun, ets-1, ets-2, fos, gil 1, rel, ski, vav,	
lyl-1, maf, myb, myc, L-myc, N-myc, evi-1	

Proto-oncogenes encode growth factors as well as membrane and cytoplasmatic receptors. These proteins transmit signals from an extracellular ligand to the nucleus and activate DNA expression. In general, proto-oncogenes stimulate cellular proliferation. Examples of proto-oncogenes include fms, which encodes the transmembrane receptor for the colony stimulating factor; erbB2, which encodes the receptor for epidermal growth factor; and sis, which encodes the receptor for transforming growth factor β. Oncogenes are a target for molecular therapies, since inhibition of oncogene overexpression has been shown to cause cell growth arrest in various cancer cell lines.
Reference: Pages 127–128

5. C (see Table 6.3)
TGF-β belongs to a family of proteins with a variety of effects on different cell systems. It mainly elicits inhibitory effects on the immune system. TGF-β inhibits stimulation and proliferation of T cells and, therefore. inhibits important immune responses against tumor cells. TGF-β is produced by a variety of cells. It is important in embryonic development and induces production of the Müllerian Inhibiting Substance (MIS). It exerts its effect via a complex of Type-I and Type-II receptors on the cell surface. Upon binding to the receptor complex, intracytoplasmatic serine kinases are activated. This activation induces a pathway, which ultimately leads to the induction of transcriptional activity. Most cells are growth inhibited by TGF-β; other cell lines, however, show growth activation with TGF-β.

TGF-β seems to play an important role in gynecologic malignancies. In ovarian cancer, TGF-β has been overexpressed. TGF-β was also a major immunosuppressive factor in ascites from patients with ovarian cancer. Ascites from ovarian cancer patients are able to inhibit the generation of lymphokine activated killer cells mainly due to the presence of high amounts of TGF-β.
Reference: Pages 129–131

Table 6.3   Growth factors that play important roles in female reproductive physiology

Growth Factor	Sources	Targets	Actions
Platelet-derived growth factor (PDGF)	Placenta, platelets, preimplantation embryo, endothelial cells	Endothelial cells Trophoblast	Mitogen
Epidermal growth factor (EGF)	Submaxillary gland, theca cells	Granulosa cells Endometrium, cervix	Mitogen
Transforming growth factor-alpha (TGF-alpha)	Embryo, placenta, theca cell, ovarian stromal cell	Placenta Granulosa cell	Mitogen
Transforming growth factor-beta (TGF-beta)	Embryo, theca cells	Endometrium Granulosa cells Theca cells	Mitogen
Insulin-like growth factor 1 (IGF-1)	Granulosa cell	Theca cell Granulosa cell	Mediates growth hormone activity
Insulin-like growth factor 2 (IGF-2)	Theca cell	Theca cell	Insulin-like effects
Fibroblast growth factor (FGF)	Granulosa cell	Granulosa cell	Angiogenic activity Mitogen

6. B

Proto-oncogenes and G-proteins participate in intracellular signal transduction. Growth factors elicit an effect on cells mainly by controlling cyclic AMP levels via activating or inhibiting adenylate cyclase. In mammalian cells, different proteins couple the activated receptor to cyclase. Transmembrane receptors interact with a ligand at the cytoplasmatic or membrane portion of the receptor. The receptor is subsequently activated and may dimerize with homologous or heterologous receptors. The cytoplasmatic portion of the activated receptor displays kinase activity, which induces a number of downstream effects on different intracytoplasmatic and intranuclear proteins. The receptor-growth factor complex activates G-proteins that undergo structural changes upon binding to GTP. Carrying the GTP, it now activates the adenylate cyclase molecule. The activated G-protein keeps the cyclase active as long as the GTP is intact. Hydrolysis of the GTP to GDP by the G-protein terminates the action of the cyclase. These are important pathways for the understanding of receptor-induced cellular changes in normal and neoplastic cells.
Reference: Pages 131–132

7. E

Normal cells and tumor cells are dividing cells, constantly producing genetic material during the cell cycle. DNA synthesis may yield various errors in the replicated DNA, altering the structure and function of the cells. A number of these aberrations have been identified in premalignant, malignant, and benign neoplasms. Amplification, point mutations, deletions, and rearrangements are all mechanisms that lead to genetic errors. Amplification is an increase in the copy number of a gene and can enhance gene expression by increasing the amount of template DNA available for transcription. Proto-oncogene amplification is a common event in gynecologic malignancies. An example of oncogene amplification is erbB2, which is found in 30% of all ovarian malignancies.

Point mutations can lead to altered code sequences and, subsequently, to gene products with modified activity. The p53 tumor suppressor gene has a number of common genetic mutations termed "hot spots." Loss of p53 activity through genetic mutation increases the likelihood of uninhibited cell proliferation.

Deletions and rearrangements yield altered proteins that may, for example, encode mutant receptors such as the epidermal growth factor receptor, which is constitutively activated and transmits signals to the cytoplasm for cellular proliferation in the absence of ligand.
Reference: Pages 131–133

8. E

A number of preclinical studies in different animal models and ongoing clinical trials are currently investigating the therapeutic effect of genetic modification of cancer cells in gynecologic malignancies. Different approaches are currently being used. However, none of these approaches have been found to be effective in patients to date.

Advances in our understanding of the biology of tumors and novel techniques in molecular biology have led to a variety of therapeutic approaches that target different tumor characteristic phenomena. Genes for the expression of cytokines have been transferred into tumor cells. The resulting tumor cells co-present tumor-associated antigen on the cell surface and produce cytokines necessary to stimulate immune effector cells. The close vicinity of tumor-associated antigen and immunostimulatory cytokine effectively stimulate a strong anti-tumor response in animals.

Inhibition of oncogene expression in cancer cells can result in reversal of the malignant phenotype. For example, the oncogene erbB2 has been blocked in ovarian cancer cells yielding tumor cells with abrogated tumorigenicity in mice. Mutated or missing p53 protein can be replaced in cancer cells by insertion of the wild type p53 gene. The genetically modified cells are growth arrested due to the cell cycle inhibitory effect of p53. Furthermore, these cells have a higher degree of apoptosis when transfected with the wild type p53 gene. In suicide cancer gene therapy, cancer cells are transfected with genes that encode an enzyme capable of converting a normal nontoxic substance into a toxic metabolite. Upon presentation of the appropriate substrate, the toxic metabolic is produced in transgene expressing tumor cells and induces cell death.
Reference: Page 126

9. E

Although a variety of tumor-associated antigens such as SCC, CA125, and CEA have been described in gynecologic malignancy, unfortunately none of these tumor markers are specific for a particular type of cancer. Tumor-associated antigens have been identified using monoclonal antibody techniques. They are useful markers in following the progression of the disease and the success of treatment. The combination of different tumor markers, for example CA125 and OVX1 in ovarian cancer, may improve the specificity and sensitivity of screening tests.

Monoclonal antibodies react with tumor-associated antigens and can be conjugated to toxins like recin, radioisotopes, or chemotherapeutic agents. These conjugated antibodies can be directed toward human ovarian carcinoma antigens to induce tumor cell killing. However, although the antitumor effects observed in animal studies have been very promising, conjugated monoclonal antibodies have not shown significant effects in patients with gynecologic malignancies. Recently, antigen-specific T cells have been used to identify novel antigens.
Reference: Pages 135–136, 1164

10. A

T cells can be distinguished from other lymphocytes by their cell surface phenotype. They express complexes of proteins on the cell surface that are responsible for various functions in the different subsets of T cells. All mature T cells express the cluster determinant CD3. In addition to CD3, T cells classified as helper T cells express CD4 and killer T cells express CD8. CD20 molecules are found on B cells. The CD56 molecule is unique to natural killer cells. Immunofluorescence is used to identify cluster determinants on T cells and subsequently identification of different subsets.
Reference: Page 136

11. C

T cells can respond to antigens only when the processed antigens are presented in association with MHC molecules on antigen-presenting cells. The CD4 helper T cell population recognizes antigens in association with MHC class II molecules. The CD8 positive T cell killer cell population recognizes antigens in association with MHC class I molecules. B cells express antibodies on their cell surface which function as receptors for antigens. These antibody receptors do not need additional molecules for effective antigen recognition and binding.

T cells belong to the cellular immune system, whereas B cells produce antibodies and are responsible for the humoral immune response. Both B and T cells are able to effectively process antigens and clonally expand. As much as B cells produce specific antibodies against antigens, T cells specific for a certain antigen can expand in a clonal fashion. Both B and T cells have been isolated from gynecologic malignancies. Tumor infiltrating T cells can be isolated from tumors and stimulated to expand *in vitro* by interleukin-2. These lymphokine-activated tumor infiltrating lymphocytes are the base for cellular immunotherapy. Reference: Pages 134–136

12. D

Cytotoxic killer T cells (or CD8 positive T cells) are considered to be the most effective mediators of tumor cell lysis. Killer T cells can recognize antigens associated with MHC class I molecules. Through antigen-specific T-cell receptors, a series of events involving cytokine production by CD4 helper T cells induces activation of cytotoxic T cells, which are able to lyse tumor cells directly.

Macrophages are professional antigen-presenting cells for CD4 positive helper T cells. Macrophages and B cells express MHC class II molecules. These cells are able to phagocytose antigen and subsequently present intracellularly processed antigen to CD4 postive helper T cells. Helper T cells possess T-cell receptors for the specific antigen and can produce a variety of cytokines.

One of the most important cytokines generated by CD4 postive T cells is interleukin-2, which is able to stimulate killer T cells. The killer T cells ultimately integrate signals from specific antigens and unspecific stimulation by differenct cytokines, mainly interleukin-2. Natural killer cells have an innate immune response. They can generate nonspecific killing of tumor cells and virus infected cells without stimulation by specific antigens. Reference: Page 136

13. B

T cells can generate a memory response. After first encounter with an antigen, specific T-cells clones are generated. These T-cell clones can be induced by a secondary presentation of the antigen to the T cells. A rapid clonal expansion upon secondary antigen recognition increases the velocity and magnitude of the immune response against the previously recognized antigen. This memory response is crucial, for instance, for the effect of immunization against viruses.

Natural killer cell activity presents an innate form of immunity that is unspecific and unable to generate a memory response. Monocytes and their tissue form (macrophages) are unspecific cytotoxic cells and are unable to mount a memory response. B cells can effectively generate immune responses particularly important in vaccination. Reference: Pages 136–137

14. A

Interleukin-2 is a T-cell produced cytokine, part of the so-called Type I T-helper cell-related immune response (TH1). TH1 and TH2 are T-helper cell subpopulations, characterized by the nature of the induced immune response. Although originally described in mice, a similar dichotomy exists in humans. TH1-type immune responses are characterized by the production of interleukin-2 (IL-2) and interferon-γ; TH2-like responses produce IL-4, IL-5, IL-6, IL-10, and granulocyte macrophage colony stimulating factor

(GM-CSF). In general, TH1-type responses generate cellular immune responses compared to TH2-type responses, which induce the production of antibodies by B cells. In ovarian cancer and other malignancies, a predominantly TH2-like response has been found that contributes to the failure of the immune system to respond adequately to the tumor disease. Immunotherapy attempts to stimulate TH1-type responses in order to generate the more effective cytotoxic T-cell population against the tumor.
Reference: Pages 139–141

15. A (see Table 6.4)

Interleukin-1 is involved in fever and inflammatory responses. Its pleiotropic effects include the stimulation of T cells and B cells to produce cytokines. Two forms of IL-1 have been described with similar biologic activity, namely IL-1a and IL-1b. The primary source of IL-1 are macrophages, some B cells, epithelial cells, brain cells, and the

Table 6.4 Sources, target cells, and biological activities of cytokines involved in immune responses

Cytokine	Cellular source	Target cells	Biological effects
IL-1	Monocytes and macrophages Tumor cells	T cells, B cells Neurons Endothelial cells	Costimulator Pyrogen activation
IL-2	T cells (TH1)	T cells B cells NK cells	Growth Activation and antibody production Activation and growth
IL-3	T cells	Immature hemopoietic stem cells	Growth and differentiation
IL-4	T cells (TH2)	B cells T cells	Activation and growth; isotype switch to IgE; increased MHC II expression Growth
IL-6	Monocytes and macrophages T cells, B cells Ovarian cancer cells Other tumors	B cells T cells Hepatocytes Stem cells Tumor cells	Differentiation, antibody production Costimulator Induction of acute-phase response Growth and differentiation Autocrine/paracrine growth and viability-enhancing factor
IL-10	T cells (TH2) Monocytes and macrophages	T cells (TH1) Monocytes and macrophages B cells	Inhibition of cytokine synthesis Inhibition of Ag presentation and cytokine production Activation
IL-12	Monocytes	NK cells, T cells (TH1)	Induction
IFN gamma	T cells (TH1) NK cells	Monocytes/macrophages NK cells, T cells, B cells	Activation Activation Activation Enhances responses
TNFα	Monocytes and macrophages T cells	Monocytes/macrophages T cells, B cells Neurons (hypothalamus) Endothelial cells Muscle and fat cells	Monokine production Costimulator Pyrogen Activation, inflammation Catabolism/cachexia

Reproduced with permission from **Berek JS, Martínez-Maza O.** Immunology and immunotherapy. In: **Lawton FG, Neijt JP, Swenerton KD.** *Epithelial Cancer of the Ovary.* London: BMJ, 1995:224.

cells lining the synovial spaces. IL-1 is important in the pathomechanism of infertility and may be inhibiting nidation of the fertilized egg.
Reference: Page 139

16. B

Interleukin-3 (IL-3) is a cytokine that enhances the early differentiation of hematopoetic cells. It has stimulatory effects on hematopoetic stem cells. Similar to granulocyte macrophage colony stimulating factor, it enhances the activation and proliferation of macrophages and granulocytes. It is used *in vitro* as growth factor for hematopoetic cells. Similar effects can be generated with granulocyte macrophage colony stimulating factor, which is currently used in preventing and treating neutropenia in chemotherapy-treated patients.
Reference: Page 140

17. C

High concentrations of interleukin-10 have been found in ascites from ovarian cancer patients. Other cytokines like IL-6, TNF-α, granulocyte colony stimulating factor, and granulocyte macrophage colony stimulating factor are also significantly increased in ascites from ovarian cancer patients when compared to peritoneal fluid in noncancer patients.

Interleukin-10 is a potentially immunosuppressive cytokine. Since high concentrations of interleukin-10 are found in the ascites of ovarian cancer patients, interleukin-10 might significantly contribute to the lack of effective immune responses against the tumor. Interleukin-6 inhibits TH2-type immuno responses and potentially inhibits the generation and activation of cytotoxic T-cell responses. Furthermore, it is an autocrine and paracrine growth factor for certain ovarian cancer cell lines.
Reference: Page 140

18. D

Vascular leak syndrome is a potentially lethal side effect of high dose interleukin-2 therapy. Interleukin-2 has been used in a variety of studies with different tumors including ovarian cancer for antitumor therapy. High doses of intravenously or intraperitoneally injected IL-2 might generate potent antitumor responses by stimulating cellular immune responses.

A number of side effects have been associated with interleukin-2 therapy. Vascular leak syndrome has been described in a number of patients. Disruption of endothelial membranes and subsequent leakage of fluids into the extravasal space may lead to brain and lung edema or lethal fluid and electrolyte imbalances. Vascular leak syndrome has been associated with high mortality.

Other side effects of IL-2 therapy, such as allergic reactions of hematopoetic side effects, are less likely to have lethal consequences. The administration of IL-2 and the associated side effects of high doses of IL-2 may be preventable by generating genetically modified tumor cells. The IL-2 gene can be transferred into tumor cells that function as a constant producer for interleukin-2 *in vivo*. However, since interleukin-2 is expressed constitutively, low levels can be maintained with subsequently diminished side effects. This concept is currently under investigation. The clinical application of recombinant IL-2 in ovarian cancer patient has not shown any significant antitumor effects. A number of studies in the last 10 years have revealed an overall response rate of 20% in ovarian cancer patients. Malignancies such as melanoma or renal cell carcinoma have been found to be more responsive to this form of immunotherapy.
Reference: Page 141

19. C

Advanced age is the single most important risk factor for the development of cancer. A possible explanation for the increase in risk of cancer with age might be the accumulation of critical genetic mutations over time with cumulation of exogenous, DNA-damaging factors.

Specific mutations have been found in cigarette smokers with a high frequency of G-T transversions in the sequence of the p53 tumor suppressor gene. Radiation exposure should be considered an environmental carcinogen since diagnostic studies are not associated with an increased risk of cancer due to the quite low doses of radiation. More recently, immune function particularly in HIV-infected patients with the obvious increase of Karposi sarcoma, B-cell lymphoma, and cervical cancer have become important risk factors. High fat diets correlate with the development of certain cancers, e.g., colon cancer. In contrast, vitamin C rich foods and green leafy vegetables seem to decrease the incidence of lung cancer. More advanced studies are needed to evaluate the importance of these factors.

Reference: Page 142

7

Reproductive Physiology

David L. Olive

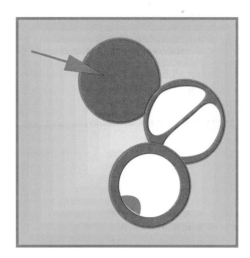

Learning Objectives

1. Understand the anatomy of the hypothalamic-pituitary-ovarian axis.

2. Be aware of the structure and function of reproductive hormones.

3. Understand menstrual cycle physiology, including endometrial changes and follicular development.

Questions

1. Feedback to the hypothalamus from the pituitary gland is referred to as:

   A. The long feedback loop
   B. The short feedback loop
   C. The ultra-short feedback loop
   D. The intracellular feedback loop

2. The blood supply to the anterior pituitary gland is via:

   A. The superior hypophysial artery
   B. The middle hypophysial artery
   C. The inferior hypophysial artery
   D. The portal venous system

3. A chemist is charged with creating a drug that binds to the GnRH receptor but is not easily or rapidly degraded. She decides to modify the basic GnRH decapeptide at which locations?

   A. Amino terminus
   B. Amino acid 3 (Trp)
   C. Amino acid 6 (Glu)
   D. Carboxy terminus

4. An assay is devised to measure LH concentrations in the blood. The method used is an immunoassay that recognizes the alpha subunit of the LH molecule. In clinical trials, there is a major discordance between this test and all commercially available tests. The reason for this apparent lack of accuracy is:

   A. The alpha subunits of FSH, LH, and TSH are identical and thus cross-react with the assay.
   B. Only assays of beta subunits will detect available hormones.
   C. All existing tests are inaccurate.
   D. Successful assays are limited to recognizing carbohydrate moieties on the pituitary hormone molecules.

5. Which of the following are the major secretory products of the posterior pituitary?

   1. Oxytocin
   2. Arginine-vasopressin
   3. Growth hormone
   4. Adrenocorticotropic hormone
   5. Prolactin

   A. 1 and 4
   B. 2 and 3
   C. 1 and 2
   D. 3 and 4
   E. 3, 4, and 5

6. Regularly timed episodes of bleeding that are excessive in amount (>80 ml) and duration of flow (>5 days) is termed:

   A. Oligomenorrhea
   B. Polymenorrhea
   C. Menorrhagia
   D. Metrorrhagia
   E. Menometrorrhagia

7. Hormonal characteristics of the luteal phase of the menstrual cycle include:

  A. High estrogen and progesterone; low FSH and LH
  B. High progesterone; low estrogen, FSH, and LH
  C. Low estrogen, progesterone, FSH, and LH
  D. High estrogen, progesterone, and LH; low FSH

8. The maximum amount of oocytes in a female's ovaries occurs at what point in her life?

  A. 8 weeks gestation
  B. 20 weeks gestation
  C. At birth
  D. At puberty
  E. At 18 years of age

9. Follicular development is a result of:

  A. LH stimulation of both theca and granulosa cells
  B. LH stimulation of theca cells, FSH stimulation of granulosa cells
  C. FSH stimulation of theca cells, LH stimulation of granulosa cells
  D. FSH stimulation of both theca and granulosa cells

Answers

1. B

Several levels of feedback to the hypothalamus exist and are known as the long, short, and ultra-short feedback loops. The long feedback loop is composed of endocrine input from circulating hormones, just as feedback of androgens and estrogens onto steroid receptors are present in the hypothalamus. Similarly, pituitary hormones may feed back to the hypothalamus and serve important regulatory functions in short- loop feedback. Finally, hypothalamic secretions may directly feed back to the hypothalamus itself in an ultra- short feedback loop.
Reference: Page 150

2. D

Blood is supplied to the posterior pituitary via the superior, middle, and inferior hypophysial arteries. In contrast, the anterior pituitary has no direct blood supply. Instead, it receives blood via a rich capillary plexus of the portal vessels that originate in the median eminence of the hypothalamus and descend along the pituitary stalk. This is not absolute, however, and retrograde flow has been demonstrated. This blood flow, combined with the location of the median eminence outside the blood-brain barrier, permits bidirectional feedback control between the two structures.
Reference: Page 151

3. C (see Figure 7.4)
As a peptide hormone, GnRH is degraded by enzymatic cleavage of bonds between its amino acids. Pharmacologic alterations of GnRH have led to the creation of agonists and antagonists. The primary sites of enzymatic cleavage are between amino acids 5 and 6, 6 and 7, and 9 and 10. Substitution of the amino acid glycine at the 6

Figure 7.4   Gonadotropin-releasing hormone (GnRH) is a decapeptide.

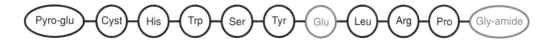

position with large, bulky amino acid analogues makes degradation more difficult and creates a form of GnRH with a relatively long half-life. Substitution at the carboxy terminus produces a form of GnRH with increased receptor affinity. These two locations are thus the most commonly modified when producing such analogues. GnRH analogues are now widely used to treat disorders dependent on ovarian hormones, such as precocious puberty, ovarian hyperandrogenism, leiomyomas, and hormonally dependent cancers.
Reference: Pages 153–154

4. A (see Figure 7.6)
Structurally, there is great similarity between FSH and LH. They are both glycoproteins that share identical alpha subunits and differ only in the structure of their beta subunits, which confer receptor specificity. TSH and hCG also share identical alpha subunits with the gonadotropins.
Reference: Pages 155–156

5. C (see Figure 7.7)
The posterior pituitary (neurohypophysis) is composed exclusively of neural tissue and is a direct extension of the hypothalamus. It lies directly adjacent to the adenohypophysis but is embryologically distinct, derived from an invagination of neuroectodermal tissue in the third ventricle. Axons in the posterior pituitary originate from neurons with cell bodies in two distinct regions of the hypothalamus—the surraoptic and paraventricular nuclei. These neurons secrete their synthetic products directly from axonal boutons into the general circulation to act as hormones. This is the

Figure 7.6   The structural similarity between FSH, LH, and TSH. The α subunits are identical and the β subunits differ.

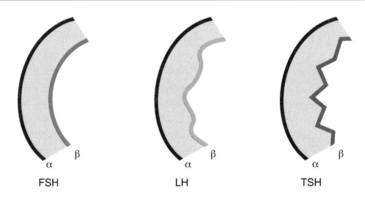

Figure 7.7   Oxytocin and arginine-vasopressin (AVP) are nine amino acid peptides produced by the hypothalamus. They differ only in two amino acids.

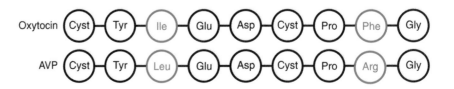

mechanism of secretion of the hormones of the posterior pituitary—oxytocin and arginine-vasopressin.
Reference: Pages 157–158

6. C (see Table 7.1)

Menstruation disorder is one of the most frequent reasons women seek medical care. A normal menstrual cycle lasts from 21 to 35 days with 2 to 6 days of flow and an average blood loss of 20 to 60 ml. The various types of disorders are listed in the accompanying table.
Reference: Pages 158–159

7. A (see Figure 7.9)

Both estrogen and progesterone levels remain elevated throughout the life span of the corpus luteum and then wane with its demise. Gonadotropins are suppressed by the elevated sex steroid levels and begin to rise with demise of the corpus luteum.
Reference: Pages 159–161

8. B (see Figure 7.11)

The number of oocytes peaks at 6 to 7 million by 20 weeks of gestation. Simultaneously, atresia of the oogonia occurs, rapidly followed by follicular atresia. At birth, only 1 to 2 million oocytes remain in the ovary, and at puberty only 300,000 are available for ovulation.
Reference: Pages 163–164

9. B (see Figure 7.12)

The fundamental tenet of follicular development is the two-cell two-gonadotropin theory. This theory states that there is a subdivision and compartmentalization of steroid hormone synthesis activity in the developing follicle. In general, most aromatase activity, for estrogen production, is in the granulosa cells. Aromatase activity is enhanced by FSH stimulation of specific receptor on these cells. However, granulosa cells lack several enzymes that occur earlier in the steroidogenic pathway and require androgens as a substrate for aromatization. Androgens, in turn, are synthesized primarily in response to stimulation by LH, and the theca cells possess most of the LH receptors at this stage. Therefore, a synergistic relationship must exist: LH stimulates the theca cells to produce androgens, which are transferred to the granulosa cells for FSH-stimulated aromatization into estrogens.
Reference: Pages 165–166

Table 7.1	Definitions of Menstrual Cycle Irregularities
Oligomenorrhea	Infrequent, irregularly timed episodes of bleeding usually occurring at intervals of more than 35 days
Polymenorrhea	Frequent but regularly timed episodes of bleeding usually occurring at intervals of 21 days or less
Menorrhagia	Regularly timed episodes of bleeding that are excessive in amount (>80 ml) and duration of flow (>5 days)
Metrorrhagia	Irregularly timed bleeding
Menometrorrhagia	Excessive, prolonged bleeding that occurs at irregularly timed, frequent intervals
Hypomenorrhea	Regularly timed bleeding that is decreased in amount
Intermenstrual bleeding	Bleeding (usually not of an excessive amount) that occurs between otherwise normal menstrual cycles

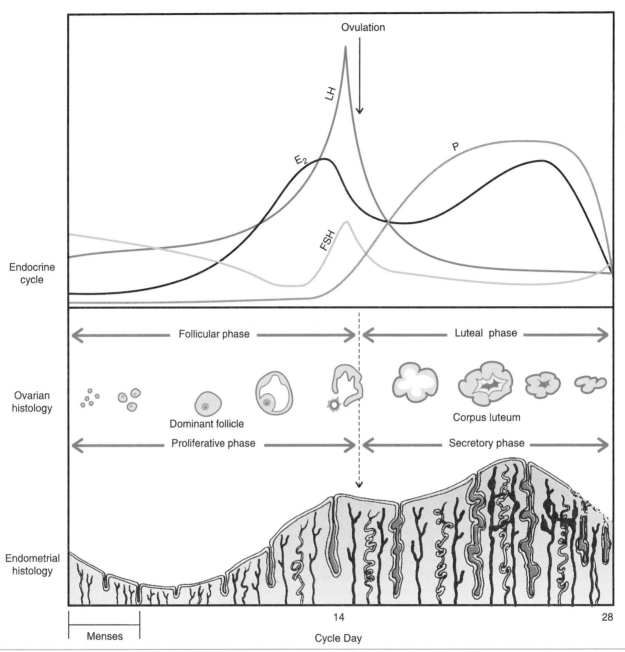

Figure 7.9   The menstrual cycle. The top panel shows the cyclic changes of FSH, LH, estradiol (E$_2$), and progesterone (P) relative to the time of ovulation. The bottom panel correlates the ovarian cycle in the follicular and luteal phases and the endometrial cycle in the proliferative and secretory phases.

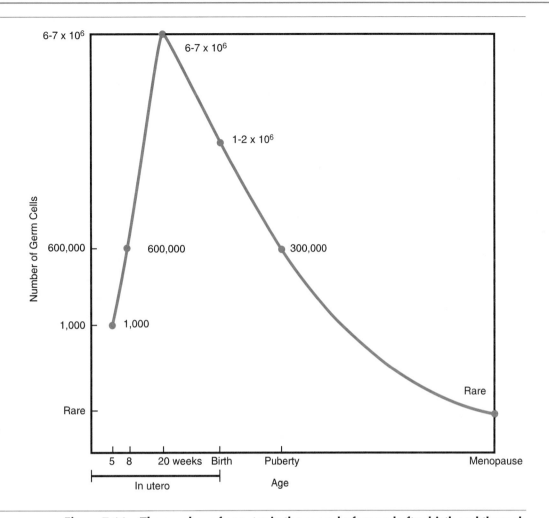

Figure 7.11   The number of oocytes in the ovary before and after birth and through menopause.

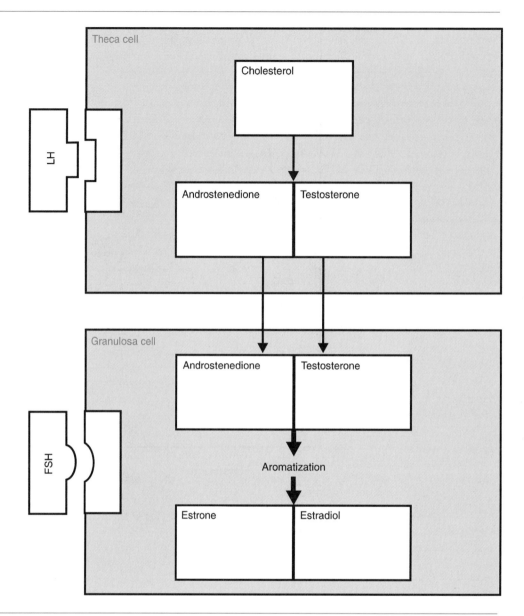

Figure 7.12 **The two-cell two-gonadotropin theory of follicular development in which there is compartmentalization of steroid hormone synthesis in the developing follicle.**

PREVENTIVE AND
PRIMARY CARE

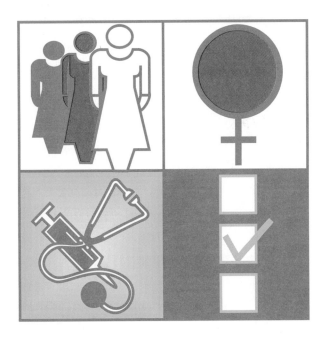

8 Preventive Health Care and Screening

Paula A. Hillard
David L. Olive

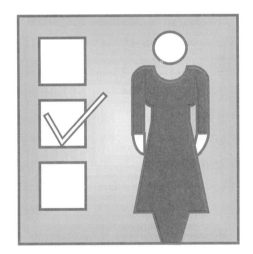

Learning Objectives

1. Be familiar with the major causes of morbidity and mortality within different age groups in order to incorporate a holistic approach to assessing patients' risks.

2. Be familiar with the quality of evidence ratings promoted by the Canadian and U.S. Task Forces on Preventive Health Services.

3. Be aware that the current health risks to adolescents are predominantly behavorial and be able to provide primary preventive services to adolescents based on the Guidelines for Adolescent Preventive Services (GAPS).

4. Be familiar with current recommendations for immunizations by age group and risk status.

5. Be able to calculate a patient's body mass index and to counsel about daily food choices based on the Food Guide Pyramid.

Questions

1. Women taking oral contraceptives and antibiotics concurrently have been reported to have had pregnancies by anecdotal report only. Individuals taking antibiotics during OC have been advised to use a back-up method during the course of antibiotic therapy, because of this risk of OC failure. The U.S. Preventive Services Task Force Quality of Evidence rating for this conclusion would be which of the following:

   A. I
   B. II-1
   C. II-2
   D. II-3
   E. III

2. A 17-year-old young woman comes for an annual gynecologic examination. She reports no current symptoms or complaints, and is currently taking combination oral contraceptives. She states that she has had no major medical problems. A sexual history reveals that she is currently sexually active with one partner. Her partner usually uses condoms. She first had intercourse at age 14, and estimates that she has had 6 lifetime partners, including 3 within the last 6 months. She is uncertain of her past immunization history, but states that she believes that she has had "all her shots." Which of the following is indicated?

   A. HBV vaccine
   B. Hepatitis A vaccine
   C. Tetanus-Diphtheria (dT) vaccine
   D. Measles, Mumps, Rubella (MMR) trivalent vaccine
   E. Varicella zoster vaccine

3. A 51-year-old woman is seen for an annual gynecologic visit. She has no current symptoms, and is having regular menses. She has no major illnesses, and her family history is negative for cardiovascular disease and malignancy. A screening mammogram is recommended. She asks how strong this recommendation is. According to the U. S. Preventive Services Task Force, the strength of this recommendation is based on good evidence. Thus, the strength of the recommendation would be:

   A. A
   B. B
   C. C
   D. D
   E. E

4. A 21-year-old young woman comes to the office for a sports physical examination. She is a distance runner. She states that she has not had a menstrual period in six months. She weighs 104 lbs (50 kg) and is 5′6″ (1.7M) tall. Her BMI (body mass index) is:

   A. 15
   B. 17
   C. 19
   D. 21
   E. 23

5. To identify a problem drinker, which of the following questionnaires can be used:

   A. T-ACE questionnaire
   B. COMCAT questionnaire
   C. BDI questionnaire

6. A 43-year-old woman asks what her target heart rate should be when she is in good condition from exercising. You tell her:

A. 120

B. 126

C. 133

D. 141

Answers

1. E

The U.S. Preventive Services Task Force has adopted a description of the quality of evidence from clinical studies from the Canadian Task Force on the Periodic Health Examination, 1979. This rating system describes three different levels of evidence (see Table 8.9).

As the data for this recommendation is based only on anecdotal, descriptive studies and several expert committee opinions, it is classified as Level III.
Reference: Pages 179, 188

2. A

Recommendations for immunization have been established by a number of national organizations. The American Academy of Pediatrics has recommended immunizations for childhood and adolescence. The American College of Obstetricians and Gynecologists has also published recommendations for immunizations as part of the Guidelines for Primary and Preventive Care. In addition, the Centers for Disease Control have suggested guidelines for the hepatitis B vaccine, which has recently become available. The consultants of The Medical Letter have made recommendations about two even newer vaccines: Hepatitis A vaccine and varicella zoster vaccine. A group of expert consultants convened as a group by the American Medical Association has issued a set of guidelines for health care of adolescents entitled the Guidelines for Adolescent Preventive Services (GAPS) (see Table 8.11).

This patient's sexual behavior clearly places her in a high-risk category for risk of hepatitis B, and thus, according to the ACOG Guidelines, would dictate that hepatitis B vaccine series be given.

The current recommendations for tetanus include the recommendation for a repeat of the bivalent dT(diphtheria/Tetanus) vaccine 10 years after the previous vaccination. The previous immunization usually occured at age 5 to 6; the booster should be given at age 15 to 16. Since pertussis is relatively benign in adolescents, re-immunization with pertussis vaccine is unnecessary.

Table 8.9   Quality of Evidence—U.S. Preventive Services Task Force

I:	Evidence obtained from at least one properly designed randomized, controlled trial.
II-1:	Evidence obtained from well-designed controlled trials without randomization.
II-2:	Evidence obtained from well-designed cohort or case-control analytic studies, preferably from more than one center or research group.
II-3:	Evidence obtained from multiple time series with or without the intervention. Dramatic results in uncontrolled experiments (such as the results of the introduction of penicillin treatment in the 1940s) could also be regarded as this type of evidence.
III:	Opinions of respected authorities, based on clinical experience, descriptive studies, or reports of expert committees.

From **Canadian Task Force on the Periodic Health Examination.** The periodic health examination. *Can Med Assoc J* 1979;121:1193–254.

Table 8.11 Guidelines For Adolescent Preventive Services (GAPS)

1. From ages 11 to 21 years, all adolescents should have an annual routine health visit.

2. Preventive services should be age and developmentally appropriate, and they should be sensitive to individual and sociocultural differences.

3. Physicians should establish office policies regarding confidential care for adolescents and how parents will be involved in that care. These policies should be made clear to adolescent and the parents.

4. Parents or other adult caregivers of adolescents should receive health guidance at least once during early adolescence, once during middle adolescence, and preferably, once during late adolescence.

5. All adolescents should receive health guidance annually to promote a better understanding of their physical growth, psychosocial and psychosexual development, and the importance of becoming actively involved in decisions regarding their health care.

6. All adolescents should receive health guidance annually to promote the reduction of injuries.

7. All adolescents should receive health guidance annually about dietary habits, including the benefits of a healthy diet, ways to achieve a healthy diet, and safe weight management.

8. All adolescents should receive health guidance annually about the benefits of exercise and should be encouraged to engage in safe exercise on a regular basis.

9. All adolescents should receive health guidance annually regarding responsible sexual behaviors, including abstinence. Latex condoms to prevent sexually transmitted diseases (STDs) (including HIV infection) and appropriate methods of birth control should be made available with instructions on how to use them effectively.

10. All adolescents should receive health guidance annually to promote avoidance of the use of tobacco, alcohol, abusable substances, and anabolic steroids.

11. All adolescents should be screened annually for hypertension according to the protocol developed by the National Heart, Lung, and Blood Institute Second Task Force on Blood Pressure Control in Children (18).

12. Selected adolescents should be screened to determine their risk of developing hyperlipidemia and adult coronary heart disease following the protocol by the Expert Panel on Blood Cholesterol Levels in Children and Adolescents (19).

13. All adolescents should be screened annually for eating disorders and obesity by determining weight and stature and asking about body image and dieting patterns.

14. All adolescents should be asked annually about their use of tobacco products, including cigarettes and smokeless tobacco.

15. All adolescents should be asked annually about their use of alcohol and other abusable substances and about their use of over-the-counter or prescription drugs for nonmedical purposes, including anabolic steroids.

16. All adolescents should be asked annually about involvement in sexual behaviors that may result in unintended pregnancies and STDs, including HIV infection.

17. Sexually active adolescents should be screened for STDs.

18. Adolescents at risk for HIV infection should be offered confidential HIV screening with the enzyme-linked immunosorbent assay and confirmatory testing.

19. Female adolescents who are sexually active or any female 18 years of age or older should be screened annually for cervical cancer by use of a Pap test.

20. All adolescents should be asked annually about behaviors or emotions that indicate recurrent or severe depression or risk of suicide.

21. All adolescents should be asked annually about a history of emotional, physical, and sexual abuse.

22. All adolescents should be asked annually about learning or school problems.

Table 8.11—*continued*

---

23. Adolescents should receive a tuberculin skin test if they have been exposed to active tuberculosis, have lived in a homeless shelter, have been incarcerated, have lived in or come from an area with a high prevalence of tuberculosis, or currently work in a health care setting.

---

24. All adolescents should receive prophylactic immunizations according to the guidelines established by the federally convened Advisory Committee on Immunization Practices: a bivalent tetanus-diphtheria vaccine 10 years after their previous diphtheria vaccination (usually 5–6 years old). All adolescents should receive a second trivalent measles–mumps–rubella vaccination, unless there is documentation of two vaccinations earlier during childhood. A measles–mumps–rubella vaccination should not be given to adolescents who are pregnant—susceptible adolescents who engage in high-risk behaviors should be vaccinated against hepatitis B virus. This includes adolescents who have had more than one sexual partner during the previous 6 months, have exchanged sex for drugs or money, are males who have engaged in sex with other males, or have used intravenous drugs. Widespread use of the hepatitis B vaccine is encouraged because risk factors are often not easily identifiable among adolescents.

From **Elster AB, Kuznets NJ.** *AMA Guidelines for Adolescent Preventive Services (GAPS): Recommendations and Rationale.* Baltimore: Williams & Wilkins, 1994:1–191.

The measles, mumps, rubella (MMR) vaccinations should be given if an adolescent, 1) has not had measles, mumps, or rubella infections documented by a physician, 2) lacks laboratory evidence of immunity, or 3) has not had two doses of MMR. Preferably, the second MMR should be given during early puberty, prior to the time when an adolescent is at risk for pregnancy. Adolescents who are sexually active should be cautioned not to become pregnant for three months following the MMR vaccination, although this remains a theoretical precaution.

A live attenuated varicella vaccine was approved in mid-1995. Chickenpox occurs mainly in children less than 8 years old; by the age of 12, less than 10% are still susceptible. Adults account for only 2% of cases of chickenpox, although they account for 50% of the deaths. The Medical Letter recommends vaccination for everyone more than one year old who is in good health and has no history of clinical varicella. It should not be given to pregnant women. It is not clear how long immunity lasts or whether a booster will be necessary in adulthood.

A vaccine to prevent hepatitis A is also now available in the United States. Many adults in the United States are immune to hepatitis A. Antibody testing costs less than the two doses, which are recommended for travelers to endemic areas and members of other high-risk groups including homosexual men and intravenous drug abusers. Thus it is *not* recommended for most adolescents.
Reference: Page 188

3. A

The U.S. Preventive Services Task Force has rated the strength of clinical recommendations; see the scale in Table 8.10. As mammography has been shown to be effective in reducing the mortality from breast cancer by randomized clinical trials, the strength of recommendation is A.
Reference: Page 189

4. B

The body mass index is calculated by dividing the weight in kilograms by the height in meters squared. This calculated value gives a good assessment of nutritional status. Tables facilitate these calculations and the conversions from pounds to kilograms and inches to meters. In addition, tables also indicate the percentiles of weight. Patients who are 20% above or below the normal range (approximately 22) should be assessed for systemic disease or eating disorder. This patient's BMI of 17 suggests further question-

---

Table 8.10   U.S. Preventive Services Task Force—Strength Of Recommendations

A.   There is good evidence to support the recommendation that the condition be specifically considered in a periodic health examination.

B.   There is fair evidence to support the recommendation that the condition be specifically considered in a periodic health examination.

C.   There is poor evidence regarding the inclusion of the condition in a periodic health examination, but recommendations may be made on other grounds.

D.   There is fair evidence to support the recommendation that the condition be excluded from consideration in a periodic health examination.

E.   There is good evidence to support the recommendation that the condition be excluded from consideration in a periodic health examination.

Modified with permission from **ACOG.** *The Obstetrician–Gynecologist and Primary-Preventive Health Care.* Washington, DC: American College of Obstetricians and Gynecologists, 1993:1–22.

Table 8.12   T-ACE Questionnaire

Do you have a drinking problem?

Experts in treating alcohol abuse use the T-ACE questions below to help them find out whether a person has a drinking problem. These questions can also apply to other drugs.

T   How many drinks does it take to make you feel high (**TOLERANCE**)?

A   Have people **ANNOYED** you by criticizing your drinking?

C   Have you ever felt you ought to **CUT DOWN** on your drinking?

E   Have you ever had a drink first thing in the morning to steady your nerves or get rid of a hangover (**EYE OPENER**)?

If your answer to the tolerance questions is *more than two drinks,* give yourself a score of 2. If you answer *yes* to any of the other questions, give yourself a score of 1 each. *If your total score is 2 or more, you may have a drinking problem.*

Modified from **Sokol RJ, Martier SS, Ager JW.** The T-ACE questions: practical prenatal detection of risk-drinking. *Am J Obstet Gynecol* 1989;160:865.

---

ing about bulimic behaviors, distorted body image, and excessive dieting or exercise is indicated. In women with anorexia nervosa, hypoestrogenism with attendant risk for osteoporosis is a concern. Menstrual disturbances are also common in these young women, and amenorrhea is one of the diagnostic criteria for anorexia nervosa. Psychiatric evaluation and treatment are indicated; hospitalization may be necessary in severe cases. Reference: Page 189

5. A (see Table 8.12)

Alcoholic beverages should be limited to less than 1 ounce of absolute alcohol per day (equivalent to two cans of beer, two glasses of wine, or two average cocktails). A simple device called the T-ACE questionnaire can be used to elicit information about alcohol use and identify problem drinkers. Women should be questioned in a nonjudgmental fashion about their alcohol use and directed to counseling services as required. Reference: Page 192

6. C

Cardiovascular fitness can be evaluated by measurement of heart rate during exercise. As conditioning improves, the heart rate stabilizes at a fixed level. The heart rate at which conditioning will develop is called the target heart rate. The formula for calculating the target heart rate is 220 minus the patient's age times 0.75. In the above example, the THR would be $(220-43) \times 0.75 = 177 \times 0.75 = 133$. Reference: Page 193

9 Primary Medical Care

David L. Olive

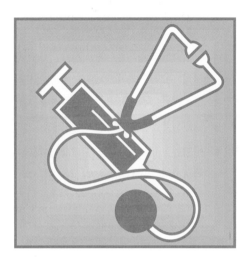

Learning Objectives

1. Be able to describe the most common respiratory diseases of women, their diagnoses, and their treatment.

2. Understand the role of hypertension in health and disease.

3. Be prepared to diagnose and treat hyperlipoproteinemia.

4. Know the classification, diagnosis, and treatment of diabetes mellitus.

5. Grasp the scope of thyroid disease in the female.

Questions

1. Most cases of acute sinusitis begin:

   A. As an allergic reaction
   B. As a result of direct bacterial invasion
   C. As a viral infection
   D. Due to genetic predisposition

2. The rate of chronic bronchitis in the adult population is:

   A. 0.1 to 0.5%
   B. 1 to 2%
   C. 3 to 5%
   D. 10 to 25%

3. Each of the following increases the risk of hypertension **except:**

   A. Being African American
   B. Lower level of education
   C. Living in the southeastern United States
   D. Higher income

4. A 44-year-old African-American presents for her annual well-patient exam. On presentation, she is noted to have a blood pressure of 130/95, pulse of 80. Further history is obtained and it is discovered she has had "borderline" blood pressure in the past. She states she was in a hurry to get to the appointment. Her current weight is 175 pounds and she is 65 inches tall. At this time, you should:

   A. Explain to her that a single elevated reading does not require therapy
   B. Explain to her that her weight is the major problem causing her hypertension
   C. Explain to her that if her blood pressure remains elevated at the next visit in two weeks, medication will be necessary
   D. Begin the laboratory workup for hypertension with a complete blood count, chemistries, chest radiograph, and electrocardiogram
   E. Begin to assess for other risk factors for cardiovascular disease

5. A 55-year-old Caucasian female presents for her annual well-patient exam and desires repeat cholesterol testing. She had a measurement two years ago with a total cholesterol of 210 mg/dL, a LDL- Cholesterol of 130, and HDL-Cholesterol of 80 mg/dL. Her triglycerides were 90 mg/dL. Her weight is normal, she is a nonsmoking normotensive individual, and she is on hormone replacement therapy. You counsel her:

   A. Cholesterol measurements are known to fluctuate and a repeated measurement is reasonable.
   B. Her HMO will not pay for it and she shouldn't be worried anyway.
   C. Individuals on hormone replacement therapy rarely have cholesterol problems.
   D. Her elevated total cholesterol is on the basis of an elevated HDL-Cholesterol and she is not at increase risk for cardiovascular disease.
   E. Cholesterol measurement should only be performed every five years.

6. Which of the following is *not* associated with an elevated risk of myocardial infarction?

   A. HDL Cholesterol
   B. LDL Cholesterol
   C. LDL (a')
   D. B-100 apoprotein

7. A patient is being evaluated for hypercholesterolemia, and you wish to perform laboratory evaluation of her cholesterol level. To minimize variations in this measurements, you should instruct the patient to do which of the following in the 12 hours prior to collection?

   A. Avoid caffeine
   B. Avoid vigorous exercise
   C. Fast
   D. Avoid excessive amounts of water consumption
   E. All of the above

8. The principal cause of hypothyroidism in women is:

   A. Latrogenic hypothyroidism
   B. Autoimmune thyroiditis
   C. Hypothalamic disease
   D. Pituitary tumors
   E. Postpartum hypothyroidism

9. The most common cause of hyperthyroidism in women is:

   A. Postpartum thyroiditis
   B. Choriocarcinoma
   C. Grave's disease
   D. Pituitary adenoma
   E. Struma ovarii

Answers

1. **C**

   Most infections begin with a viral agent in the nose or nasopharynx that causes inflammation to block the draining ostia. The location of symptoms varies by anatomic site: maxillary sinus over the cheeks, ethmoid sinuses across the nose, frontal sinus in the supraorbital area, and sphenoid sinus to the vertex of the head. Viral agents impede the sweeping motion of cilia in the sinus and, in combination with edema from inflammation, lead to superinfection with bacteria.
   Reference: Page 196

2. **D**

   Chronic bronchitis is defined as a productive cough from excessive secretions for at least three months in a year for two consecutive years. It is estimated that between 10 and 25% of the adult population is affected by chronic bronchitis. Contributing factors include cigarette smoking, chronic infections, and environmental pathogens in dust.
   Reference: Pages 197–198

3. **D**

   The incidence of hypertension is twice as high in African Americans than in Caucasians. Geographic variations are present: the southeastern United States has a higher prevalence of hypertension and stroke, regardless of race. One multi-institutional study confirmed an increase of incidence not only among African Americans but also among persons with lower levels of education. Preventive measures can be most effective in those at highest risk, such as in African-American women and individuals from the lowest socioeconomic levels. The influence of genetic predisposition is poorly understood. Studies of women have been limited to those that determine side effects of medication and the impact of certain medications on long-term lipid status.
   Reference: Page 201

4. A

The diagnosis of hypertension is never made with a single measurement (see Figure 9.2). The error in diagnosis with a single measurement may be greater that 35% and is probably related to "white coat" hypertension. Most patients, when blood pressure is repeated at a less stressful time, will be normotensive. The incidence of white coat hypertension is probably more prevalent in the gynecologist office with the expectation of a pelvic examination. First-line therapy for mild (140–159 mm Hg systolic and 90–99 mm Hg diastolic) to moderate (160–179 mm Hg systolic and 100–109 mm Hg diastolic) hypertension is not medication, but lifestyle adjustments (see Table 9.2). Therefore, answer B would be appropriate after the diagnosis of high blood pressure was established. In addition to weight loss, exercise, elimination of tobacco use, and reduction of salt and dietary fats intake are important. The issue of alcohol use remains an enigma. The use of 2 to 5 ounces of alcohol daily is associated with an increase in

Figure 9.2   Algorithm for the treatment of uncomplicated hypertension.

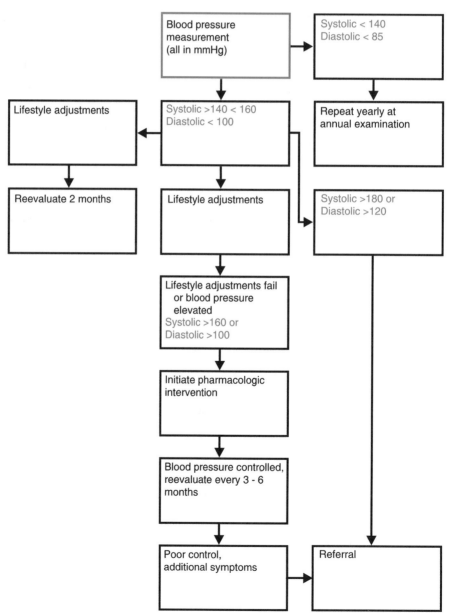

Table 9.2   Life-style Adjustment for Cardiovascular Risk Reduction and Hypertensive Therapy

Weight reduction if overweight

Limit alcohol use to less than 1 ounce of absolute alcohol per day (2 beers, 8 ounces of wine, 2 ounces of 100-proof whiskey)

Regular aerobic exercise (30 minutes fast walking 3 times/week)

Decrease salt intake to less than 6 g/day

Stop cigarette smoking

Reduce dietary saturated fat and cholesterol

Maintain adequate intake of calcium, potassium, and magnesium

If diabetic, control glucose

HDL-Cholesterol, but has the addition of calories and potential for abuse and risk-taking behaviors such as drunk driving. Answer C would only be appropriate if after six months, lifestyle adjustments had failed to control the hypertension. Finally, laboratory workup is only appropriate after the diagnosis is established and other risk factors for cardiovascular disease become known.
Reference: Pages 202–207

5. D (see Figure 9.4)
The role of cholesterol testing in women is undergoing extensive review and unfortunately, multiple guidelines exist depending on the sponsoring organization. The role of cholesterol testing in women without known risk factors (family history of cardiovascular disease [i.e., myocardial infraction or stroke] prior to age 55 in men and 65 in women, tobacco use, obesity, diabetes, and lack of hormone replacement therapy) has become increasingly controversial. Guidelines for screening are currently undergoing revisions. The American College of Obstetricians and Gynecologists in the past have used the United States Preventative Services Task Force (USPSTF) guidelines published in 1988. Guidelines recommended by the National Cholesterol Education Program are for total cholesterol testing to be initiated at age 20 and performed every 5 years. The newest recommendations (1996) by the USPSTF are to test every 5 years between the ages of 45 and 65, but the effectiveness of this protocol in women has been questioned.

This question was designed to demonstrate several key points. Many patients, especially the more educated and affluent, demand that certain "trendy" tests be performed. This patient knew her total cholesterol was elevated, but did not realize this was because her HDL-Cholesterol was extremely high. As a matter of fact, in certain communities (Finnish communities in the upper peninsula of Michigan, for example) where HDL-Cholesterols have been found to be elevated (HDL-Cholesterol in the 80 mg/dL-range), the members of the community have very long lives and lack cardiovascular disease. Additionally, diet may have no influence on these individuals.
Reference: Pages 209–216

6. A (see Figure 9.3)
The major lipid in the LDL-Cholesterol group is the cholesterol ester, which is associated with B-100 apoprotein. Approximately 60 to 70% of total cholesterol consists of LDL-Cholesterol. Elevated levels of LDL-Cholesterol have been associated with increased risk of myocardial infarction in women over 65 years of age. There is a structural class called LDL(a') that is associated with myocardial infarction. Several families with structurally abnormal B-100 apoprotein have been described. Individuals with this abnormal protein are at high risk of myocardial infarction, as a result of lipid buildup and premature atherosclerosis. The density of these particles ranges from 1.019

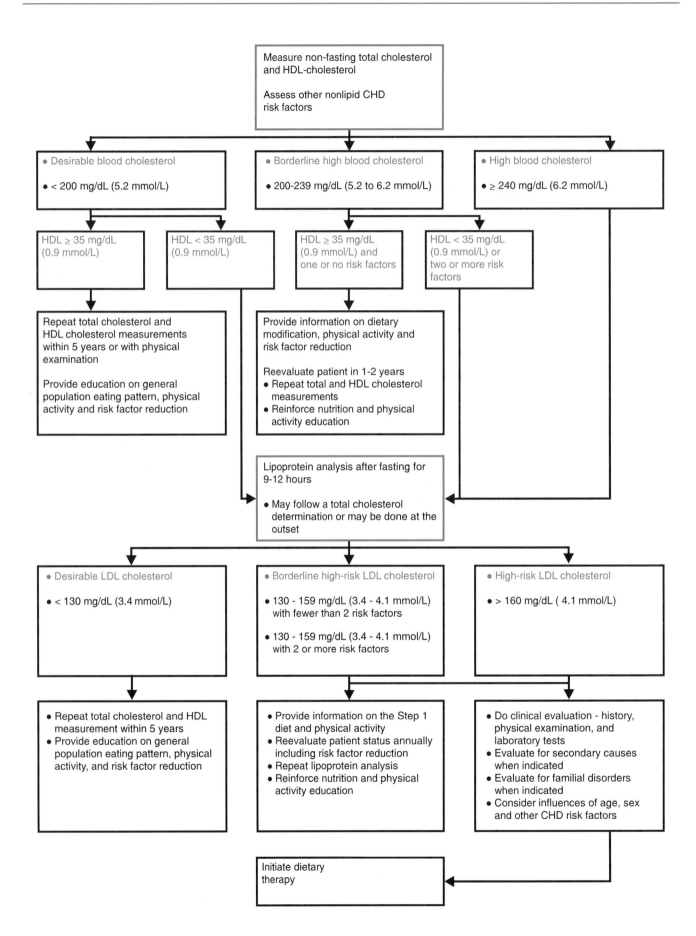

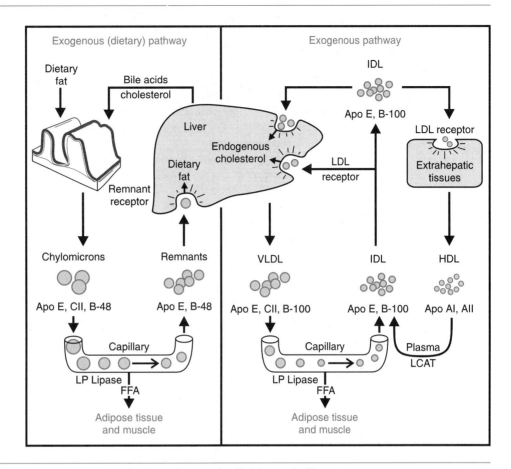

Figure 9.3   Metabolic pathways for lipid metabolism.

to 1.063 g/ml, and they have a diameter of 180 to 280 nm. High-density cholesterol is composed of cholesterol esters with apoproteins A-I and A-II. These particles make up 20 to 30% of total cholesterol and are the most dense, with a weight of 1.063 to 1.120 g/ml. The diameter of this group of proteins is 50 to 120 nm.
Reference: Pages 210–211

7. E
To minimize variations in cholesterol measurement, patients should be instructed as follows:
1. Avoid caffeine
2. Avoid vigorous exercise
3. Continue to smoke the usual number of cigarettes
4. Fast for 12 hours prior to testing
5. Avoid consuming excessive quantities of water.

Caffeine has mixed effect on lipoprotein measurements but should be avoided in the 12 hours prior to blood collection.

Moderate levels of exercise are as important in overall cardiovascular health as control of hypertension and cessation of cigarette smoking. Strenuous exercise lowers the concentration of triglycerides and LDL and increases HDL in the serum. Vigorous exercise should not be performed within 12 hours of blood collection because of these acute changes.

Figure 9.4   Classification of total cholesterol, HDL cholesterol, and LDL cholesterol.

Because of the diurnal variation of blood triglycerides, blood samples should be collected in the morning after a 12-hour fast. The following technique can be used for the collection of blood for cholesterol measurements:

1. Request that the patient sit quietly for 15 minutes prior to testing
2. Minimize tourniquet time (less than 5 minutes)
3. Collect cholesterol sample first, if multiple samples are required
4. Use blood collection tubes with ethylenediaminetetraacetic acid (EDTA) as anticoagulant
5. If samples are not to be analyzed immediately
   - store at 0°C for up to 4 days
   - at −20°C for 6 months
   - at −50°C to −80°C indefinitely

6. Transport by mail on dry ice

Alcohol and cigarette smoking are well-known modifiers of cholesterol. Moderate alcohol intake (defined as approximately 2 ounces of absolute alcohol per day) is noted to increase HDL-Cholesterol and decrease LDL-Cholesterol; however, there is a complimentary increase in triglycerides. Higher intake negates this effect. The increase in HDL-Cholesterol is in the HDL^3 fraction, which is important to the scavenger mechanism of removing LDL-Cholesterol. Smoking (more than 15 to 20 cigarettes per day) has the opposite effect: increasing LDL-Cholesterol and triglyceride levels and decreasing HDL-Cholesterol. HDL^3 decreases with cigarette smoking.
Reference: Pages 213–214

8. B

Overt hypothyroidism occurs in 2% of women, and at least an additional 5% of women develop subclinical hypothyroidism. This is especially true in elderly individuals, in whom many of the signs and symptoms are subtle. The principal cause of hypothyroidism is autoimmune thyroiditis (Hashimoto's thyroiditis). A familial predisposition is observed in many cases, but the specific genetic or environmental trigger is unknown. The incidence of autoimmune thyroiditis increases with age, affecting up to 15% of women over 65 years of age. Many have subclinical hypothyroidism, which is defined as an elevated serum TSH concentration with a normal serum free T4 level. Thyroid replacement therapy usually reverses this condition. Autoimmune thyroiditis may be associated with other endocrine (e.g., type I diabetes, primary ovarian failure, adrenal insufficiency, and hypoparathyroidism) and nonendocrine (e.g., vitiligo and pernicious anemia) autoimmune disorders. Therefore, when autoimmune diseases are present, there should be a high degree of suspicion for concurrent thyroid disorders. Iatrogenic causes of hypothyroidism include surgical removal of the thyroid gland or radioactive iodine therapy for hyperthyroidism or thyroid cancer. Thirty years ago, radiation was used to treat acne and other dermatologic disorders; these patients have an increased risk of thyroid cancer and require close monitoring. Hypothyroidism rarely occurs secondary to pituitary or hypothalamic diseases from TSH or TRH deficiency but must be considered if symptoms occur after neurosurgical procedures.
Reference: Page 221

9. C

Hyperthyroidism affects 2% of women during their lifetime, most often during their childbearing years. The most common disorder is Graves' disease, which is associated with orbital inflammation causing the classic exophthalmus associated with the disease and a characteristic dermopathy, pretibial myxedema. The etiology of Graves' disease in genetically susceptible women is unknown. Autonomously functioning benign thyroid neoplasias are less common causes of hyperthyroidism and are associated with toxic adenomas and toxic multinodular goiter. Transient thyrotoxicosis may be the result of

unregulated glandular release of thyroid hormone in postpartum (painless, silent, or lymphocytic) thyroiditis and subacute (painful) thyroiditis. Other rare causes of thyroid overactivity include: human chorionic gonadotropin-secreting choriocarcinoma, TSH-secreting pituitary adenoma, and struma ovarii. Factitious ingestion or iatrogenic over-prescribing of thyroid hormones should be considered in patients with eating disorders.
Reference: Page 222

10 Family Planning

Phillip G. Stubblefield

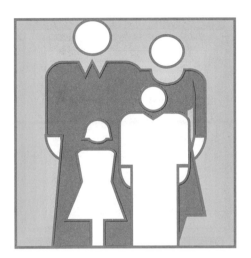

Learning Objectives

1. Describe the pattern of use of fertility control methods in the United States.

2. Discuss the mechanism of action contraceptive methods.

3. Describe the efficacy of contraceptive methods under best-results and usual-results conditions.

4. List the health risks of each method and describe the evidence.

5. List the health benefits of each and describe the evidence.

6. Describe the common methods for inducing legal abortion, their complications, and prevention and management of complications.

7. Describe male and female methods of sterilization and their complications.

8. Be able to adequately counsel couples as to choice of and method of use of contraception, abortion, and sterilization.

Questions

1. Your patient wants some idea of the amount of risk reduction for some of the serious sexually transmitted conditions she can expect if she uses condoms with every act of intercourse. You tell her there is good evidence that:

   A. It does not really matter
   B. Infertility is reduced by about 40% and invasive cancer of the cervix is reduced by about 60% by long term use of condoms.
   C. Condom use provides complete protection against all sexually transmitted diseases.
   D. Infertility is reduced by 10%, invasive cancer by about 30%.
   E. Condom use decreases risk of vaginitis but has little effect on more serious conditions.

2. Your 18-year-old patient will be starting to use the diaphragm. She wants to know the conditions when the diaphragm is likely to fail. You say:

   A. If she puts the diaphragm in correctly, she will have no problems.
   B. Diaphragms are pretty unreliable for young women.
   C. Under laboratory conditions, the female superior positions and multiple re-insertions of the penis just prior to orgasm were associated with the penis being inserted between the diaphragm and the vaginal wall, where conception would be likely.
   D. It depends upon the relative size of the genital organs of the man and the woman.
   E. The lowest pregnancy rate that can be expected with the diaphragm is 6 pregnancies per 100 women per year.

3. You've been asked by an attorney to review a case of possible malpractice in which pelvic inflammatory disease developed in a woman wearing a TCU 380A intrauterine device approximately 18 months after the device was inserted. You note that according to current literature, the risk of PID developing in women wearing this specific IUD is:

   A. PID is increased only during the first 20 days after insertion, and that thereafter PID occurs no more frequently in women wearing this IUD than in women not wearing IUDs.
   B. The number of cases of PID with copper IUDs is three to four times greater than in women not using contraception.
   C. It is more than 50% probable that PID in an IUD-wearing woman is related to the IUD.
   D. PID risk is increased measurably during the first year after insertion, then gradually declines to that of women not wearing IUDs.
   E. When it comes to PID risk, all IUDs are the same.

4. You've been referred to a woman who is pregnant with a Progestasert IUD. Her last menstrual period was seven weeks ago. The strings of the IUD are visible at the cervical os. What is the best advice you can give her?

   A. Caution the patient about risks, but do not remove the IUD because it will provoke loss of the pregnancy.
   B. Administer a broad spectrum antibiotic.
   C. Advise termination of the pregnancy because of infection risk.
   D. Present the options to the patient—removal of the device, leaving the device in, or terminating the pregnancy—as equal possibilities and let the patient decide.
   E. Advise immediate removal of the device by gentle traction on the string.

5. You are seeing for the first time a 30-year-old woman who has been on an oral contraceptive containing 50 mcg of ethinyl estradiol. She wants to know if a lower dose pill would significantly reduce risk of thrombosis. You tell her:

   A. It will make little difference.
   B. By going from a 50 mcg estrogen pill to a lower dose pill, her risk of thrombosis is reduced by about half.
   C. Women on lower dose oral contraceptives have no increased risk of thrombosis unless they smoke cigarettes.
   D. While 50 mcg estrogen pills clearly have less risk than the older, higher dose pills, no evidence exists to show that still lower dose pills are safer.
   E. Risk of thrombosis is unacceptably high for her and she should select a different contraceptive method.

6. Mutation of which of the clotting factors has been recently determined to be the most frequently occurring of the inherited predispositions to clotting:

   A. Factor X
   B. Von Willebrand factor
   C. Fibrinogen
   D. Fibronectin
   E. Factor V

7. Based on current literature, the effect of oral contraceptive use on gynecologic malignancies is best described as follows:

   A. All oral contraceptives are known to increase the risks for breast cancer.
   B. Endometrial cancer is reduced, ovarian cancer is reduced, overall breast cancer risk is unchanged, cervical cancer risk may be modestly increased.
   C. Oral contraceptives protect against breast cancer, ovarian cancer, and cervical cancer, but increase risk for endometrial cancer.
   D. Endometrial cancer is reduced, ovarian cancer is increased, overall breast cancer risk is increased.

8. Your 25-year-old patient has just had laparoscopic surgery for her third symptomatic functional ovarian cysts. Her internist has suggested treatment with a triphasic oral contraceptive to prevent cyst recurrence, but seeks your opinion. You state:

   A. Oral contraceptives cause ovarian cysts.
   B. Oral contraceptive therapy will reduce risk for recurrent functional cysts, but the protection is dose related; a monophasic, 50 mcg estrogen pill would offer the best protection against recurrent cysts.
   C. Any combination estrogen-progestin oral contraceptive can be expected to reduce the risk of functional ovarian cysts. No convincing evidence indicates that the particular preparation is important.
   D. Multiphasic oral contraceptives are considerably safer in all respects and, therefore, are the first choice for this patient.
   E. A patient who has had three recurrent ovarian cysts is best advised to have her ovaries removed to prevent later ovarian cancer.

9. You've been consulted by a 28-year-old woman who wishes to conceive. What is the probability of pregnancy after discontinuing depot medroxyprogesterone acetate?

   A. Ninety percent will have conceived by 24 months after discontinuation of DMPA.
   B. Only fifty percent will have conceived by 24 months after discontinuation of DMPA.
   C. Virtually all women who will conceive again after discontinuing DMPA do so by 12 months. Those who do not will be permanently sterile.
   D. The probability of pregnancy depends upon too many factors to allow estimation.
   E. Thirty percent will have conceived by one year.

10. Your 21-year-old patient has been using the levonorgestrel implant for two years. Initially she had irregular bleeding several days each month, but now she has had no bleeding at all for eight weeks and wonders if this means anything. You tell her:

    A. Irregular bleeding and episodes of amenorrhea are both commonly seen with the implant. She should not be alarmed.
    B. The implants should be removed and replaced with new ones.
    C. This bleeding pattern requires discontinuation of implants and selection of a new method of contraception.
    D. She should come into the office for a pregnancy test.
    E. About 20% of implant users have this bleeding pattern. Additional low-dose oral estrogen should be given to produce more endometrial proliferation and restore a normal bleeding pattern.

11. It is 2 am. Your 18-year-old patient just paged you to report that she was having intercourse at approximately 4 pm, the condom broke, and she is so worried she cannot sleep. She is using no other contraception now, but she used *Ovral,* a combination oral contraceptive containing levonorgestrel and ethinyl estradiol until six months ago. Her last menstrual period started 12 days ago. What is the best advice you can give her?

    A. She should use a postcoital contraceptive. High-dose estrogen, a combination oral contraceptive, a copper IUD, danazol, or misoprostol have all been used for this purpose.
    B. She should wait to see if she misses her period and then come in for a pregnancy test.
    C. Postcoital contraception should be considered an abortion and should not be proposed.
    D. If she still has her levonorgestrel/ethinyl estradiol pills around, she could take 2 now and 2 more in 12 hours.
    E. Douching might help prevent pregnancy.

12. Your patient is eight weeks pregnant and feels she cannot continue the pregnancy. She asks about serious risk for her from a legal abortion at this point compared with risk if she continues the pregnancy. You answer:

    A. Interruption of pregnancy is always wrong. She should not consider it.
    B. Risk of death is about 0.4 per 100,000 legal abortions in the United States, compared with a maternal mortality rate of 7 to 8 per 100,000 live births.
    C. Risk of death from early abortion exceeds that of childbirth.
    D. Risk of death is about 5.4 per 100,000 legal abortions in the United States, compared with a maternal mortality rate of 3 per 100,000 live births.
    E. Serious risk is so rare with either that it is not important.

Answers

1. B

Condoms and other barriers reduce risk of sexually transmitted disease. Gonorrhea, ureaplasma, and pelvic inflammatory disease and its sequela (tubal infertility) are reduced with consistent use of barriers. A comparison of infertile women to postpartum women showed a 40% reduction in infertility with past use of condoms or the diaphragm. The greatest benefit was for methods that combined a barrier with a spermicide.

Condoms also offer some protection from cervical neoplasia. In one study, the relative risk of severe dysplasia among users of condoms or diaphragms was 0.4 at 5 to 9 years of use and only 0.2 when the barriers had been used for 10 years or more, which is a 60 to 80% reduction. Another study compared women with invasive cervical cancer to controls. The risk of invasive cervical cancer was 0.4 whenever users of condoms or diaphragms were compared to none users. With the worldwide epidemic of acquired

immune deficiency disease, there is intense interest in the ability of condoms to prevent transmission of the human immunodeficiency virus (HIV). Tested *in vitro, C. trachomatis,* herpes virus type 2, HIV virus, and hepatitis B did not penetrate latex condoms but did cross through condoms made from animal intestine. Additional protection is provided by the addition of the spermicide *nonoxynol-9.* Follow-up of sexual partners of HIV-infected people has shown considerable protection when condoms are used. Studies of HIV-negative, high-risk women given both condoms and spermicidal suppositories of *nonoxynol-9* demonstrated a high degree of protection from HIV seroconversion during follow-up. Vaginal spermicide should be used in addition to condoms when prevention of infection is of prime concern.
Reference: Pages 234–235

2. C

Studies of simulated and actual intercourse under laboratory conditions by Johnson and Masters discovered elevation of the uterus and expansion of the vaginal barrel with normal sexual excitement, which can allow slippage of the diaphragm. Female superior position and multiple mountings just prior to orgasm are likely to result in the penis being reinserted in front of the diaphragm, which would cause failure of contraception.
Reference: Pages 235–237

3. A

The large World Health Organization study found increased risk for PID with copper IUDs during only the first 20 days after insertion. IUDs are not all the same. The Dalkon shield, with its tail composed of a sheath of fibers, could act as a wick and pull vaginal microorganisms up into the uterine cavity. Other IUDs have much less risk of infection. Actinomyces pelvic abscesses can be seen in women wearing plastin IUDs long term, but the addition of copper to the IUD appears to markedly reduce this possibility.

A still larger, prospective World Health Organization study found PID increased during only the first 20 days after insertion. Thereafter the rate of diagnosis of PID was about 1.6 cases per 1000 women per year, the same as in the general population. Exposure to sexually transmitted pathogens is the more important determinant of PID than is the wearing of an IUD.
Reference: Pages 238–242

4. E

A risk of spontaneous loss of the pregnancy does exist when the device is removed, but most pregnancies will continue after removal of the device. If the device is not removed, the patient is at risk for premature rupture of the membranes in the midtrimester, extremely premature birth, and septic abortion with possible loss of maternal life.

If the IUD strings are visible, the IUD should be removed as soon as pregnancy is diagnosed in order to prevent later septic abortion, premature rupture of the membranes, and premature birth. If the strings are not visible, an ultrasound exam should localize the IUD and determine whether an unnoticed expulsion has occurred. If the IUD is present, there are three options for management: therapeutic abortion, ultrasound-guided intrauterine removal of the IUD, and continuation of the pregnancy with the device left in place. If the patient wishes to continue the pregnancy, we advise ultrasound evaluation of the location. If the IUD is not in a fundal location, ultrasound-guided removal using small alligator forceps is advised. If the location is fundal, the IUD should be left in place. If pregnancy will continue with an IUD in place, the patient must be warned of the symptoms of intrauterine infection and be cautioned to seek care promptly for fever or flu-like symptoms, abdominal cramping, or bleeding. At the earliest sign of infection, high-dose intravenous antibiotic therapy should be begun and the pregnancy promptly evacuated.
References: Pages 238–242

Table 10.5   Oral Contraceptive Estrogen Dose and Risk of Deep Vein Thrombosis (DVT)

Estrogen (dose)	(Rate/10,000 person years)	Relative Risk (all cases)	Relative Risk (proven diagnosis)
<50 μg	4.2	1.0	1.0*
50 μg	7.0	1.5	2.0 (0.0–4.0)
>50 μg	10.0	1.7	3.2 (2.4–4.3)

*Base line risk used to calculate risk for higher doses.
From **Gerstman BB, Piper JM, Tomita DK, Ferguson WJ, Stadel BV, Lundin FE.** Oral contraceptive dose and the risk of deep venous thrombosis. *Am J Epidemiol* 1991;133:32–7.

5. B (see Table 10.5)

A large U.S. study described in the *American Journal of Epidemiology* showed that risk of proven deep-vein thrombosis was twofold greater in women using 50 mcg pills compared with those who had used oral contraceptives containing less than 50 mcg of estrogen. Reference: Page 246

6. E

A mutation of Factor V, called Factor V Leidin, resists attack-activated protein C and, therefore, thrombosis is promoted. Women with familial deficiency of antithrombin III, protein C, or protein S are highly likely to suffer thromboembolic episodes if given estrogen-containing OCs. These abnormalities are rare, but recently a mutation of the gene for blood clotting Factor V (Factor V Leidin) has been identified in 3 to 5% of the population. The abnormal Factor V resists cleavage by the natural anticoagulant protein C, producing a syndrome described as "activated protein C resistance." A 1994 study estimated increased risk of a first thromboembolic episode among women using OCs who do not have the Factor V mutation to be 2.2 per 10,000 women years, 4.9 per 10,000 women years for women homozygous or heterozygous for the mutation who do not use OCs, and 27.7 per 10,000 women years for women with the mutation who also take OCs. Effect of estrogen dose was not examined. Cigarette smoking did not effect risk of thrombosis. Pregnancy is an even greater challenge for women with inherited defects of anticoagulation. Reference: Pages 245–246

7. B

Indisputable evidence exists to show that endometrial cancer and ovarian cancer are significantly reduced by a history of use of combination oral contraceptives, and the benefit increases with increased years of past use. Overall breast cancer risk is not increased, but may be increased for some subgroups. Cervical cancer may be somewhat increased, but this is difficult to sort out because of confounding by other risk factors, most especially age at first intercourse, exposure to multiple partners, and exposure to human papilloma virus.

Combination OCs reduce risk for subsequent endometrial cancer and ovarian cancer providing a very important health benefit. Two years of OC use reduces risk of subsequent endometrial cancer by 40% and four or more years use reduce risk by 50%. A 50% reduction in ovarian cancer risk was observed for women who took OCs for 3 to 4 years, and an 80% reduction with 10 or more years of use. There was some apparent benefit from as little as 3 to 11 months of past use. The benefit continues for at least 15 years since last use and does not diminish, even at 15 years. National vital statistics data from England support these observations. Ovarian cancer mortality is declining in England and Wales for women under 55 and this has been attributed to OC use.

Squamous cancer of the cervix may be weakly associated with OC use. The important risk factors are early sexual intercourse and exposure to human papilloma virus. Women who have used OCs typically started sexual relations at younger ages and, in some studies, will report more partners. Alternative choices for contraception make it harder to resolve the question because barrier contraceptives reduce risk for cervical cancer. A comparison of IUD wearers to OC users found that preneoplastic lesions of the cervix progressed more rapidly among OC users. Most cervical cancers are of the squamous cell type. Adenocarcinomas of the cervix are rare, but are not as well detected by screening cervical cytology, and appear to be increasing. A 1994 study found a doubling of risk with OC use, which increased with duration of use, reaching a relative risk of 4.4 (95% confidence interval 1.8 to 10.8) if total use of OCs exceeded 12 years. This study adjusted for history of genital warts, number of sexual partners, and age at first intercourse. Because adenocarcinoma of the cervix is rare, absolute risk is low. The cumulative risk to age 55 of long-term OC use would be about 1 in 1000 patients, if this apparent association is real. Use of OCs is at most a minor factor in causation of cervical cancer; however, women who have used OCs should have annual cervical cytology, as should any sexually active woman.

The prevalence of breast cancer in the United States has increased, but the increase is seen among women too old to have taken OCs. A very large study showed no overall relation between OC use and breast cancer. Another large study, the U.S. Nurses Health study, reported on 1,127,415 person years of observation and found no increase among OC users compared to nonusers overall. Some studies have found apparent risk to subgroups of users, for example, young women, nulligravid women, and women who used OCs before a first-term pregnancy. A British study that found a small but statistically stable increase in breast cancer diagnosed before age 36 among OC users, found that risk was less for OCs with less than 50 mcg of estrogen. Progestin-only OCs appeared to have a protective effect. Significantly, OC users who developed breast cancers had somewhat lower stage tumors and were less likely to have positive lymph nodes than controls. One explanation for the apparent paradox of no overall increase but possible increased risk for small subgroups of young women is that OC use may promote growth of preexisting breast cancers, allowing early diagnosis, but not increasing the lifetime risk. A small increase for diagnosis of breast cancer prior to age 44 may be offset by decreased risk for women developing breast cancer at an older age, when there are many more cases. Hence the potential exists that future studies may show that OCs have prevented many breast cancers. OC use by women with a first-degree relative who had breast cancer does not increase risk regardless of duration of use before first-term pregnancy.
Reference: Pages 250–251

8. B

While there is still controversy, a population-based study found all combination oral contraceptives decrease the risk of ovarian cyst formation, but higher-dose pills provided the best protection.

All combination OCs offer some protection from functional ovarian cysts, but this protection is less with multiphasic preparations.
Reference: Page 251

9. A

Women treated with *DMPA* experience disruption of the menstrual cycle and have initial spotting and bleeding at irregular intervals, but eventually most develop total amenorrhea—50% by one year and 80% by three years of continued administration. Persistent irregular bleeding can be treated by giving the next dose of *DMPA* ahead of schedule, or by adding low-dose estrogen temporarily, as for example conjugated estrogens 1.25 mg per day for 10 to 21 days at a time. *DMPA* persists in the body several months in women who have used it for long-term contraception, and return to fertility may be delayed; however, in a large study, 70% of former users desiring pregnancy had conceived within 12 months, and 90% within 24 months.
Reference: Pages 253–255

10. D

Implant-related amenorrhea is more likely early in the use of a set of implants, when release rates for the *levonorgestrel* are highest. Women who continue cyclic bleeding are those more likely to conceive, even though conception is rare with the implants. The pattern described, of cyclic bleeding followed later by amenorrhea, is worrisome for pregnancy.

Norplant produces endometrial atrophy. The normal menstrual cycle is disrupted, resulting in a range of possible bleeding patterns, from reasonable regular monthly bleeding, to frequent spotting and almost daily bleeding, to complete amenorrhea. Bleeding patterns change over time and tend to become more like a normal menstrual pattern. Women who have monthly bleeding are more likely to be ovulating, and if they become amenorrheic must be evaluated for pregnancy.
Reference: Pages 255–256

11. D

While A is true, it does not give the patient a specific plan of help at 2 am. Since several hours have elapsed since intercourse, and she is at midcycle, prompt action is advisable. Until mifepristone becomes available, the regimen using oral contraceptives offers acceptable efficacy with few side effects. This patient may already have what she needs at home, and can begin immediately. As to whether postcoital contraception should be regarded as termination of pregnancy, that is a philosophical debate, not a medical one. It is the physician's responsibility to make the information available and let the patient decide. Use of postcoital contraception markedly reduces the possibility of unwanted pregnancy that may lead to need for induced abortion.

Implantation of the fertilized ovum is thought to occur on the sixth day after fertilization. This interval provides an opportunity to prevent pregnancy even after fertilization. High-dose estrogen taken within 72 hours of coitus prevents pregnancy. The mechanism of action of postcoital estrogens may involve altered tubal motility, interference with corpus luteum function medicated by prostaglandins, or alteration of the endometrium. In an analysis of over 3000 women treated after coitus with 5 mg of *ethinyl estradiol* daily for 5 days, the pregnancy rate was 0.15%.

The single most used regimen is the combination of *ethinyl estradiol* 200 mcg and d,l *norgestrel* 2 mg (2 *Ovral* tablets followed by 2 more 12 hours later). The average pregnancy rate with this method is 1.8%, but is 1.2% if taken within 12 hours of intercourse. Estrogens appear more effective; however, a randomized trial concluded that the *Ovral* method was just as effective. Nausea and vomiting are common with both regimens and an antiemetic is usually prescribed. There are no placebo-controlled trials of postcoital contraception.

Postcoital insertion of a copper IUD within 72 hours appears even more effective than sex steroids. Of 879 patients treated in this fashion, only one pregnancy occurred. Haspells reported inserting copper IUDs as long as seven days after coitus and reports no pregnancies have occurred during the first month after insertion. Copper is toxic to the embryo.

Danazol, a weak androgen, has also been used for emergency contraception. The pregnancy rate was 2% among 998 women reported.

The antiprogesterone *mifepristone* (*RU486*) is also highly effective for emergency contraception, and appears to have no significant side effects. A three-way trial of the *Ovral* method, *danazol* (600 mg repeated after 12 hours), and *mifepristone* (600 mg as a single dose) yielded pregnancy rates of 2.62, 4.66, and 0%, respectively. *Mifepristone* is also highly effective in inducing menstruation when taken on day 27 of the menstrual cycle, well beyond the 72-hour window usually considered for postcoital contraception. Of 62 women treated in this fashion, only one conceived.
Reference: Pages 256–257

Table 10.11 Death to Case Rates for Legal Abortion Mortality by Weeks of Gestation,
United States, 1972–1987

Weeks of Gestation	Deaths	Abortions	Rate*	Relative Risk
≤8	33	8,673,759	0.4	1.0
9–10	39	4,847,321	0.8	2.1
11–12	33	2,360,768	1.4	3.7
13–15	28	962,185	2.9	7.7
16–20	74	794,093	9.3	24.5
≥21	21	175,395	12.0	31.5

*Legal abortion deaths per 100,000 procedures, excludes deaths from ectopic pregnancies or pregnancy with gestation length unknown.
From **Lawson HW, Frye A, Atrash HK, Smith JC, Shulman RB, Ramick M, et al.** Abortion mortality, United States, 1972–1987. *Am J Obstet Gynecol* 1994;171:1365–72.

12. B (see Table 10.11)

Physicians who feel abortion is wrong under all circumstances still have a responsibility as health professionals to "put health first" and tell the patient factual information about abortion risk when requested.

The risk of death from legal abortions is 0.4 per 100,000 induced abortions, while total maternal mortality runs 7 to 8 per 100,000 live births. The risk of death from legal abortion prior to 16 weeks is 5- to 10-fold less than that from continuing the pregnancy on to delivery.
Reference: Pages 266–267

11 Sexuality and Sexual Function

David A. Baram

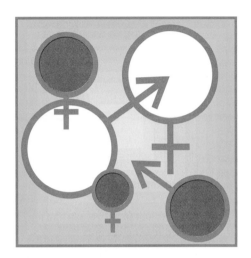

Learning Objectives

1. Understand the rationale for and barriers to obtaining a good sexual history.

2. Be able to identify the variations in sexual practices of men and women.

3. Understand the sexual response cycle in women.

4. Enumerate the factors affecting sexual response.

5. Understand the types and causes of sexual dysfunction.

6. Be able to evaluate and treat sexual assault in children and adults.

Questions

1. Compared to the sexual response cycle in women, the unique feature of the sexual response cycle in men is the presence of the:

   A. desire phase
   B. excitement phase
   C. plateau phase
   D. resolution phase
   E. refractory phase

2. Vaginal lubrication formed during the arousal phase of the sexual response cycle in women comes from the:

   A. bartholin glands
   B. skene glands
   C. transudate from the walls of the vagina
   D. cervix
   E. periurethral glands

3. Correct statements regarding the effect of aging on sexuality in women include each of the following **except:**

   A. Vaginal lubrication in older women takes longer to appear.
   B. Orgasmic contractions in older women are less intense and less frequent.
   C. Frequency of intercourse decreases as women age.
   D. Older women are more likely to experience dyspareunia.
   E. Women lose interest in sex at an earlier age than men.

4. A 27-year-old women has never been able to insert a tampon or have a pelvic examination. She has no difficulty becoming sexually aroused. She is orgasmic, but has never been able to have intercourse. When she and her partner attempt intercourse, she becomes anxious and experiences involuntary spasmodic contractions of the muscles surrounding her introitus. This conditions is known as:

   A. vaginismus
   B. dyspareunia
   C. inhibited sexual desire
   D. phobic avoidance of sex
   E. impaired arousal

5. Adult survivors of childhood sexual abuse, when compared to women who have not been sexually abused, are at increased risk for each of the following conditions **except:**

   A. depression
   B. eating disorders
   C. schizophrenia
   D. sexual dysfunction
   E. chronic pelvic pain

6. A woman who has been raped is most likely to have been raped by:

   A. a stranger
   B. her teacher
   C. an acquaintance
   D. her minister
   E. her husband

7. A 25-year-old woman presents to the emergency department five hours after she was sexually assaulted. The assailant ejaculated in her vagina. Which of the following antibiotic regimens would be most effective in treating this patient for sexually transmitted diseases that may have been acquired during the assault?

    A. ampicillin and doxycycline
    B. penicillin and doxycycline
    C. ceftriaxone and doxycycline
    D. ampicillin and metronidazole
    E. ceftriaxone and metronidazole

8. A 20-year-old woman presents to her family physician 30 hours after she was sexually assaulted. The assailant ejaculated in her vagina. She uses no birth control. Her last menstrual period started two weeks ago. The most appropriate way to prevent pregnancy in this patient is to:

    A. insert an intrauterine device
    B. administration of a combination birth control pill followed by a second dose 12 hours later
    C. administration of diethylstilbestrol
    D. administration of depomedroxyprogesterone acetate
    E. administration of misoprostol suppositories

9. The percentage of women who will be forcibly raped during their lifetime is:

    A. 1%
    B. 3%
    C. 13%
    D. 20%
    E. 25%

10. Each of the following medications interferes with sexual functioning **except:**

    A. antihypertensives
    B. antidepressants
    C. oral contraceptives
    D. antihistamines
    E. digoxin

11. The best predictor of sexual functioning and satisfaction following surgery for breast cancer is:

    A. the type of mastectomy
    B. precancer sexual functioning
    C. the presence or absence of metastatic disease
    D. the size of the scar
    E. the degree of postsurgical pain

12. A woman presenting with the recent onset of inhibited sexual desire should have which of the following laboratory tests performed?

    A. TSH and prolactin
    B. TSH and testosterone
    C. testosterone and prolactin
    D. estrogen and FSH
    E. FSH and prolactin

13. A 36-year-old woman noted the recent onset of superficial dyspareunia. Prior to this episode of dyspareunia, she never experienced painful intercourse. Which of the following is the most likely cause of her dyspareunia?

   A. vulvar vestibulitis
   B. partially imperforate hymen
   C. candida vaginitis
   D. urinary tract infection
   E. episiotomy scar

Answers

1. **E**

   Orgasm is a myotonic response mediated by the sympathetic nervous system and is experienced as a sudden release of the tension that has built up during the arousal and plateau stages. Orgasm is the most intensely pleasurable of the sexual sensations. Orgasm consists of multiple (3 to 15) 0.8-second reflex rhythmic contractions of the muscles surrounding the vagina, perineum, anus, and orgasmic platform. Many women who are orgasmic prefer to have orgasms prior to intercourse, during the time when clitoral stimulation is most intense. Unlike men, who are unresponsive to sexual stimulation after orgasm (refractory period), woman are potentially multiorgasmic and capable of experiencing more than one orgasm during a single sexual cycle. Thus, they can experience orgasms both prior to and during intercourse, provided enough clitoral stimulation is provided.
   Reference: Pages 280–282

2. **C**

   The arousal phase is mediated by the parasympathetic nervous system and is characterized by erotic feelings and the appearance of vaginal lubrication. Sexual arousal increases blood flow to the vagina, and the resulting vasocongestion and possible changes in capillary permeability create a condition that increases the capillary filtration fraction. The filtered capillary fluid transudates between the intercellular spaces of the vaginal epithelium causing droplets of fluid to form on the walls of the vagina.
   Reference: Pages 280–281

3. **E (see Tables 11.1 and 11.2)**

   Aging and the cessation of ovarian function accompanying menopause has a significant effect on the sexual response cycle of women. Sexual desire and the frequency of intercourse decrease as women age, although women retain interest in sex and continue to have the potential for sexual pleasure for their entire lives. The need for closeness, love, and intimacy does not change with age. The way women function sexually as they grow older is largely dependent on partner availability and how frequently they had sex and how much they enjoyed sex when they were younger. Anatomical changes that accompany aging include reduced vaginal size, thinning and decreased elasticity of the vaginal walls, shrinkage of the labia majora and thinning of the labia minora, decreased clitoral sensitivity and size, reduced perineal muscle tone, and a thinner orgasmic platform. Breast atrophy, decreased breast engorgement during arousal, and sensory changes in the nipple and areola are also noted. These physiologic changes predispose women to more frequent episodes of vulvovaginitis and urinary tract infections, which, along with decreased vaginal lubrication, may cause dyspareunia. Women, as they age, require more time to become sexually aroused, take longer to lubricate, produce less vaginal lubrication, have less intense orgasms, and need more stimulation to become orgasmic. The ability to have orgasms does not change significantly with aging, but older women are less likely to be multiorgasmic. Interestingly, women who remain coitally active after menopause have less vulvar and vaginal atrophy than abstinent women.
   Reference: Pages 282–283

Table 11.1 Anatomic Changes of Aging
Reduced vaginal size
Thinning of vaginal walls
Decreased elasticity of vaginal walls
Shrinkage of the labia majora
Thinning of the labia minora
Decreased clitoral sensitivity
Decreased clitoral size
Reduced perineal muscle tone
Thinner orgasmic platform
Breast atrophy
Decreased breast engorgement during arousal
Sensory changes in the nipple and areola

From **Masters WH, Johnson VE.** *Human Sexual Response.* Boston: Little, Brown and Company, 1966.

Table 11.2 Sexual Physiology—Effects of Aging
Increased time required to become sexually aroused
Longer time needed to lubricate
Production of less vaginal lubrication
Less intense orgasms
Increased need for stimulation to become orgasmic
No change in the ability to have orgasms
Less likely to be multiorgasmic

From **Mooradian AD, Greiff V.** Sexuality in older women. *Arch Intern Med* 1990;150:1033–8.

4. A

Vaginismus is the recurrent or persistent involuntary contraction of the perineal muscles surrounding the outer third of the vagina when vaginal penetration with a penis, finger, tampon, or speculum is attempted. Vaginismus is an involuntary reflex precipitated by real or imagined attempts at vaginal penetration and can be *global* (the woman is unable to place anything inside her vagina) or *situational* (she is able to use a tampon and can tolerate a pelvic examination but cannot have intercourse). Many women with vaginismus have normal sexual desire, experience vaginal lubrication, and are orgasmic but are unable to have intercourse.. Vaginismus can be *primary* (the woman has never been able to have intercourse) or *secondary* (often due to acquired dyspareunia). Some couples may cope with this situation for years before they decide to seek help. They usually seek treatment because they desire children or decide they would like to consummate their relationship. Vaginismus is relatively rare, affecting approximately 1% of women.
Reference: Pages 288–289

5. C

Women who have been sexually abused as children or sexually assaulted as adults often experience sexual dysfunction and difficulty with intimate relationships and parenting. Compared to women who have not been sexually assaulted, they are more likely

to experience depression, chronic anxiety, anger, substance abuse problems, multiple personality disorder, borderline personality disorder, fatigue, low self-esteem, feelings of guilt, and sleep disturbance. They often experience social isolation, phobias, and feelings of vulnerability and loss of control. Survivors of sexual assault represent a disproportionate number of patients with chronic headaches and chronic pelvic pain. They may develop posttraumatic stress disorder. They are more likely to commit suicide. The cognitive sequelae include flashbacks, nightmares, disturbances in perception, and dissociative experiences. These women may not be able to tolerate pelvic examinations and may avoid seeking routine gynecologic care, yet they are more likely to utilize the medical care system for nongynecologic concerns. They are at greater risk for being overweight and for having gastrointestinal disturbances.
Reference: Pages 290–291

6. C (see Table 11.5)

There are many myths about rape. Perhaps the most common is that women are raped by strangers. In fact, only about 20 to 25% of women are raped by someone they do not know. Most women are raped by a relative or acquaintance (9% by husbands or ex-husbands, 11% by father or stepfather, 10% by boyfriend or ex-boyfriend, 16% by other relatives, and 29% by other nonrelative). While acquaintance rape may seem to be less traumatic than stranger rape, survivors of acquaintance rape often take longer to recover.
Reference: Pages 291–294

7. C (see Table 11.6)

The risk of acquiring a sexually transmitted disease is difficult to assess, as the prevalence of preexisting sexually transmitted diseases is high (43%) in rape survivors. STD prophylaxis should be offered to all survivors and should cover infections with N. gonorrhoeae, C. trachomatis, and incubating syphilis. Current recommendations include ceftriaxone 250 mg intramuscularly or cefixime 400 mg orally (if allergic to cephalosporins, spectinomycin 2 mg intramuscularly may be used), followed by doxycycline 100 mg twice a day or tetracycline 500 mg four times a day for seven days.
Reference: Pages 295–296

8. B

Approximately 5% of fertile rape survivors will become pregnant. Options include: 1) awaiting the next expected menses; 2) repeating the serum pregnancy test in one to two weeks; and 3) postcoital contraception. If the patient desires postcoital contraception, a preexisting pregnancy can usually be ruled out by performing a sensitive human chorionic gonadotropin assay. Pregnancy prophylaxis can be provided by the immediate administration of two tablets of ethinyl estradiol-norgestrel (Ovral birth control pills), followed by two more tablets 12 hours later. This regimen will only be effective

---

Table 11.5 Physician Responsibilities in Treating Sexual Assault Survivors

1.	Obtaining an accurate gynecologic history, including a recording of the sexual assault.
2.	Assessing, documenting, and treating physical injuries.
3.	Obtaining appropriate cultures (including samples for forensic tests), treating any existing infection, and providing prophylaxis for sexually transmitted diseases.
4.	Providing therapy to prevent unwanted pregnancy.
5.	Providing counseling for the patient and her partner and/or family.
6.	Arranging for follow-up medical care and counseling.
7.	Reporting to legal authorities as required by state law.

From **American College of Obstetricians and Gynecologists.** *Sexual Assault.* Technical Bulletin. Washington, DC: ACOG, 1992:172.

Table 11.6 Laboratory Studies in the Evaluation of Sexually Assaulted Adults

Cultures of the cervix, mouth, and rectum for:
Neisseria gonorrhoeae
Chlamydia trachomatis
Herpes simplex
Cytomegalovirus
Serologic test for syphilis
Wet prep for trichomonas
Hepatitis B surface antigen
Human immunodeficiency virus antibody
Pregnancy test

if it is administered within 72 hours following the sexual assault. Some patients experience nausea and vomiting when given postcoital contraception, and this can be controlled with an antiemetic agent like promethazine, 12.5 mg every four to six hours. Postcoital contraception has a small failure rate (about 1%) and potential teratogenicity which should be explained to the patient.
Reference: Page 295

9. C

The National Women's Study provides the best statistics about the incidence of forcible rape in America. This study found that 13%, or one out of eight adult women, are survivors of at least one completed rape during their lifetime. Of the women they surveyed, 0.7% had been raped in the past year, equating to an estimated 683,000 adult women who were raped during a 12-month period. Thirty-nine percent of the women they surveyed were raped more than once. Most disturbing, however, is their finding that the majority of rapes occurred during childhood and adolescence, with 29% of all forcible rapes occurring when the survivor was less than 11 years old, and 32% occurring between the ages of 11 and 17. Indeed, rape in America is a tragedy of youth. Twenty-two percent of rapes occurred between the ages of 18 and 24, 7% between the ages of 25 and 29, and only 6% when the survivor was older than 30.
Reference: Pages 291–292

10. E (see Table 11.3)

Drugs that interfere with sexual functioning include the following:

- Antihypertensives
- Thiazide diuretics
- Antidepressants
- Antipsychotics
- Antihistamines
- Barbiturates
- Narcotics
- Benzodiazepines
- Hallucinogens
- Amphetamines
- Cocaine
- Oral contraceptives

Reference: Pages 283–284

Table 11.3 Drugs That Can Interfere With Sexual Functioning

Antihypertensives

Thiazide diuretics

Antidepressants

Antipsychotics

Antihistamines

Barbiturates

Narcotics

Benzodiazepines

Hallucinogens

Amphetamines

Cocaine

Oral contraceptives

Table 11.4 Assessment of Dyspareunia

Behavior	Faulty technique
Affect	Guilt, anger, fear and shame
Sensation	Where is the pain?
Imagery	Do intrusive thoughts or negative images disrupt sexual enjoyment?
Cognition	Are there dysfunctional beliefs or misinformation that play a role in undermining sexual participation?
Interpersonal	How do the partners communicate and relate in both sexual and nonsexual settings?
Drugs	Is the patient on any medication that would diminish vaginal lubrication?

From **Lazarus AA.** Dyspareunia: a multimodal psychotherapeutic perspective. In: **Leiblum SR, Rosen RC,** eds. *Principles and Practice of Sex Therapy.* 2nd ed. New York: The Guilford Press, 1989:89–112.

11. B

Breast cancer diagnosis and treatment impacts women's sexuality. However, most women cope well with the stress of treatment and do not develop major psychiatric disorders or significant sexual dysfunction. A number of studies have compared women who undergo mastectomies to women who have conservative surgery with breast conservation, and have found little difference between the two groups in postoperative marital satisfaction, psychological adjustment, frequency of sex, or incidence of sexual dysfunction. The frequency of breast stimulation with sexual activity does decrease after mastectomy. Women who undergo lumpectomy do have more positive feelings about their bodies, especially their appearance in the nude, than do women who have mastectomies. The strongest predictor of postcancer sexual satisfaction is not the extent of her surgery but rather the woman's overall psychological health, relationship satisfaction, and precancer sexual functioning.
Reference: Page 284

12. C

Physiological causes of hypoactive sexual desire include medications, chronic medical illnesses, depression, stress, substance abuse, aging, and hormonal alterations. Any patient presenting with the recent onset of a desire phase disorder should have serum testosterone and prolactin titers evaluated, as an elevated prolactin titer (from a pituitary adenoma) or a low testosterone titer (sometimes following natural or surgical menopause) could be responsible.

Reference: Pages 285–286

13. C (see Table 11.4)

Causes of pain on stimulation of the external genitalia include chronic vulvitis and clitoral irritation and hypersensitivity. Pain at the introitus caused by penile entry can be caused by a rigid hymenal ring, scar tissue in an episiotomy repair, a Müllerian abnormality, vaginitis caused by one of the many common vaginal pathogens such as candida, trichomonas, or Gardnerella, or by irritation from over-the-counter vaginal sprays, douches, or contraceptive devices. Vaginal infection is the most common cause of successfully treated dyspareunia. Another common cause of dyspareunia is friction due to inadequate sexual arousal. This can be treated by counseling the couple to spend more time with foreplay, ensuring that the woman has adequate lubrication prior to intercourse. Use of a water-soluble lubricant such as KY Jelly is also helpful.. Vaginal atrophy resulting from hypoestrogenic states (menopause and lactation) can be treated with systemic or vaginal estrogen replacement.

Reference: Pages 289–290

12 Common Psychiatric Problems

Nada L. Stotland

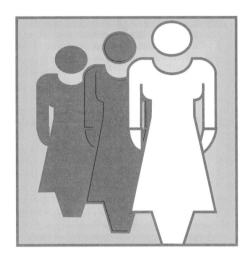

Learning Objectives

1. Be able to identify the indications and techniques of psychiatric referral.

2. Be able to identify the signs and symptoms of depression.

3. Understand the pitfalls in the diagnosis and treatment of premenstrual dysphoria.

4. Recognize the characteristics and dangers of anorexia nervosa.

Questions

1. Which of the following is a significant concern in the referral of a patient to a psychiatrist?

   A. The anxiety provoked by the discussion of psychiatric referral may precipitate suicidal behavior in the susceptible patient.

   B. The patient may perceive the referral as a statement that she is "crazy."

   C. The patient may fail to return for follow-up gynecologic care.

   D. The patient will be disturbed when she discovers that the doctor she has been referred to is a psychiatrist.

   E. The patient will become more demanding of the gynecologist's attention.

2. Which of the following is a criterion for the diagnosis of depression?

   A. fluctuating mood

   B. increased dependency

   C. decreased energy

   D. presence of a precipitating trauma

   E. delusions of persecution

3. Which of the following is not a risk in the diagnosis and treatment of premenstrual dysphoria?

   A. A diagnosis of depression may be overlooked.

   B. The patient will attempt to treat her symptoms by adopting a healthier lifestyle.

   C. Retrospective reporting may reinforce a patient's misattribution of her symptoms to the menstrual cycle.

   D. The clinician will attempt to identify the hormonal aberration causing the symptoms.

   E. The disorder will be overdiagnosed.

4. Which of the following statements is true of anorexia nervosa?

   A. It is evenly distributed between males and females.

   B. It can be appropriately managed in the gynecologist's office.

   C. It often resolves without treatment.

   D. It rarely presents to the gynecologist.

   E. It poses significant medical risks.

Answers

1. **B (see Table 12.1)**

   Uneasiness with the referral process stems logically from stigmas and misconceptions. Clinicians fear that patients will be insulted, alienated, or alarmed by a recommendation to seek psychiatric care.

   Many physicians fear that discussion of suicide or homicide will precipitate an enactment of this behavior that otherwise would not have taken place. The opposite is the case.

   Although becoming less prevalent, some patients believe that any mention of mental health intervention implies either that they are crazy or that the referring physician is convinced that their physical symptoms are imaginary or even deliberately manufactured. The gynecologist may wish to state explicitly that this is not the case. Clearly stating the real reason for the referral and explaining the signs and symptoms known to the patient will usually allay anxiety over a psychiatric referral.

   Under no circumstances is it acceptable to refer the patient to a psychiatrist without informing her in advance.
   Reference: Pages 302–303

Table 12.1   Practitioners' Negative Reactions Toward Patients with Psychiatric Problems

1. Social stigma attached to psychiatric diagnoses, patients, and practitioners.

2. Belief that individuals with psychiatric disorders are weak, unmotivated, manipulative, or defective.

3. Belief that the criteria for psychiatric diagnoses are intuitive rather than empirical.

4. Belief that psychiatric treatments are ineffective and unsupported by medical evidence.

5. Fear that patients with psychiatric problems will demand and consume inordinate and limitless time from a medical practice.

6. Precipitation in others, including doctors, of feelings that are complementary to the strong and unpleasant emotions experienced by patients with psychiatric disorders.

7. Gynecologists' own uncertainty about their skills at psychiatric diagnosis, referral, and treatment.

8. Failure to view psychiatric problems as legitimate grounds for medical attention.

---

2. C

Depression is characterized by:

1. sad mood, crying
2. irritability
3. hopelessness and helplessness
4. decreased ability to concentrate
5. decreased energy
6. interference with sleep, early awakening
7. decreased appetite
8. withdrawal from social relationships
9. inability to enjoy previously gratifying activities
10. guilt
11. decreased libido
12. speeding or slowing of speech and activity
13. thoughts of death or suicide

The patient who has five or more of the signs and symptoms of depression for a significant part of each day for two weeks or more has clinical depression.
Reference: Page 305

3. B

No specific hormonal levels, treatments, or markers associated with premenstrual symptoms have been identified. Women who have premenstrual symptoms may be suffering from a specific psychiatric illness such as depression or personality disorder. Therefore, women who experience premenstrual symptoms should undergo a thorough psychologic evaluation to identify any other underlying disorders that can be treated. They also must rate their symptoms prospectively on forms, separate from the record of their menses, for at least two consecutive cycles before the diagnosis of premenstrual dysphoria can be confirmed by a clear association with symptoms during the luteal phase of the cycle. A small percentage of patients who describe premenstrual changes qualify for the strict diagnosis of premenstrual dysphoric disorder. In these cases, the premenstrual dysphoria interferes with the patient's ability to function in her daily activities. Initial treatment of premenstrual symptoms that are not disabling should be directed at lifestyle changes. Nonpharmacologic treatments with few or no negative side effects and the potential for overall positive effects include the following:

- elimination of caffeine intake
- smoking cessation
- regular exercise
- regular, nutritious diet
- adequate sleep
- active stress reduction

Reference: Pages 306–307

4. E

Anorexia nervosa is associated with severe restrictions on food intake, often accompanied by excessive physical exercise and the use of diuretics or laxatives. Clinical features include menstrual irregularities; intense, irrational fear of becoming fat; preoccupation with body weight as an indicator of self-worth; and inability to acknowledge the realities and dangers of the condition.

More than 90% of cases of anorexia and bulimia occur in females; the prevalence is 0.5 to 1.0% in late adolescence and 1 to 3% in early adulthood. Some cases of anorexia are diagnosed when patients seek care from gynecologists for infertility or amenorrhea. Untreated anorexia poses significant risk of death, often from cardiac complications of electrolyte abnormalities.

Patients with anorexia should be treated by mental health professionals, preferably individuals with specific expertise in this area. A specific contract for weight gain must be made with the patient; if she fails to comply, hospitalization may be required. Patients sometimes resort to elaborate subterfuges to conceal their failure to eat and gain weight. Eating disorders should be treated by a mental health professional before instituting gynecologic interventions such as ovulation induction. Attention to the risks of osteopenia or osteoporosis is essential in amenorrheic patients with anorexia nervosa, and warrants a collaborative effort between the psychiatrist and gynecologist.
Reference: Pages 322–323

IV

GENERAL
GYNECOLOGY

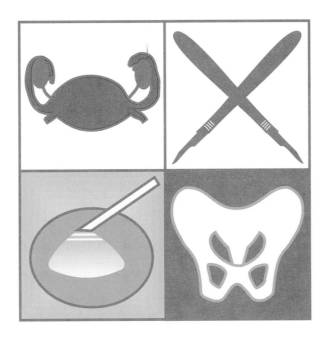

13 Benign Diseases of the Female Reproductive Tract: Symptoms and Signs

Paula A. Hillard
David L. Olive

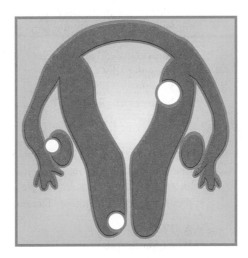

Learning Objectives

1. Be able to state two causes of abnormal bleeding in each of the following age groups: prepubertal girls, adolescents, reproductive age women, perimenopausal women, and postmenopausal women.

2. Be able to state two causes of a pelvic mass in each of the following age groups: prepubertal girls, adolescents, reproductive age women, perimenopausal women, and postmenopausal women.

3. Be able to describe the technique of office endometrial sampling.

4. Be able to describe the technique of office vulvar biopsy.

Questions

1. A 3-year-old girl is brought to the office because of a foul-smelling vaginal discharge. Common causes of this symptom that should be investigated include each of the following **except:**

    A. Bacterial infection
    B. Candidal vaginitis
    C. Vaginal foreign body
    D. Sexual abuse

2. A 12-year-old girl is brought to the emergency department because of very heavy vaginal bleeding with the onset of her first menstrual period. Her hemoglobin level is 9.0 mg/dl. Each of the following diagnoses should be considered **except:**

    A. Anovulatory, dysfunctional bleeding
    B. Coagulopathy
    C. Pregnancy
    D. Endometrial polyps
    E. Thyroid dysfunction

3. A 27-year-old woman is found to have a 5-centimeter, left adnexal mass during a routine pelvic examination. She denies symptoms. She is sexually active, but is not using any method of contraception. Her last menstrual period was 27 days earlier. A urine pregnancy test is negative. The most likely diagnosis is:

    A. Follicular cyst
    B. Corpus luteal cyst
    C. Ectopic pregnancy
    D. Pedunculated leiomyoma
    E. Pelvic kidney

4. Which of the following characteristics is considered abnormal in a 16-year-old girl who underwent menarche at age 12?

    A. Cycle length of 38 days
    B. Cycle length of 23 days
    C. Bleeding for 8 days
    D. 65-ml blood loss per cycle
    E. Bleeding for 1 day

5. The first line of treatment for cystic glandular hyperplasia is:

    A. Hysterectomy
    B. Endometrial ablation
    C. Progestin therapy
    D. Estrogen therapy
    E. Anti-fibrinolytic therapy

6. A 6-year-old girl comes to your office with lower abdominal pain. Ultrasonography reveals an enlarged ovary on the right side. The most likely diagnosis is:

    A. Benign epithelial neoplasm
    B. Malignant germ cell tumor
    C. Benign germ cell tumor
    D. Malignant epithelial neoplasm
    E. Follicular cyst

7. In which of the following situations is surgery for uterine leiomyomata *not* indicated?

   A. Anemia, abnormal uterine bleeding, unresponsive to hormonal management
   B. Asymptomatic, uterus enlarged to 14-week size
   C. Asymptomatic, hydronephrosis on IVP
   D. Urinary frequency and a 14-week size uterus
   E. Prolapsing submucus myoma

8. A 23-year-old woman presents to your office with a small, raised area on her vulva. You perform a biopsy. The most likely diagnosis is:

   A. Epidermal inclusion cyst
   B. Lentigo
   C. Carcinoma *in situ*
   D. Melanocytic nevi
   E. Hidradenoma

Answers

1. B

Vulvovaginitis is the most common gynecologic problem in prepubertal girls. Girls are often unable to adequately describe their symptoms, but parents may notice that the child cries during urination, scratches herself repeatedly, or complains of vague symptoms in the genital area. Consideration should be given to a possible urinary tract infection or pinworms, as these can lead to vulvar symptoms. Chronic skin conditions such as lichen sclerosus can occur in prepubertal girls, but the symptoms are usually vulvar symptoms of itching or burning, rather than a *vaginal* discharge. Vulvovaginal symptoms of any sort in a young child should prompt the consideration of possible sexual abuse. Evaluation should include questioning the child herself; parents rarely object, if an appropriate explanation is given prior to questioning. If the child answers negatively, the opportunity can be used as a "teachable moment" to ensure that the child knows what she should do if she encounters inappropriate touching. A vaginal discharge in a prepubertal child should be cultured for STDs. The most common cause of vaginal discharge in this age group is that of a multibacterial origin due to the presence of perineal organism, the proximity of the anus to the vaginal introitus, and hormonal factors rendering the hypoestrogenic vagina and vestibule more susceptible to infection. Candida vaginitis is uncommon in prepubertal children who are out of diapers. A foreign body may cause a foul-smelling discharge that is persistent in spite of appropriate therapy with topical estrogen cream and a broad-spectrum antibiotic. The most common foreign body is a small piece of toilet paper within the vagina. Irrigation can be performed in the office using a small catheter, flushing small foreign bodies from the vagina.
Reference: Page 390

2. D

Anovulatory cycles are common during the first one to two gynecologic years. The mechanism relates to a failure of the feedback mechanism in which rising estrogen levels result in a decline of FSH with subsequent decline of estrogen levels. Thus, estrogen secretion continues, resulting in endometrial proliferation with subsequent unstable growth and incomplete shedding. The clinical result is irregular, prolonged, and heavy bleeding. Dysfunctional bleeding is a diagnosis of exclusion, and testing for other causes of abnormal bleeding should be performed. The possibility of a pregnancy-related complication must be considered when an adolescent presents with abnormal bleeding. A pregnancy test is indicated in all adolescents with excessive bleeding, regardless of her statements about whether she has had intercourse. The medical consequences of failing to diagnose a pregnancy are too severe to risk missing the diagnosis. Exogenous hormone usage may be a cause of abnormal bleeding and should be

excluded by history. In the adolescent age group, the possibility of a hematologic cause of abnormal bleeding must be considered. Several studies have shown that coagulopathies such as von Willebrand's disease or ITP may be causative, particularly in the youngest age group or those presenting at menarche. Patients who present with menorrhagia have been found to have a higher incidence of STDs, and subclinical endometritis may be causative. Structural lesions such as endometrial polyps or uterine leiomyomata are rare in adolescents.
Reference: Pages 336–340

3. A

It is difficult to determine the frequency of diagnoses of pelvic mass in women of reproductive age because many pelvic masses are not ultimately treated with surgery. Non-ovarian or nongynecologic conditions should be considered and excluded, although a pelvic kidney is an infrequent diagnosis. Pedunculated leiomyoma may be asymptomatic, but an isolated pedunculated fibroid is uncommon in the absence of fibroids palpable within the uterine wall. Nonneoplastic functional ovarian masses are common, and comprise follicular cysts, corpus luteum cysts, and theca lutein cysts. All are benign, and the most common functional cyst is the follicular cyst, which is usually found incidentally during the pelvic exam, although they may rupture, causing pain and peritoneal signs. Corpus luteum cysts are less common than follicular cysts and are typically a complex mass, rather than a simple, unilocular cyst. Given the sensitivity of the currently available urine pregnancy tests, a negative urine pregnancy virtually excludes the possibility of ectopic pregnancy.
Reference: Pages 358–373

4. C

To assess vaginal bleeding during adolescence, it is necessary to have an understanding of the range of normal menstrual cycles. During the first two years after menarche, most cycles are anovulatory. Despite this, they are somewhat regular, within a range of approximately 21 to 40 days. In more than one-quarter of girls, a pattern of +10 days and a cycle length of 20 to 40 days are established within the first three cycles; in one-half of girls, the pattern is established by the seventh cycle; and in two-thirds of girls, such a pattern is established within two years of menarche.

The mean duration of menses is 4.7 days; 89% of cycles last 7 days or less. The average blood loss per cycle is 35 ml, and the major component of menstrual discharge is endometrial tissue. Recurrent bleeding in excess of 80 ml per cycle results in anemia. The transition from anovulatory to ovulatory cycles takes place during the first several years after menarche. It results from the so-called "maturation of the hypothalamic-pituitary-ovarian axis," characterized by positive feedback mechanisms in which a rising estrogen level triggers a surge of luteinizing hormone and ovulation. Most adolescents have ovulatory cycles by the end of their second year of menstruation, although most cycles (even anovulatory ones) remain within a rather narrow range of 21 to 42 days.

Cycles that are longer than 42 days, cycles that are shorter than 21 days, and bleeding that lasts more than 7 days should be considered out of the ordinary, particularly after the first two years from the onset of menarche. The variability in cycle length is greater during adolescence than adulthood; thus, greater irregularity is acceptable if significant anemia or hemorrhage is not present. However, consideration should be given to an evaluation of possible causes of abnormal menses (particularly underlying causes of anovulation such as androgen excess syndromes) for girls whose cycles are consistently outside normal ranges.
Reference: Pages 336–337

5. C (see Figure 13.10)

The terminology that has been used to describe endometrial hyperplasia is confusing, and the clinician must consult with the pathologist to ensure an understanding of the diagnosis. The following lesions are considered to be benign: anovulatory, proliferative, cystic

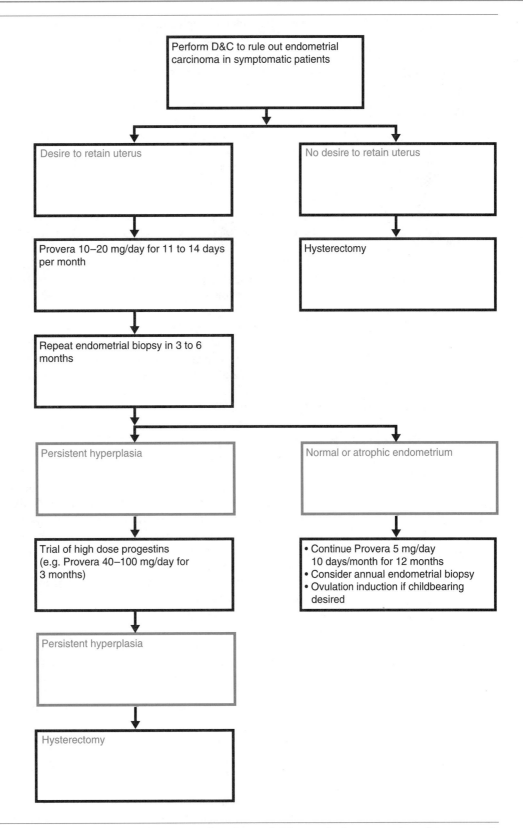

Figure 13.10 Management of endometrial hyperplasia. (Reproduced from **Berek JS, Hacker NF.** *Practical Gynecologic Oncology.* 2nd ed. Baltimore: Williams & Wilkins, 1994:299.)

glandular hyperplasia, simple cystic hyperplasia, simple hyperplasia, and adenomatous hyperplasia without atypia. These terms reflect and describe an exaggerated proliferative response of the endometrium. In most cases, benign endometrial hyperplasia is resolved with D&C or progestin therapy. Repeat surveillance with endometrial biopsy may be warranted.

The presence of atypia with abnormal proliferation, including features of "back-to-back" crowding of the glands, with epithelial activity demonstrated by papillary projections into the glands, is associated with an increased risk of progression to endometrial carcinoma. These architectural abnormalities may be associated with individual cellular atypia (enlarged, irregular nuclei, chromatin clumping, and prominent nucleoli). The presence of mitotic activity also can be variable.

The management of endometrial hyperplasia rests on an understanding of the natural history of the lesion involved. In one study, only 2% of 122 patients with hyperplasia without cytologic atypia progressed to carcinoma, whereas 23% of those with atypical hyperplasia subsequently developed carcinoma. Architectural complexity and crowding appears to place patients at greater risk for progression than does the presence of cytologic atypia alone.

These data suggest that most women with endometrial hyperplasia will respond to progestin therapy and are not at increased risk of developing cancer. Patients who do not respond are at a significantly increased risk of progressing to invasive cancer and should be advised to have a hysterectomy. Patients who are unlikely to respond can be identified on the basis of cytologic atypia.
Reference: Pages 351–352

6. B

Fewer than 5% of ovarian malignancies occur in children and adolescents. Ovarian tumors account for approximately 1% of all tumors in these age groups. Germ cell tumors make up one-half to two-thirds of ovarian neoplasms in individuals younger than 20 years of age. A review of studies conducted from 1940 through 1975 concluded that 35% of all ovarian neoplasms occurring during childhood and adolescence were malignant. In girls younger than nine years of age, approximately 80% of the ovarian neoplasms were found to be malignant. Germ cell tumors account for approximately 60% of ovarian neoplasms in children and adolescents, compared with 20% of these tumors in adults. Epithelial neoplasms are rare in the prepubertal age group.
Reference: Pages 352–353

7. B

Determining potential indications for surgical treatment requires careful judgment and assessment of the degree of associated symptoms. Asymptomatic leiomyomas do not usually require surgery. Some indications for surgery include the following:

1. Abnormal uterine bleeding with resultant anemia, unresponsive to hormonal management
2. Chronic pain with severe dysmenorrhea, dyspareunia, or lower abdominal pressure and/or pain
3. Acute pain, as in torsion of a pedunculated leiomyoma, or prolapsing submucosal fibroid
4. Urinary symptoms or signs such as hydronephrosis after complete evaluation
5. Rapid enlargement of the uterus during the premenopausal years, or any increase in uterine size in a postmenopausal woman, because of inability to exclude a uterine sarcoma
6. Infertility, with leiomyomas as the only abnormal finding
7. Enlarged uterine size with compression symptoms or discomfort

Reference: Pages 374–375

8. A

A vulvar biopsy is essential in distinguishing benign from premalignant vulvar lesions, especially because many lesions may have a somewhat similar appearance. Vulvar biopsies should be performed liberally to ensure that these lesions are diagnosed and treated appropriately. A prospective study of vulvar lesions biopsied in a gynecologic clinic found lesions occurring in the following order of frequency: epidermal inclusion cyst, lentigo, Bartholin duct obstruction, carcinoma *in situ,* melanocytic nevi, acrochordon, mucous cyst, hemangiomas, postinflammatory hyperpigmentation, seborrheic keratoses, varicosities, hidradenomas, verruca, basal cell carcinoma, and unusual tumors such as neurofibromas, ectopic tissue, syringomas, and abscesses. Clearly, the frequency with which a lesion would be reported on biopsy is related to the frequency with which all lesions of a given pathology are biopsied. Thus, the above listing probably underrepresents such common lesions as condylomas.

Reference: Pages 380–381

14 Pelvic Pain and Dysmenorrhea

David L. Olive

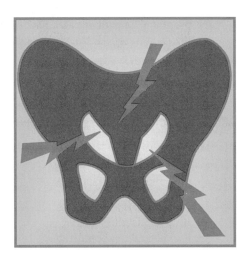

Learning Objectives

1. Know the differential diagnosis of acute pelvic pain.

2. Be aware of the pathophysiologic mechanisms of acute pelvic pain.

3. Understand the causes and treatments of dysmenorrhea.

4. Know the definition and differential diagnosis of chronic pelvic pain.

5. Be aware of the method of evaluation for chronic pelvic pain.

6. Understand the causes and treatments of chronic pelvic pain.

7. Be able to define vulvar vestibulitis syndrome.

Questions

1. A patient presents to the emergency room with acute pain. The pain is intermittent, and began just after an episode of exercise. The patient has nausea, emesis, and is quite apprehensive. Examination shows the abdomen to be tender with localized rebound tenderness in the lower quadrants. A large pelvic mass is present on the left, where the patient is most tender. Mild temperature elevation and leukocytosis are present. The patient has a past history of laparoscopic removal of a dermoid from the right ovary, and she claims she is not currently sexually active. Her most likely diagnosis is:

   A. Ectopic pregnancy
   B. Acute salpingo-oophoritis
   C. Adnexal torsion
   D. Uterine leiomyoma
   E. Endometriosis

2. Each of the following may cause acute pelvic pain **except:**

   A. Acute poryphyria
   B. Diverticulitis
   C. Pelvic thrombophlebitis
   D. Ureteral lithiasis
   E. Ovarian remnant syndrome

3. A woman presents with acute pain, and after a careful history and physical examination, you decide the most likely diagnosis is diverticulitis. A leukocytosis is noted, further increasing your suspicion. Which test should be performed to confirm the diagnosis?

   A. CT scan
   B. Barium enema
   C. Gastrografin enema
   D. Pelvic MRI

4. Which of the following is *not* a characteristic of primary dysmenorrhea:

   A. Usually appears one to two years after menarche
   B. The cause is increaed endometrial prostaglandin production
   C. Is associated with endometriosis
   D. Pain begins with the onset of menses

5. What percentage of women who suffer from primary dysmenorrhea will obtain relief from birth control pills?

   A. 10%
   B. 25%
   C. 50%
   D. 75%
   E. 90%

6. The presence of endometrial glands within the myometrium is termed:

   A. Endometriosis
   B. Adenomyosis
   C. Primary dysmenorrhea
   D. Endometriosis interna

7. While examining a patient with chronic lower abdominal and pelvic pain, you ask her to tense her rectus muscle with a straight leg raised. This maneuver exacerbates the pain. Possible diagnosis includes:

   A. Myofascial pain
   B. Interstitial cystitis
   C. Ovarian remnant syndrome
   D. Endometriosis
   E. Pelvic adhesions

8. A patient presents with urinary frequency and urgency, as well as nocturia and dysuria. A cystoscopy under anesthesia shows submucosal hemorrhages and cracking of the mucosa. The diagnosis is:

   A. Diabetes melitus
   B. Urethral syndrome
   C. Interstitial cystitis
   D. Chronic cystitis

9. The presacral neurectomy is designed to treat pain from what area of the pelvis?

   A. Adnexal structures
   B. Uterus and fallopian tubes
   C. Sigmoid colon
   D. Ureters and kidneys

10. Appropriate treatments for vulvar vestibulitis syndrome include:

    A. Sitz baths, lubrication with intercourse, and 1% hydrocortisone cream with calcium carbonate
    B. Tricyclic antidepressants
    C. Pelvic floor muscle relaxation exercises
    D. Surgical excision of minor vestibular glands
    E. All of the above

Answers

1. **C**
   Torsion (twisting) of the vascular pedicle of an ovary, fallopian tube, paratubal cyst, or rarely just a fallopian tube results in ischemia and rapid onset of pelvic pain. A benign cystic teratoma is the most common neoplasm to undergo torsion. Because adhesions are usually involved with ovarian carcinoma and inflammatory masses, these conditions are rarely affected by torsion. Torsion occludes the lymphatic and venous drainage of the involved adnexa; therefore, the mass will rapidly increase in size and it will not be difficult to palpate or to visualize with ultrasonography.
   Reference: Pages 403–404

2. **E**
   A wide variety of conditions can produce acute pelvic pain; that is, pain characterized by sudden onset, sharp rise, and short course (see Table 14.1). Conversely, ovarian remnant syndrome is a chronic pain generally occuring with ovulation or the luteal phase.
   Reference: Pages 399–400, 417–418

3. **A**
   Acute diverticulitis is a condition in which there is inflammation of a diverticulum or outpouching of the wall of the colon. Diverticulitis typically affects postmenopausal women, but it can occur rarely in women in their thirties and forties. A

Table 14.1   Differential Diagnosis of Acute Pelvic Pain

Gynecologic Disease or Dysfunction

Acute Pain

1. Complication of pregnancy
   a. Ruptured ectopic pregnancy
   b. Abortion, threatened or incomplete
   c. Degeneration of a leiomyoma
2. Acute infections
   a. Endometritis
   b. Pelvic inflammatory disease (acute PID)
   c. Tubo-ovarian abscess
3. Adnexal disorders
   a. Hemorrhagic functional ovarian cyst
   b. Torsion of adnexa
   c. Twisted para ovarian cyst
   d. Rupture of functional or neoplastic ovarian cyst

Recurrent Pelvic Pain

1. Mittelschmerz (midcycle pain)
2. Primary dysmenorrhea
3. Secondary dysmenorrhea

Gastrointestinal

1. Gastroenteritis
2. Appendicitis
3. Bowel obstruction
4. Diverticulitis
5. Inflammatory bowel disease
6. Irritable bowel syndrome

Genitourinary

1. Cystitis
2. Pylonephritis
3. Ureteral lithiasis

Musculoskeletal

1. Abdominal wall hematoma
2. Hernia

Other

1. Acute poryphyria
2. Pelvic thrombophlebitis
3. Aneurysm
4. Abdominal angina

CT scan is a useful adjunct to the history and physical examination. Enemas, however, are contraindicated.
Reference: Page 407

4. C

Primary dysmenorrhea is menstrual pain without pelvic pathology, wheras secondary dysmenorrhea is painful menses with underlying pathology. Primary dysmenorrhea usually appears within one to two years of menarche, when ovulatory cycles are established. The disorder affects younger women but may persist into a woman's forties. The cause of primary dysmenorrhea is increased endometrial prostaglandin production. Women with primary dysmenorrhea have higher uterine tone, and high amplitude contractions result in decreased uterine blood flow.
Reference: Pages 410–412

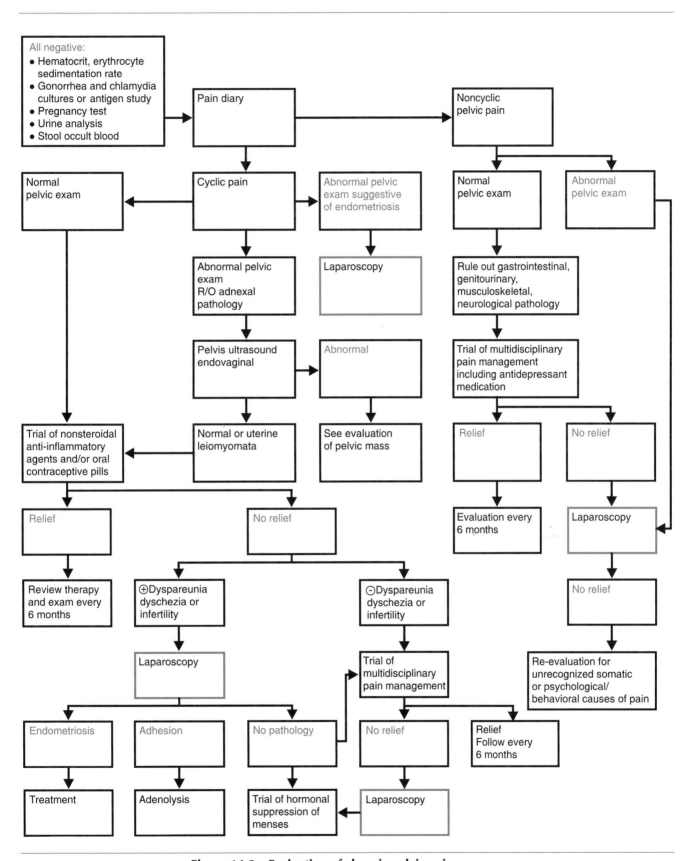

Figure 14.3   Evaluation of chronic pelvic pain.

5. E

For the patient with primary dysmenorrhea who has no contraindications to oral contraceptive agents or who desires contraception, the birth control pill is the treatment of choice. Oral contraceptives decrease endometrial proliferation and create an endocrine milieu similar to the early proliferative phase when prostaglandins are lowest. More than 90% of women with primary dysmenorrhea will have relief from birth control pills.
Reference: Page 412

6. B

Adenomyosis is ingrowth of the endometrium into the uterine musculature. Dysmenorrhea associated with this disorder often begins up to one week prior to menses. The average age of diagnosis is roughly 40 years. However, this may be because the most common method of diagnosis is hysterectomy. An alternative method, MRI, is gaining in popularity as a method of diagnosing the disorder.
Reference: Pages 412–413

7. A (see Figure 14.3)

Examination of a woman with pelvic pain should include evaluation of the abdomen with muscles tensed (head raised off the table or with straight leg raised) to differentiate abdominal wall and visceral sources of pain. Abdominal wall pain is augmented and visceral pain is diminished with these maneuvers.
Reference: Page 415

8. C

Interstitial cystitis is more frequent in women than in men. Most patients are between 40 and 60 years of age. The cause of interstitial cystitis is unknown, although an autoimmune basis is generally accepted. Symptoms include urinary frequency and urgency, nocturia, dysuria, and occasional hematuria. Pain is common and can be relieved by emptying the bladder. The diagnosis is made on the basis of these symptoms and the above cystoscopic findings.
Reference: Page 420

9. B

Presacral neurectomy is a treatment designed to combat dysmenorrhea. The neurectomy will only relieve pain derived from the cervix, uterus, and proximal fallopian tube. The nerve supply to adnexal structures bypasses the hypogastric nerve. Therefore, lateralizing visceral pain is unlikely to be relieved by presacral neurectomy.
Reference: Page 423

10. E

Vulvar vestibulitis syndrome is defined as severe pain on vestibular or vaginal entry, tenderness to pressure localized within the vulvar vestibule, and physical findings confined to vestibular erythema of varying degrees. The etiology is unknown. It is often associated with preceeding candidal infections and may be a hypersensitivity reaction or possibly an irritant or allergic reaction. Nonspecific chronic inflammatory infiltrate within the vestibular glands is the most frequent histologic finding. All of the above are potentially helpful treatments, although surgery is generally utilized as a last resort.
Reference: Pages 424–425

15 Genitourinary Infections and Sexually Transmitted Diseases

Jonathan S. Berek

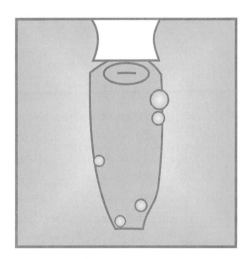

Learning Objectives

1. Be able to identify the causes, diagnosis, and treatment of vaginal infections.

2. Know the causes, diagnosis, and treatment of pelvic inflammatory disease.

3. Be aware of the differential diagnosis of genital ulcers.

4. Understand the impact of human immunodeficiency virus in women.

5. Be able to enumerate the types of urinary tract infection.

Questions

1. The normal vaginal flora is:

   A. aerobic, pH < 4.5
   B. aerobic, pH > 4.5
   C. anaerobic, pH < 4.5
   D. mixed aerobic/anaerobic, pH > 4.5

2. A 21-year-old woman complains of vaginal discharge that she states has a fishy odor. It is particularly noticeable following coitus. You examine her and find the pH is 5. The most likely diagnosis is:

   A. *candida albicans*
   B. bacterial vaginosis
   C. *trichomonas vaginalis*
   D. normal postcoital discharge

3. A 28-year-old complains of a "cottage cheese" discharge that has not responded to over- the-counter *clotrimazole*, which she self-administered. The most likely reason for the condition is:

   A. vaginal injury
   B. hypersensitivity reaction
   C. colonization resistance
   D. autoimmune reaction

4. A 22-year-old woman presents with a purulent vaginal discharge one week after having sexual intercourse for the first time with a new boyfriend. She states that he informed her in retrospect that he had felt burning with urination. She is asymptomatic. At the time of pelvic examination, cervical cultures are taken for *Neisseria gonorrhea* and for *Chlamydia trachomatis*. The gonorrhea culture is positive. She has no known allergies. You should prescribe:

   A. *doxycycline*
   B. *erythromycin*
   C. *azithromycin*
   D. *ceftriaxone*
   E. *gentamicin*

5. A 25-year-old woman presents with diffuse acute pelvic and lower abdominal pain, fever, chills, and nausea. There is lower abdominal guarding and cervical motion tenderness. A "fullness" in the pelvis is appreciated, and therefore, a tubo-ovarian abscess is suspected. The diagnosis of acute salpingitis (pelvic inflammatory disease) is made. The patient is admitted to the hospital for antibiotic therapy. Of the following, which is the most appropriate antibiotic therapy:

   A. *cefoxitin* and *doxycycline*
   B. *ceftriaxone* and *erythromycin*
   C. *amoxicillin* and *trimethoprim*
   D. *clindamycin* and *clotrimazole*

6. A 34-year-old woman presents with a painful vulvar ulceration. The ulcer has irregular margins and is deep with undermined edges. The ipsilateral inguinal lymph nodes are swollen and tender. The most likely diagnosis is:

   A. syphilis
   B. herpes
   C. chanchroid
   D. lymphogranuloma venereum

7. The most common human papillomavirus (HPV) subtype associated with genital warts are:

A. HPV 1 and 2
B. HPV 4 and 7
C. HPV 6 and 11
D. HPV 18 and 24
E. HPV 22 and 33

8. A 22-year-old woman presents with symptoms of dysuria. She has a new sex partner. The physical examination reveals some mucopurulent discharge of the cervix. Urinalysis shows some pyuria, but no hematuria. Urinary cultures are negative. The most likely diagnosis is:

A. cystitis with false negative culture
B. ureterolithiasis and pyelitis
C. urethritis associated with chlamydia
D. vulvovaginitis caused by fungi

Answers

1. A

The normal vaginal flora is predominately aerobic, with an average of six different species of bacteria, the most common of which is hydrogen peroxide producing lactobacilli. The pH of the normal vagina is lower than 4.5, which is maintained by the production of lactic acid. Estrogen-stimulated vaginal epithelium are rich in glycogen. Vaginal epithelial cells break down glycogen to monosaccharides, which can then be converted by lactobacilli to lactic acid.
Reference: Pages 429–430

2. B

Bacterial vaginosis (BV) has previously been called "nonspecific vaginitis" or *Gardnerella* vaginitis. The condition is an alteration of the normal vaginal flora that results in the loss of normal lactobacilli and the associated hydrogen-peroxide production. This situation encourages the overgrowth of the anaerobic bacteria, which normally account for less than 1% of normal vaginal flora, and produces the infection. It is the most common form of vaginitis in the United States. The fishy odor and the exacerbation of the condition by coitus are characteristic of the infection. The vaginal pH is typically between 4.7 and 5.7. The treatment is typically *metronidazole* or *clindamycin*. The infection can be distinguished for the other conditions by the use of a vaginal "wet mount," as trichomonas are seen in normal saline and candida species are seen in potassium hydroxide.
Reference: Pages 430–434

3. C

Development and persistence of vaginal infections with candida species is known as colonization resistance. This phenomenon results from conditions that predispose to the infection, such as antibiotic use, pregnancy, and diabetes. Lactobacilli normally prevent the overgrowth of fungi in the vagina. With the disruption of the normal flora, an overgrowth of the fungi occurs. The most appropriate alternatives to therapy of candida vaginal infections are presented in Table 15.1.
Reference: Pages 432–434

4. D

As presented in Table 15.2, the standard treatment for asymptomatic women with a positive culture for *Neisseria gonorrhea* is a single intramuscular dose of *ceftriaxone*.

Table 15.1   Vulvovaginal Candidiasis—Topical Treatment Regimens

---

Butoconazole

2% cream 5 g intravaginally for 3 days[†]

Clotrimazole

1% cream 5 g intravaginally for 7–14 days[†]
100 mg vaginal tablet for 7 days[†]
100 mg vaginal tablet, two tablets for 3 days
500 mg vaginal tablet, single dose

Miconazole

2% cream 5 g intravaginally for 7 days[*†]
200 mg vaginal suppository for 3 days[*]
100 mg vaginal suppository for 7 days[*†]

Ticonazole

6.5% ointment 5 g intravaginally, single dose[*]

Terconazole

0.4% cream 5 g intravaginally for 7 days
0.8% cream 5 g intravaginally for 3 days
80 mg suppository for 3 days[*]

---

[*]Oil-based, may weaken latex condoms.
[†]Available over-the-counter
Morbidity and Mortality Weekly Report. Centers for Disease Control and Prevention. *MMWR* 1993;42: 72–3.

Table 15.2   Treatment Regimens for Gonococcal and Chlamydial Infections

---

***Neisseria gonorrhoeae* endocervicitis**

Ceftriaxone 125 mg intramuscularly (single dose), or
Ofloxacin 400 mg orally (single dose), or
Cefixime 400 mg orally (single dose), or
Ciprofloxacin 500 mg orally (single dose)

***Chlamydia trachomatis* endocervicitis**

Doxycycline 100 mg orally b.i.d. for 7 days, or
Azithromycin 1 gram orally (single dose), or
Ofloxacin 300 mg orally b.i.d. for 7 days, or
Erythromycin base 500 mg orally 4 times a day for 7 days, or
Erythromycin ethylsuccinate 800 mg orally 4 times a day for 7 days

---

Morbidity and Mortality Weekly Report. Centers for Disease Control and Prevention. *MMWR* 1993;42: 51–57.

Alternatively, *ofloxacin*, *cefixime*, or *ciprofloxacin* are recommended. *Doxycycline* or *erythromycin* would be appropriate if chlamydia were identified.
Reference: Pages 435–437

5. A (see Tables 15.3 and 15.4)
The appropriate treatment of pelvic inflammatory disease with a suspected tubo-ovarian abscess is combination antibiotic therapy administered in the hospital. The CDC-recommended treatment is either *cefoxitan* plus *doxycycline* or *clindamycin* plus *gentamicin*.
Reference: Pages 437–438

Table 15.3 Clinical Criteria for the Diagnosis of Pelvic Inflammatory Disease (PID)

Symptoms

None necessary

Signs

Pelvic organ tenderness
Leukorrhea and/or mucopurulent endocervicitis

Additional criteria to increase the specificity of the diagnosis

Endometrial biopsy showing endometritis
Elevated C-reactive protein or erythrocyte sedimentation rate
Temperature higher than 38°C
Leukocytosis
Positive test for gonorrhea or chlamydia

Elaborate criteria

Sonography documenting tubo-ovarian abscess
Laparoscopy visually confirming salpingitis

Table 15.4 CDC Guidelines for Treatment of PID

Outpatient treatment

Regimen A:

Cefoxitin 2 g intramuscularly, plus *probenecid,* 1 g orally concurrently, or *ceftriaxone,*
    250 mg intramuscularly, or equivalent cephalosporin
        <PLUS>
Doxycycline 100 mg orally 2 times daily for 14 days

Regimen B:

Ofloxacin 400 mg orally 2 times daily for 14 days
        <PLUS>
Clindamycin 450 mg orally 4 times daily, or *metronidazole* 500 mg orally 2 times daily
    for 14 days

Inpatient treatment

Regimen A:

Cefoxitin 2 g intravenously every 6 hours, or
Cefotetan 2 g intravenously every 12 hours,
        <PLUS>
Doxycycline 100 mg intravenously or orally every 12 hours

Regimen B:

Clindamycin 900 mg intravenously every 8 hours
        <PLUS>
Gentamicin loading dose intravenously or intramuscularly (2 mg/kg of body weight) fol-
    lowed by a maintenance dose (1.5 mg/kg) every 8 hours

Morbidity and Mortality Weekly Report. Centers for Disease Control and Prevention. *MMWR* 1993;42:
78–80.

---

6. **C (see Figure 15.2)**
   The differential diagnosis of genital ulcers is often difficult without appropriate tests. Although the pattern described is most likely to be chanchroid, syphilis must be excluded by the performance of VDRL, FTA-ABS, and/or dark-field examination. The appropriate treatment of the condition is *azithromycin, ceftriaxon*e, or *erythromycin*.
   Reference: Pages 438–441

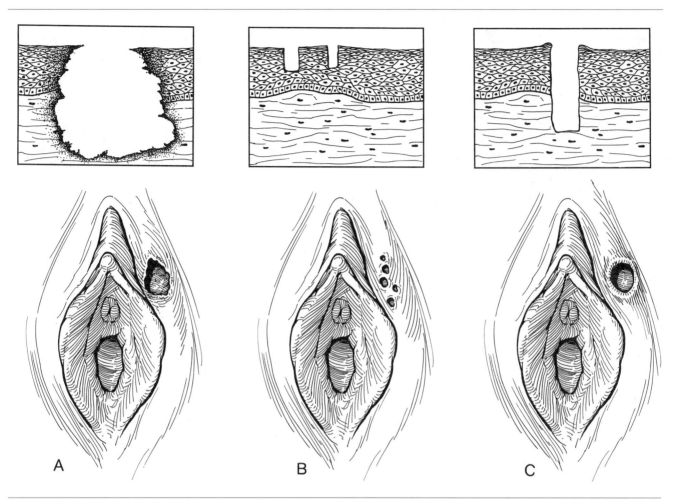

Figure 15.2   Showing the appearance of the ulcers of chancroid (A), herpes (B), and syphilis (C). The ulcer of chancroid has irregular margins and is deep with undermined edges. The syphilis ulcer has a smooth, indurated border and a smooth base. The genital herpes ulcer is superficial and inflamed. (Modified from **Schmid GP, Shcalla WO, DeWitt WE.** Chancroid. In: **Morse SA, Moreland AA, Thompson SE,** eds. *Atlas of Sexually Transmitted Diseases.* Philadelphia: JB Lippincott, 1990.)

7. C

The most common subtypes of HPV associated with genital warts are HPV 6 and 11. Most often these are nononcogenic. They tend to occur in the areas most directly affected by coitus. Exophytic genital warts are highly contagious.
Reference: Page 441

8. C

In patients with a negative urine culture, pyuria, and no hematuria, the most likely diagnosis is urethritis associated with a sexually transmitted disease. Appropriate cultures of the cervix should identify the specific organism that should be treated as discussed above in question 4.
Reference: Page 443

16 Intraepithelial Disease of the Cervix, Vagina, and Vulva

Anne P. Shapter
Jonathan S. Berek

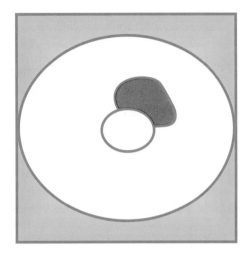

Learning Objectives

1. Understand the pathophysiology of cervical intraepithelial neoplasia.

2. Know the role of diagnostic methods for cervical intraepithelial neoplasia.

3. Have an algorithm for the evaluation, treatment, and follow-up of an abnormal Pap test.

4. Know the treatment options for cervical intraepithelial neoplasia.

5. Know the diagnosis and treatment of vaginal intraepithelial neoplasia.

6. Be able to identify vulvar intraepithelial disease and know its differential diagnosis.

Questions

1. Which of the following statements regarding cervical intraepithelial neoplasia (CIN) is incorrect?

   A. CIN 1 refers to the situation in which immature or dysplastic cells are present in the lower one-third of the epithelium.
   B. CIN is more likely to develop in the anterior lip of the cervix than in the posterior lip.
   C. The transformation zone refers to the zone between the active squamocolumnar junction and the columnar epithelium.
   D. Nabothian cysts may be useful in determining the location of the original squamo-columnar junction (SCJ).
   E. In neonates, the SCJ is located on the exocervix.

2. Which of the following human papillomavirus (HPV) types is most common in patients with invasive cervical cancer, CIN 3, and CIN 2?

   A. HPV type 6
   B. HPV type 11
   C. HPV type 16
   D. HPV type 18
   E. HPV type 31

3. Which of the following HPV types is most common in women with normal cervical cytology?

   A. HPV type 6
   B. HPV type 11
   C. HPV type 16
   D. HPV type 18
   E. HPV type 31

4. Which of the following statements regarding the Bethesda system is false?

   A. The category "ASCUS" refers to cells described as reactive, inflammatory, or reparative.
   B. The "HSIL" category includes cells consistent with carcinoma *in situ* (CIS) by the CIN system.
   C. Ideally, when standardized diagnostic criteria are used, the rate of ASCUS cytology should be 3 to 5%.
   D. Cellular changes associated with HPV (koilocytosis and CIN 1) should be classified as "LSIL."

5. Which of the following factors has been associated with an increased chance of failure of cryotherapy in the treatement of CIN?

   A. Treatment of higher grade lesions such as CIN 3 by this method
   B. Large lesion size
   C. Positive endocervical curettage (ECC)
   D. Endocervical glandular involvement
   E. All of the above

6. Which of the following statements regarding glandular cell abnormalities is false?

   A. AGUS (atypical glandular cells of undetermined significance) is more predictive of significant underlying disease than is ASCUS.
   B. Microinvasive adenocarcinoma of the cervix is a well established phenomenon.
   C. Fifty percent of women with adenocarcinoma *in situ* (AIS) will also have squamous CIN.

D. A patient with negative margins after conization for AIS should be counselled that there is a significant chance she may still have residual AIS.

E. Any patient with AIS and positive margins after conization should undergo repeat cone biopsy at a minimum and should be offered hysterectomy if fertility is not desired.

7. The most appropriate initial treatment for a 70-year-old female diagnosed with vaginal intraepithelial neoplasia 3 (VAIN 3) near the vaginal cuff is:

A. Cryosurgery
B. Fulguration with the electrosurgical ball under colposcopic guidance
C. Surgical excision
D. Laser therapy
E. 5-fluorouracil (*Efudex* cream)

8. Histologically, Paget's disease of the vulva:

A. is primarily a squamous cell lesion.
B. arises in melanocytes.
C. is a type of sarcoma of the vulva.
D. arises primarily in Bartholin gland.
E. is a disease of the apocrine sweat glands.

9. Which of the following statements regarding vulvar intraepithelial disease is true?

A. The malignant potential of VIN is similar to that of CIN.
B. VIN lesions should always be treated by superficial vulvectomy.
C. Most cases of Paget's disease of the vulva are intraepithelial.
D. Mucicarmine staining may assist in differentiating melanoma from Paget's disease as melanocytes stain postive.
E. Paget's disease of the vulva is primarily a disease of premenopausal women.

10. Which of the following situations provide indications for cervical conization?

A. Endocervical curettage positive for CIN 2–3
B. Lack of correlation between cytology, biopsy, and colposcopy with persistent high-grade (HSIL) cytology
C. Suspicion for microinvasion
D. Inadequate colposcopy in the setting of persistent HSIL
E. All of the above

Answers

1. C

In the neonatal period, the SCJ is indeed located on the ectocervix and the SCJ at this time is termed the original SCJ. During menarche, metaplasia occurs inward over the columnar cells and a new or active SCJ forms (Figure 16.2). The transformation zone actually refers to the area between the original SCJ and the physiologically active SCJ. Nabothian cysts may aid in the identification of the original SCJ. The importance of the transformation zone is that this is the area in which CIN is likely to develop. The anterior cervix is twice as likely as the posterior lip to develop CIN. CIN rarely develops in the lateral angles. CIN 1 refers to the situation in which immature cells are present in the lower one-third of the epithelium whereas CIN 2 and CIN 3 refer to involvement of the middle and upper thirds respectively in addition to the lower one-third (Figure 16.1).
Reference: Pages 448–450

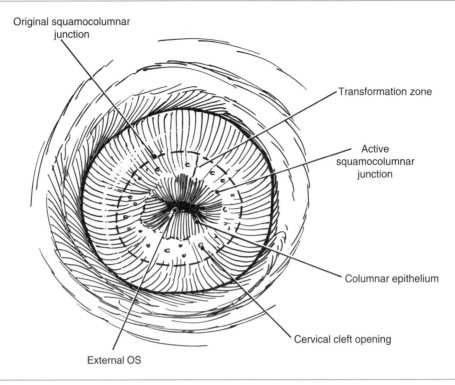

Original squamocolumnar junction

Transformation zone

Active squamocolumnar junction

Columnar epithelium

Cervical cleft opening

External OS

Figure 16.2   The cervix and the transformation zone.

Figure 16.1   Diagram of the different grades of CIN.

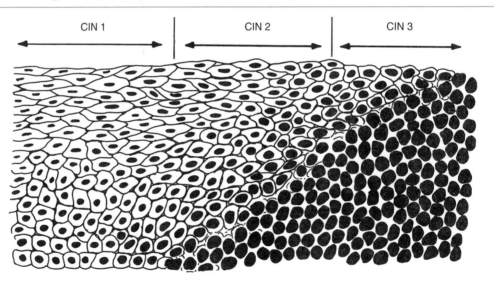

CIN 1   CIN 2   CIN 3

2. C

The transformation zone is an area established as metaplasia advances from the original squamocolumnar junction (SCJ) inward toward the external os and over the columnar villi. The transformation zone extends from the original SCJ to the physiologically active SCJ.

Reference: Page 448

3. C

The percent of intraepithelial neoplasia associated with HPV infection approaches 90%. The number of known genital HPV types is greater than 20 but certain subtypes account for the majority of high-grade and cancerous lesions of the cervix: HPV types 16, 18, 31, 33, 35, 39, 45, 51, 52, 56, and 58. Type 16 is the most common subtype found in CIN 2, CIN 3, and invasive carcinoma, and is present in nearly 50% of women with these lesions. Interestingly, it is also the most common subtype found in women with normal cytology and it is, therefore, not very specific. By contrast, HPV type 18 is found in 23% of women with invasive cancers and in only 5% of women with CIN 1, CIN 2, and CIN 3. It is found in less than 2% of women with normal cytology and is, therefore, more specific than HPV 16 for invasive lesions. Most women exposed to HPV do not subsequently develop CIN. Any factor (such as cigarette smoking) which influences incorporation of HPV-DNA into the host genome may contribute to the development of CIN and ultimately to the development of invasive cancer.
Reference: Pages 451–453

4. A (see Table 16.1)

In 1989, the Bethesda System for cervical cytology was developed in an attempt to standardize the reporting of cytology. According to this system, premalignant conditions of the cervix fall into three categories: atypical squamous cells of undetermined significance (ASCUS); low-grade squamous intraepithelial lesions (LSIL); and high-grade squamous intraepithelial lesions (HSIL). Cytologic smears that exhibit reactive, reparative, or inflammatory changes alone are not classified as ASCUS and, in fact, are reported separately. LSIL lesions include those classified as CIN 1 by the "CIN" system as well as those which exhibit changes consistent with HPV infection such as koilocytosis. Lesions that fall into the category of CIN 2, CIN 3, and CIS by the "CIN" system are grouped together under the category of HSIL by the Bethesda system. The reason for incorporating the majority of abnormal Pap smears into two broad categories (HSIL and LSIL) is that all lesions falling into one or the other category will be managed similarly depending on the particular category. High-risk HPV subtypes such as 16 and 18 are not limited to HSIL lesions and, in fact, may be associated with CIN 1. Ideally, "ASCUS" cytologic cervical Pap smears should comprise approximately 3 to 5% of all cytologic smears within a given laboratory.
Reference: Pages 453–454

Table 16.1 Comparison of Cytology Classification Systems

Bethesda System	*Dysplasia/CIN System*	*Papanicolaou System*
Within normal limits	Normal	I
Infection (organism should be specified)	Inflammatory atypia (organism)	II
Reactive and reparative changes		
Squamous cell abnormalities Atypical squamous cells of undetermined significance	Squamous atypia	IIR
Low-grade squamous intraepithelial lesion (LSIL)	HPV atypia	
High-grade squamous intraepithelial lesion (HSIL)	Mild dysplasia CIN 1 Moderate dysplasia CIN 2	III
	Severe dysplasia Carcinoma *in situ* CIN 3	IV
Squamous cell carcinoma	Squamous cell carcinoma	V

CIN, cervical intraepithelial neoplasia.
From **Berek JS, Hacker NF**, eds. *Practical Gynecologic Oncology.* 2nd ed. Baltimore: Williams & Wilkins, 1994: 205.

5. E (see Figure 16.9)

Cryotherapy is a most effective method for the treatment of CIN when certain specific criteria are met. It is also a relatively safe procedure with very few complications. Cryotherapy is most appropriate for lower grade lesions (CIN 1–2) which are small and are located on the ectocervix. CIN 3 lesions have a relatively higher chance of failure (Table 16.4) in comparison to CIN 1 or CIN 2 lesions. Cryotherapy should not be used to treat lesions which are not fully visualized or which extend into the endocervical canal. If there is a positive ECC or if there is documented endocervical glandular involvement, an alternative method of treatment should be undertaken. Lesion size

Figure 16.9   An algorithm for the evaluation, treatment, and follow-up of an abnormal Pap test.

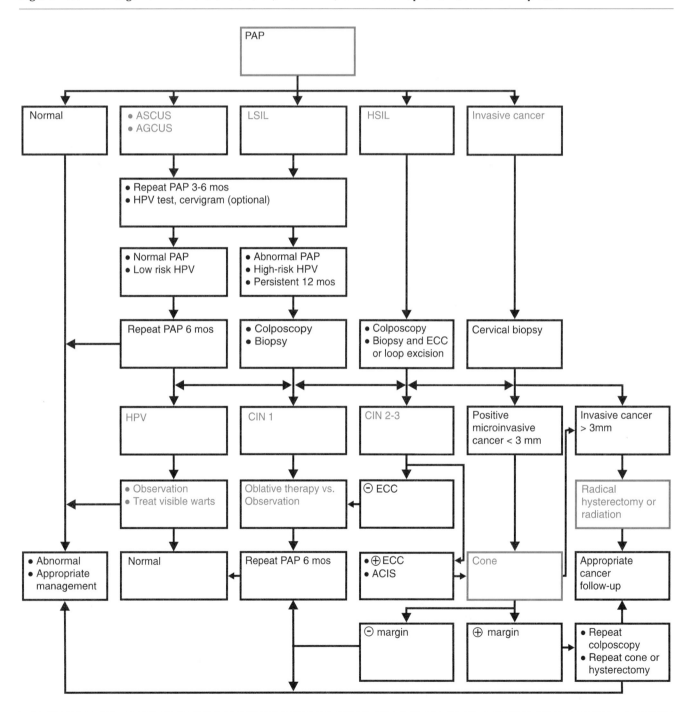

Table 16.4   Results of Cryotherapy for Cervical Intraepithelial Neoplasia (CIN) Compared to Grade of CIN

Author (Ref. No.)	CIN 1		CIN 2		CIN 3	
	No.	% Failure	No.	% Failure	No.	% Failure
Ostergard (42)	13/205	6.3%	7/93	7.5%	9/46	19.6%
Creasman (43)	15/276	5.4%	17/235	7.2%	46/259	17.8%
Andersen (41)	—	—	9/123	7.3%	17/74	23.0%
Benedet (44)	7/143	4.9%	19/448	4.2%	65/1003	6.5%
Total	35/624	5.6%	50/899	5.6%	137/1382	9.9%

should also influence the choice of treatment as lesions less than 1 centimeter are associated with a significantly lower failure rate with cryotherapy. In summary, cryotherapy is an excellent option for the treatment of CIN when there is adherence to the above criteria but may be associated with significant failure rates when used to treat higher grade lesions or those which involve the endocervix.
Reference: Pages 464–466

6. A

The Bethesda system has a separate category for reporting glandular cell abnormalities. AGUS is more likely than ASCUS to reflect significant underlying pathology. In a recent study of 63 patients with AGUS, approximately 50% were found to have significant abnormalities, including two patients with invasive adenocarcinoma. Therefore, a Pap smear read as AGUS should be given serious consideration and appropriate biopsies taken depending on the patient's age and clinical scenario. The phenomenon of microinvasive adenocarcinoma of the cervix has been proposed but has not been proven to exist. Therefore, the term should be avoided and such tumors should be classified as AIS or invasive adenocarcinoma. Several recent publications have addressed the issue of conization margins in the setting of AIS. Negative margins are not necessarily reassuring as a high percentage of patients may have residual AIS. A scant 40% of patients with positive margins after cone biopsy are found to have residual disease at repeat conization or hysterectomy. Treatment of AIS should be individualized and hysterectomy should be considered if fertility is not desired.
Reference: Pages 473–474

7. C

Patients with VAIN 1 need not be treated as these lesions will often regress spontaneously. VAIN 2 lesions are usually treated with laser therapy. The malignant potential of VAIN appears to be less than that of CIN but, nevertheless, VAIN 3 lesions have a significant chance of harboring an occult invasive lesion. Therefore, surgical excision, as opposed to one of the ablative procedures, should be undertaken initially to rule out an invasive carcinoma. Once invasion has been ruled out, consideration may be given to treating VAIN 3 with laser ablation.
Reference: Pages 474–477

8. E

(See answer to question 9 below)

9. C

Paget's disease of the vulva is an intraepithelial lesion involving cells of the apocrine sweat glands but may be associated with an underlying adenocarcinoma. This disease must be differentiated from superficial spreading melanoma. Mucicarmine stains may assist in this determination as melanocytes stain negative. Interestingly, a synchronous or metachronous primary neoplasm is associated with extramammary Paget's disease in 30% of patients. Treatment is wide surgical excision, as this disease frequently extends beyond the gross lesion, and positive margins are associated with a significant chance of recurrence. Paget's disease is seen primarily in post-menopausal Caucasian women.

The malignant potential of VIN is felt to be significantly lower than that of CIN and progression to invasive carcinoma is uncommon. Smaller lesions may be treated with simple excision or recurrent VIN.
Reference: Pages 479–482

10. E
All of the above scenarios are situations in which cervical conization should be performed. Conization provides a pathologic specimen for review and, therefore, is preferable over the ablative therapies in the evaluation and treatment of higher grade lesions or if an occult carcinoma is suspected. All of the above situations should raise a concern for severe dysplasia, microinvasion, or possibly invasive cancer, and cervical cone biopsy should be performed in order to exclude these diagnoses.
Reference: Pages 469–472

17 Early Pregnancy Loss and Ectopic Pregnancy

Jonathan S. Berek

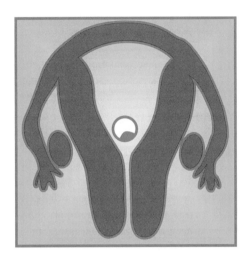

Learning Objectives

1. Know the different types of abnormal intrauterine pregnancy, including their definitions and sequelae.

2. Know the epidemiology of ectopic pregnancy, including risk factors.

3. Understand the methods of diagnosis of ectopic pregnancy, and be able to provide an algorithm for diagnosis.

4. Know the medical and surgical treatment options for ectopic pregnancy, including the relative merits of each.

Questions

1. If one uses serial human chorionic gonadotropin (hCG) measurements to detect early subclinical pregnancy losses, the percentage of pregnancies that terminate in spontaneous abortion is:

    A. 5%
    B. 10%
    C. 20%
    D. 30%
    E. 50%

2. After an ectopic pregnancy, there is an increased risk of subsequent ectopic pregnancy. The risk is increased by how many fold:

    A. 2
    B. 5
    C. 10
    D. 20
    E. 50

3. A 27-year-old woman presents with a copper-T intrauterine devise (IUD) in place, right lower quadrant abdominal pain, and an adnexal mass. The hCG is positive, and an ultrasound documents a right tubal pregnancy. Compared with the risk of ectopic pregnancy in patients without the IUD, the risk is:

    A. higher
    B. lower
    C. the same

4. A 19-year-old woman who is known to have an early pregnancy presents with some vaginal "spotting." She is suspected of having either a threatened abortion or an ectopic pregnancy. At the time of initial presentation five weeks from her last menstrual period, the hCG is just <2000. The ultrasound does not yet document an intrauterine pregnancy. An ectopic pregnancy is not seen. After 48 hours, the patient remains asymptomatic. In order to distinguish an intrauterine pregnancy from an ectopic pregnancy, the change in the hCG over 48 hours is observed. The hCG is now 2450. What percentage rise in hCG represents the lower limit of normal values for viable intrauterine pregnancies?

    A. 33%
    B. 50%
    C. 66%
    D. 80%
    E. 100%

5. The earliest ultrasonographic sign of an intrauterine pregnancy is:

    A. a small fluid space and the gestational sac surrounded by a thick echogenic ring
    B. a fetal heart with evidence of pulsatile activity
    C. a large decidual sac with a very thick concentric ring
    D. a fetal neural tube sign

6. At what level of hCG will essentially all intrauterine pregnancies be identifiable by transvaginal ultrasonography?

    A. 2500 mIU/ml
    B. 4500 mIU/ml
    C. 6500 mIU/ml
    D. 8500 mIU/ml

7. A 31-year-old woman presents with vaginal bleeding six weeks from her last menstrual period. Her hCG is 4860 mIU/ml. An ultrasonogram of the pelvis shows a tubal gestation measuring 4 centimeters with cardiac activity. The surgical treatment of choice for this tubal pregnancy, which cannot be treated with *methotrexate* is:

   A. salpingectomy
   B. salpingostomy
   C. salpingotomy
   D. salpingoplasty

8. A good candidate for the use of *methotrexate* to treat an ectopic pregnancy is:

   A. no intrauterine gestational sac or fluid collection, hCG levels < 2000 mIU/ml, ectopic < 3.5 cm
   B. equivocal intrauterine sac, hCG levels 2000 to 4500 mIU/ml, ectopic < 5 cm
   C. no intrauterine gestational sac, ectopic 3 to 5 cm, with cardiac activity, regardless of hCG level
   D. any patient with an unruptured ectopic

9. A 28-year-old woman presents with a positive pregnancy test and vaginal bleeding six weeks from her last menstrual period. On pelvic examination, the uterus feels small while the cervix is expanded. On ultrasound, the cervix appears to contain a gestational sac. The best management of this presumed case of cervical pregnancy is:

   A. dilation and curettage
   B. hysterectomy
   C. embolization
   D. *methotrexate*

Answers

1. D (see Table 17.1)
Although 15 to 20% of known pregnancies terminate in spontaneous abortion, if the serial follow-up with hCG is added, the percentage increases to 30%, as there are many losses that otherwise go undetected. About 80% of spontaneous abortions occur in the first trimester, and the incidence decreases with each gestational week. Spontaneous pregnancy losses include anembryonic gestations, inevitable abortions, and incomplete abortions.
Reference: Page 487

2. C
After an ectopic pregnancy, there is a 7- to 13-fold increase in the risk of subsequent ectopic pregnancy. The chance that a subsequent ectopic pregnancy will be intrauterine is 50 to 80%, and the chance that the pregnancy will be tubal is 10 to 25%; the remaining patients will be infertile. However, many variables make the accurate assessment of the risk very difficult.
Reference: Pages 490–491

3. A
Women who conceive with an IUD in place are 0.4 to 0.8 times more likely to have a tubal pregnancy than those not using contraceptives. However, because IUDs prevent implantation more effectively in the uterus than in the tube, a woman conceiving with an IUD is 6 to 10 times more likely to have a tubal pregnancy than if she conceives without contraception.
Reference: Page 492

Table 17.1   Definitions of Types of Abnormal Intrauterine and Extrauterine Pregnancies

Extrauterine Pregnancy

Tubal pregnancy	A pregnancy occurring in the fallopian tube — most often these are located in the ampullary portion of the fallopian tube.
Interstitial pregnancy	A pregnancy that implants within the interstitial portion of the fallopian tube.
Abdominal pregnancy	Primary abdominal pregnancy — the first and only implantation occurs on a peritoneal surface. Secondary abdominal pregnancy — implantation originally in the tubal ostia, subsequently aborted, and then reimplanted onto a peritoneal surface.
Cervical pregnancy	Implantation of the developing conceptus in the cervical canal.
Ligamentous pregnancy	A secondary form of ectopic pregnancy in which a primary tubal pregnancy erodes into the mesosalpinx and is located between the leaves of the broad ligament.
Heterotopic pregnancy	A condition in which ectopic and intrauterine pregnancies coexist.
Ovarian pregnancy	A condition in which an ectopic pregnancy implants within the ovarian cortex.

Abnormal Intrauterine Pregnancy

Incomplete abortion	Expulsion of some but not all of the products of conception before 20 completed weeks of gestation.
Complete abortion	Spontaneous expulsion of all fetal and placental tissue from the uterine cavity before 20 weeks of gestation.
Inevitable abortion	Uterine bleeding from a gestation of <20 weeks accompanied by cervical dilation but without expulsion of placental or fetal tissue through the cervix.
Anembryonic gestation	An intrauterine sac without fetal tissue is present at more than 7.5 weeks of gestation.
First trimester fetal death	Death of the fetus in the first 12 weeks of gestation.
Second trimester fetal death	Death of the fetus between 13 and 24 weeks of gestation.
Recurrent spontaneous abortion	The loss of more than three pregnancies before 20 weeks.

4. C (see Figure 17.4)

A 66% rise in the hCG level over 48 hours (85% confidence level) represents the lower limit of normal values for viable intrauterine pregnancies. Approximately 15% of patients with viable intrauterine pregnancies will have a less-than-66% rise in hCG level over 48 hours, and a similar percentage with an ectopic pregnancy will have a more-than-66% rise. The hCG pattern most predictive of an ectopic pregnancy is one that has reached a plateau over one week. These serial measurements are usually required when the initial ultrasound examination is indeterminate.

Reference: Pages 496–497

5. A

The earliest ultrasonographic finding of an intrauterine pregnancy is usually located eccentrically within the endometrial cavity. The earliest normal gestational sac is seen at five weeks of gestation with transabdominal ultrasonography and at four weeks of

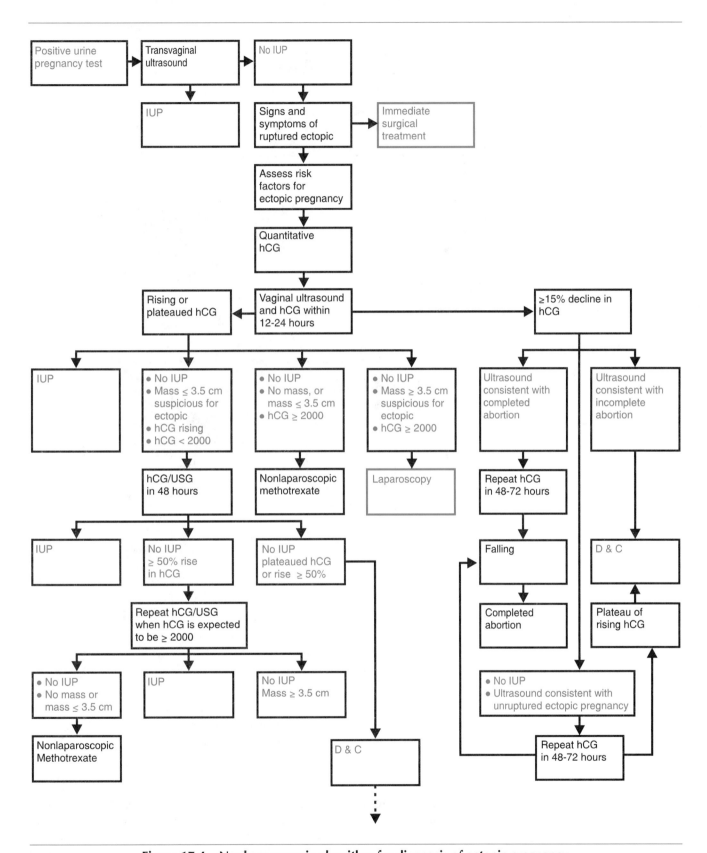

Figure 17.4 Nonlaparoscopic algorithm for diagnosis of ectopic pregnancy.

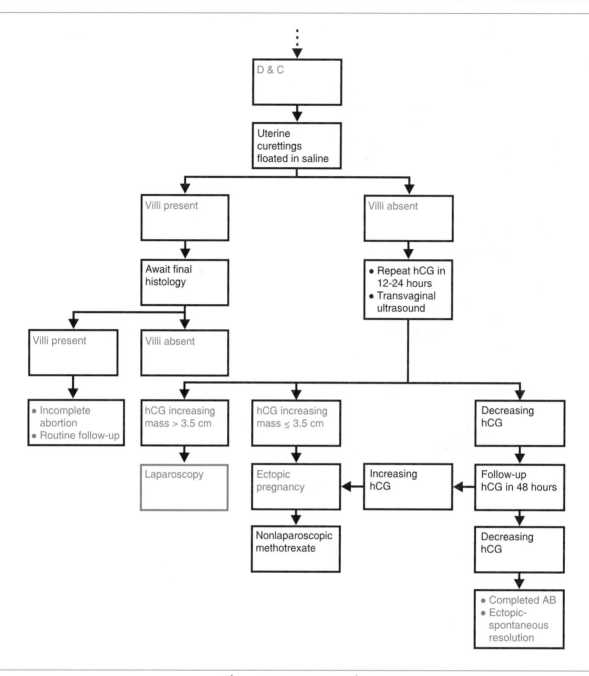

Figure 17.4—*continued*

gestation with transvaginal ultrasonography. As the gestational sac grows, a yolk sac is seen within it, followed by an embryo with cardiac activity.
Reference: Page 492

6. C

Accurate interpretation of ultrasonographic findings to determine the location of a pregnancy (intrauterine versus extrauterine), requires a correlation with the hCG level. This is called the "discriminatory zone." All viable intrauterine pregnancies can be visualized by transabdominal sonography correlated with serum hCG levels of greater than 6500 mIU/ml. Nonvisualization at that level indicates an abnormal pregnancy, either an ectopic or incomplete spontaneous abortion. Intrauterine sacs seen at lower

levels of hCG are abnormal and represent aborting intrauterine pregnancies or the pseudogestational sac of an ectopic pregnancy.
Reference: Page 500

7. B

Linear salpingostomy is currently the procedure of choice when the patient has an unruptured ectopic pregnancy and wishes to retain her potential for future fertility. It can be accomplished either via the laparoscope or via laparotomy. The salpingostomy is left open to heal spontaneously.
Reference: Pages 503–506

8. A

Based on current data, a conservative approach to the use of medical therapy is warranted. *Methotrexate* is best used in women whose ectopic pregnancies are small and have no cardiac activity. The treatment protocol for such patients is presented in Table 17.3, and a method for the initiation of *methotrexate* is presented in Table 17.4.
Reference: Pages 506–509

Table 17.3   Single–Dose *Methotrexate* Protocol for Ectopic Pregnancy

Day	*Therapy*
0	D&C, hCG
1	CBC, SGOT, BUN, creatinine, blood type and Rh
4	*Methotrexate* 50 mg/M² I.M.
7	hCG

If <15% decline in hCG level between days 4 and 7, give second dose of *methotrexate* 50 mg/m² on day 7.
If >15% decline in hCG level between days 4 and 7, follow weekly until hCG <10 mIU/ml.
In patients not requiring D&C (hCG >2000 mIU/ml and no gestational sac on transvaginal ultrasonography), days 0 and 1 are combined.
D&C, dilation and curettage; hCG, human chorionic gonadotropin; CBC, complete blood count; SGOT, serum glutamic-oxaloacetic transaminase; BUN, blood urea nitrogen; MTX, *methotrexate*.

Table 17.4   Initiation of *Methotrexate:* Physician Checklist and Patient Instructions

Physician Checklist:

Obtain hCG level.
Perform transvaginal ultrasound within 48 hours.
Perform endometrial curettage if hCG level <2000 mIU/ml.
Obtain normal liver function (SGOT), normal renal function (BUN, creatinine), and a normal CBC (WBC <2000/ml and platelet count >100,000)
Administer *Rhogam* if patient is Rh-negative.
Identify unruptured ectopic pregnancy <3.5 cm.
Obtain informed consent.
Prescribe FeSO₄ 325 mg PO bid if hematocrit <30%.
Schedule follow-up appointment on days 4, 6, and 7.

Patient Instructions:

Refrain from alcohol use, multivitarnins containing folic acid, and sexual intercourse until hCG level is negative.
Call your physician:
If you experience prolonged or heavy vaginal bleeding.
The pain is prolonged or severe (lower abdomen and pelvic pain is normal during the first 10–14 days of treatment).
Use oral contraception or barrier contraceptive methods.

Approximately 4–5% of women experience unsuccessful *methotrexate* treatment and require surgery.
hCG, human chorionic gonadotropin; SGOT, serum glutamic-oxaloacetic transaminase; BUN, blood urea nitrogen; CBC, complete blood count; WBC, white blood cell.

Table 17.5   Ultrasound Criteria for Cervical Pregnancy

---

1. Echo-free uterine cavity or the presence of a false gestational sac only.
2. Decidual transformation of the endometrium with dense echo structure.
3. Diffuse uterine wall structure.
4. Hourglass uterine shape.
5. Ballooned cervical canal.
6. Gestational sac in the endocervix.
7. Placental tissue in the cervical canal.
8. Closed internal os.

Reproduced with permission from **Hofmann HMH, Urdl W, Hofler H, Honigl W, Tamussino K.** Cervical pregnancy: case reports and current concepts in diagnosis and treatment. *Arch Gynecol Obstet* 1987;241:63–9.

9. D

Cervical pregnancy is rare (incidence 1:2,400 to 1:50,000 pregnancies), and therefore, optimal management has not been clearly defined. However, the surgical manipulation of the cervix, e.g., with dilation, can be risky because of the chance of hemorrhage.

Methotrexate offers the chance to treat the condition nonsurgically and hopefully to avoid hysterectomy. Ultrasonographic criteria for the diagnosis of cervical pregnancy are presented in Table 17.5.

Reference: Pages 511–512

18 Benign Breast Disease

Armando E. Giuliano

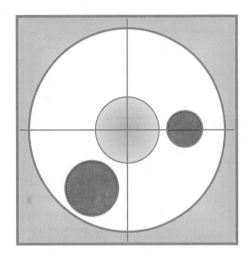

Learning Objectives

1. Know the methods of detection of breast disease.

2. Be aware of the recommendations for breast cancer screening.

3. Be able to provide an algorithm for the management of breast masses in premenopausal and postmenopausal women.

4. Know the benign breast conditions that can and do occur and their differential diagnoses.

5. Be able to identify which breast conditions require evaluation.

Questions

1. Of the following statements, which is true regarding breast tumors, especially cancerous ones:

   A. They are asymptomatic and are discovered only by physical examination or screening mammography

   B. They are typically symptomatic and, therefore, are more likely to be discovered by the patient

   C. They are most likely to be discovered by routine palpation by the physician at the time of an annual physical examination, but not by mammography

   D. They are most likely to go undetected until disease has spread when they produce symptoms in other organs

2. All of the following statements are true regarding mammography **except:**

   A. Approximately one-third of the abnormalities detected on screening mammography prove malignant when biopsy is performed.

   B. Mammography should be performed before biopsy so other suspicious areas can be noted and the contralateral breast can be checked.

   C. The specificity of mammography is approximately 85 to 90% for nonpalpable mammographic abnormalities.

   D. Biopsy must be performed on patients with a dominant or suspicious mass despite mammographic findings.

   E. The value of mammography in women aged 40 to 50 years remains controversial.

3. A 65-year-old postmenopausal female presents with a 1.5 centimeter breast mass in the left upper outer quadrant. The most appropriate management is:

   A. Lumpectomy and axillary node dissection based on a suspicious mammographic finding

   B. Observation based on a negative fine-needle aspiration cytology

   C. A two-week period of observation

   D. Lumpectomy and axillary node dissection based on a fine-needle aspiration cytology

   E. Fine-needle aspiration followed by mammography

4. A 35-year-old female presents with a 2.0 centimeter-diameter breast mass in the left lower outer quadrant. She complains of breast pain that varies with her menstrual cycle. The lesion has not changed in size for the past three months. The most appropriate management is:

   A. Decrease intake of caffeine and start Vitamin E (400 IU daily)

   B. Take *danazol* (100–200 mg twice daily orally)

   C. Observation through two menstrual cycles

   D. Biopsy the lesion

   E. Mammography

5. A fibroadenoma of the breast is most likely to:

   A. Behave in a benign manner

   B. Need to undergo surgical excision because they become symptomatic

   C. Predispose the patient to malignancy

   D. Undergo malignant transformation if the women takes exogenous estrogen

6. A 36-year-old nonlactating female presents with a two-month history of bloody-nipple discharge from her left breast. No mass is palpable on physical examination. The most appropriate management is:

A. Measure serum prolactin and thyroid-stimulating hormone levels
B. Obtain cytologic examination of the bloody nipple discharge
C. Obtain ductography
D. Observation alone
E. Excision of the involved duct

Answers

1. A

Most tumors of the breast, particularly those that are malignant, are asymptomatic and are detected either by physical examination or by screening mammograph. While the value of breast self-examination is controversial, some lesions are detected by the patient, undoubtably before they have a chance to metastasize.
Reference: Pages 526–529

2. C

About one-third of the abnormalites detected on screening mammography prove malignant when biopsy is performed. Mammography should be performed prior to biopsy so that other suspicious lesions and the contralateral breast can be examined. The specificity of mammograpy is about 30 to 40%, not 85 to 90%, for nonpalpable mammographic abnormalities. Biopsy must be performed on patients with a dominant mass or suspicious mass despite mammographic findings. Mammography is never a substitute for biopsy because it may not reveal clinical cancer.

The value of mammography in women aged 40 to 50 years will remain controversial because of the difficulty in showing a beneficial effect among patients in whom the disease has a low incidence.
Reference: Pages 527–531

3. C (see Figure 18.5)

A breast mass in a 65-year-old postmenopausal female is cancer until proven otherwise. A tissue diagnosis must be made before undertaking a definitive operative procedure. There is no role for observation in the patient described. Fine-needle aspiration cytology is a useful technique whereby cells from a breast tumor are aspirated with a small (usually 22-gauge) needle and examined by a pathologist. However, it requires the availability of a pathologist skilled in the cytologic diagnosis of breast cancer to interpret the results and it is subject to sampling problems, particularly when lesions are deep. The incidence of false-positive diagnosis is only about 1 to 2%, but the rate of the false-negative is as high as 10% in some series. Mammography should be performed before biopsy so other suspicious areas can be noted and the contralateral breast can be checked.
Reference: Pages 528, 534

4. D (see Figure 18.4)

Pain, fluctuation in size, and multiplicity of lesions are the features most helpful for differentiating fibrocystic change from carcinoma. However, if a dominant mass is present, as in this patient, the diagnosis of cancer should be suspected until it is disproved by biopsy. Final diagnosis of the mass usually depends on biopsy. Mammography may be helpful, but there are no mammographic signs diagnostic of fibrocystic change. Danazol a synthetic androgen, has been used for patients with severe pain. This treatment suppresses pituitary gonadotropins, and its androgenic effects (acne, edema, hirsutism) are usually intolerable; therefore, it probably should not be used. The role of caffeine consumption in the development and treatement of fibrocystic change is controversial. Observations about these effects have been difficult to confirm and are anecdotal
Reference: Pages 534–535

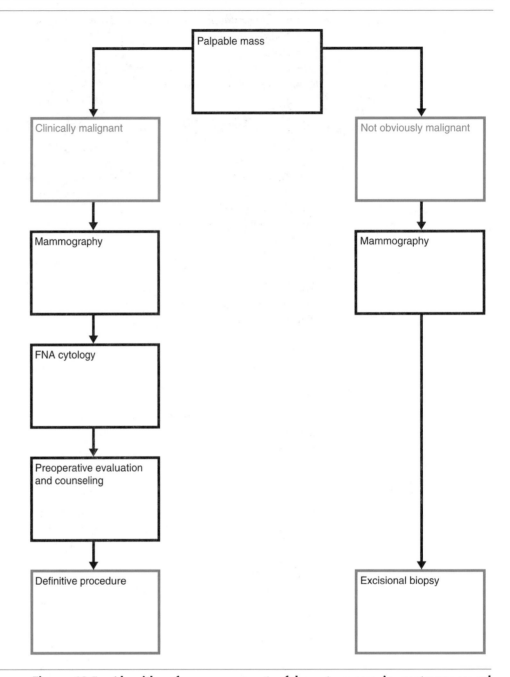

Figure 18.5 Algorithm for management of breast masses in postmenopausal women. (Adapted from **Giuliano AE.** Breast disease. In: **Berek JS, Hacker NF,** eds. *Practical Gynecologic Oncology.* 2nd ed. Baltimore: Williams & Wilkins, 1994:493.)

5. A

Fibroadenomas are the most common benign tumors of the breast. They are usually found in young women. In general, they do not predispose to the development of malignancy. Only large or growing fibroadenomas need to be excised, and this represents the minority of these lesions.
Reference: Page 536

6. E

Unilateral, spontaneous, bloody, or serosanguineous discharge from a single duct is usually caused by an intraductal papilloma or, rarely, by an intraductal cancer. Cyto-

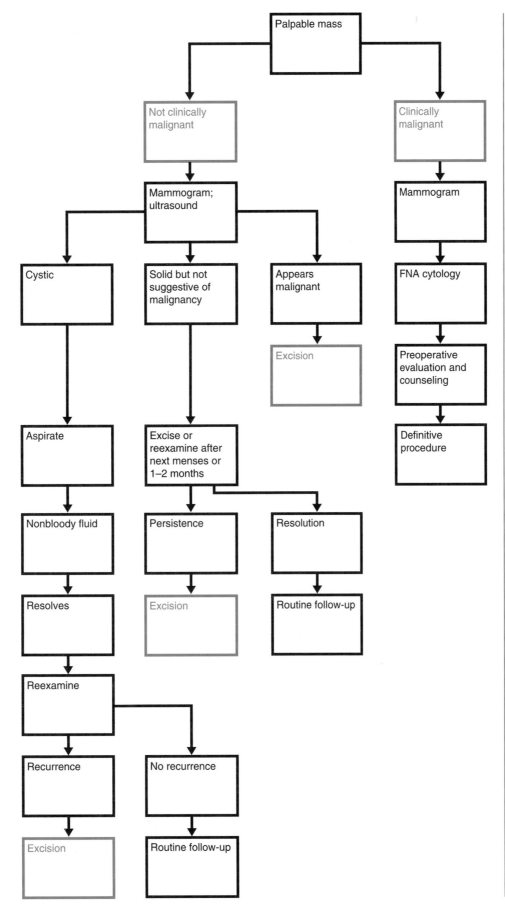

Figure 18.4 **Algorithm for management of breast masses in premenopausal women.** (Adapted from **Giuliano AE.** Breast disease. In: **Berek JS, Hacker NF,** eds. *Practical Gynecologic Oncology.* 2nd ed. Baltimore: Williams & Wilkins, 1994:492.)

147

logic examination is usually of no value but may identify malignant cells. Negative findings do not rule out cancer, which is more likely in women over 50 years of age. In any case, the involved duct—and a mass, if present—should be excised. Although ductography may identify a filling defect prior to excision of the duct system, this study is of little value. Serum prolactin and thyroid-stimulating hormone levels should be obtained to search for a pituitary tumor or hypothyroidism. In this case, a milky discharge would be present.

In order of increasing frequency, the following are the most common causes of nipple discharge in nonlactating women: carcinoma, intraductal papilloma, and fibrocystic change with ectasia of the ducts. The important characteristics of the discharge and other factors to be evaluated by history and physical examination are as follows:

- Nature of discharge (serous, bloody, or milky)
- Association with a mass
- Unilateral or bilateral
- Single or multiple ducts
- Discharge that is spontaneous (persistent or intermittent) or expressed by pressure at a single site or on entire breast
- Relation to menses
- Premenopausal or postmenopausal
- Hormonal medication (contraceptive pills or estrogen)

Reference: Page 537

19 Preoperative Evaluation and Postoperative Management

Jonathan S. Berek
Daniel L. Clarke-Pearson

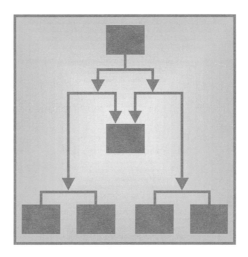

Learning Objectives

1. Provide cost-effective treatment of postoperative deep-vein thrombosis.

2. Identify the level of thromboembolism prophylaxis required in high-risk patient populations.

3. Identify patients at high risk for necrotizing fascitis and describe appropriate management.

4. Understand the appropriateness, as well as the risks, of preoperative imaging studies in patients with potential gynecologic malignancies.

5. Understand which preoperative factors are independently related to increased rates of postoperative myocardial infarction.

Questions

1. The principal purpose of the preoperative consent is:

   A. to establish a trust relationship with the patient
   B. to clarify the goals of the proposed procedure
   C. to outline the expected outcome of the procedure
   D. to outline the risks, benefits, and alternatives to the procedure

2. Weight loss prior to surgery potentially can have an adverse affect on outcome. Below what percentage of ideal body weight is a patient at risk for higher postoperative morbidity?

   A. 6%
   B. 12%
   C. 18%
   D. 24%

3. The normal daily fluid requirement in the average adult is:

   A. 1000 to 1500 ml
   B. 2000 to 3000 ml
   C. 3000 to 4000 ml
   D. 4000 to 5000 ml

4. The most common fluid and electrolyte disorder in the postoperative period is:

   A. hypovolemia from too little fluid
   B. hypernatremia
   C. fluid overload
   D. hyperkalemia

5. The most common electrolyte problem seen in the immediate postoperative period is:

   A. acidosis
   B. alkalosis
   C. hyperkalemia
   D. hyponatremia

6. The best means of maintaining postoperative pain control is to keep the level of pain reliever above the MEAC (minimum effective analgesic concentration) by using:

   A. intermittent intramuscular injections
   B. scheduled intravenous bolus infusions
   C. scheduled oral administration
   D. patient-controlled analgesia

7. Antibiotic prophylaxis should be used in:

   A. vaginal hysterectomy
   B. abdominal hysterectomy
   C. vaginal and abdominal hysterectomy
   D. vaginal and selected abdominal hysterectomy

8. Febrile morbidity is defined as:

   A. higher than or equal to 38 degrees Celcius on 2 occasions 4 hours apart after first 24 hours
   B. higher than or equal to 39 degrees Celcius on 2 occasions 4 hours apart after first 24 hours
   C. higher than 39.5 degrees Celcius at any time after 24 hours
   D. higher than 40 degrees Celcius

150

9. The most common source of postoperative infection is the:

    A. urinary
    B. incision
    C. respiratory
    D. vaginal cuff

10. Wound infection rates can be decreased by all of the following, **except:**

    A. shaving of the wound site
    B. shorten postoperative stay
    C. meticulous surgical technique
    D. *hexachlorophene* showers prior to surgery
    E. bringing drains out through sites other than the incision

11. The most common infectious agent responsible for necrotizing fasciitis is:

    A. *hemolytic streptococcus*
    B. *clostridia perfringes*
    C. *staphylococcus aureus*
    D. *Escherichia Coli*

12. The primary purpose of a preoperative "intestinal preparation" is to:

    A. empty the contents of the bowel
    B. accelerate postoperative bowel recovery
    C. reduce the postoperative infectious morbidity
    D. minimize the risk of intraoperative colorectal injury

13. The principal thrust of management of postoperative ileus is:

    A. instillation of hypertonic radiological contrast material to stimulate function
    B. pharmacological agents to stimulate gastrointestinal function
    C. gastrointestinal decompression and intravenous fluids
    D. surgical intervention to correct intestinal blockage

14. Immediate surgical decompression of the rectosigmoid colon is warranted if the colonic diameter reaches:

    A. 4 to 5 cm
    B. 6 to 8 cm
    C. 10 to 12 cm
    D. 13 to 14 cm

15. Of the following techniques for the prevention of deep venous thrombosis, which one is preferable for most patients undergoing major gynecologic operations?

    A. elastic stockings
    B. low-dose *heparin*
    C. standard-dose *heparin*
    D. external pneumatic compression

16. When acute deep venous thrombosis of the lower extremity has been diagnosed, the optimal number of days of therapeutic levels of heparin is:

    A. 3
    B. 5
    C. 7
    D. 10

17. Of the following, which is most likely to predispose to a postoperative myocardial infarction?

    A. emergency operation
    B. age older than 70 years
    C. poor general medical condition
    D. myocardial infarction in the preceding six months

18. In the management of perioperative congestive heart failure, the measurement of which variable with a pulmonary artery catheter is most helpful in guiding fluid management?

    A. left ventricular pressure (LVP)
    B. right ventricular filling pressure (RVFP)
    C. left ventricular end-diastolic pressure (LVEDP)
    D. pulmonary capillary pressure (PCP) during systole

19. The standard regimen for prophylactic antibiotics in patients with any valvular abnormality to prevent subacute bacterial endocarditis is:

    A. *ampicillin/gentamicin*
    B. *vancomycin/gentamicin*
    C. *amoxicillin* alone
    D. *vancomycin* alone

20. In patients with extensive intraoperative blood loss, in addition to the replacement of red blood cells, replacement with which of the following will most likely be necessary?

    A. albumin
    B. cryoprecipitate
    C. white blood cells
    D. fresh-frozen plasma

21. The greatest risk factor for the development of postoperative pulmonary complications is the presence of underlying:

    A. asthma
    B. malignancy
    C. bronchiectasis
    D. chronic obstructive pulmonary disease

22. The most common postoperative pulmonary complication is:

    A. atelectasis
    B. pneumothorax
    C. pulmonary edema
    D. bronchopneumonia

23. A pulmonary complication of septicemia, which is the result of damage to the capillary side of the alveolar-capillary membrane resulting in an increase in pulmonary capillary permeability, is known as:

    A. pulmonary edema
    B. pulmonary hypertension
    C. respiratory permeability defect
    D. adult respiratory distress syndrome

24. A 45-year-old woman without other complicating medical conditions undergoes abdominal hysterectomy and bilateral salpingo-oophorectomy for stage II ovarian carcinoma. On the fifth postoperative day, she develops femoral, deep-vein thrombosis. What is the proper medical management of this patient?

    A. intravenous *streptokinase* for 72 hours followed by oral *Coumadin* for 3 months

    B. intravenous *heparin* therapy for 24 hours followed by oral *Coumadin* therapy for 3 months

    C. intravenous *heparin* therapy for 10 days followed by *Coumadin* for 3 months

    D. intravenous *heparin* for 5 days followed by oral *Coumadin* for 3 months

    E. bed rest with leg elevation and immediate initiation of oral *Coumadin* therapy for 3 months

25. A 65-year-old woman with clinical stage I, grade 3 endometrial adenocarcinoma is being prepared for surgical therapy to include total abdominal hysterectomy, bilateral salpingo- oophorectomy, and pelvic and periaortic lymphadenectomy. What is the most cost-effective prophylactic regimen available to prevent postoperative venous thromboembolic complications?

    A. low-dose *heparin* (5,000 units preoperatively and every 12 hours postoperatively)

    B. low-dose *heparin* (5,000 units preoperatively and every 8 hours postoperatively)

    C. intermittent pneumatic leg compression intraoperatively and for 24 hours postoperatively

    D. intermittent pneumatic leg compression intraoperatively and for five days postoperatively

    E. graded compression stockings intraoperatively and for two weeks postoperatively

26. A 65-year-old obese female, with hypertension and insulin-dependent diabetes mellitus, has undergone a total abdominal hysterectomy and bilateral salpingo-oophorectomy for a benign pelvic mass. After an unremarkable initial postoperative course, the patient develops a fever of 102.8° Fahrenheit on postoperative day number three. On physical examination, the patient appears ill. Vital signs include a blood pressure 95/60 and heart rate of 108 beats per minute. Physical examination findings are remarkable for cold and clammy skin. The patient's wound is very tender. On palpation the incision is intact but has some purulent drainage. The left aspect of the incision has a brown discoloration and significant erythema with edema of the superficial skin that fades gradually into the normal surrounding skin. Upon opening the incision, purulent material is evacuated and digital palpation of the wound reveals an intact fascia. The subcutaneous fat overlying the fascia can easily be undermined digitally. The appropriate management of this patient would include:

    A. evacuation of the purulent material, irrigation with half-strength peroxide, re-approximation of the skin edges using staples or sutures, and initiation of broad spectrum antibiotic therapy

    B. initiation of wound care including three times daily irrigation with half-strength peroxide and packing of the wound with saline soaked gauze, and initiation of broad spectrum antibiotic therapy

    C. same as B, but no antibiotic therapy is required because this wound abscess has been adequately drained

    D. aggressive IV hydration, initiation of broad spectrum antibiotic therapy, aggressive surgical debridement in the operating room to remove all necrotic and infected tissue until healthy skin margins are achieved, and consideration of postoperative hyperbaric oxygen therapy

27. A 60-year-old black female with a long-standing history of hypertension and insulin-dependent diabetes presents to your office with a history of stage IV ovarian carcinoma. She initially presented at an outside medical center approximately five months earlier with a large left- sided malignant pleural effusion, massive intra-abdominal ascites, and a relatively small asymptomatic 5 to 6 centimeter left adnexal mass, but no other soft tissue or retroperitoneal abnormalities. After a paracentesis was performed, which revealed cells suspicious for papillary serous adenocarcinoma with psammoma bodies (likely ovarian origin), she was treated with six cycles of *cisplatin* and *paclitaxel*. Her

153

ascites and her pleural effusion resolved and her CA125, previously over 2000, is now in the normal range. A CT scan (without contrast) was normal after the third cycle of chemotherapy with the exception of a solid pelvic mass. Unfortunately, her pelvic mass had persisted on examination and she presents at your office at this time for consideration of an interval debulking surgery. Her physical examination is unremarkable with the exception of the solid pelvic mass, which is compressing the rectum. You have discussed with her the palliative roll of the surgery but in your discussion, you explain your concern about the compression on the rectum and the probable need for continued chemotherapy, should, in fact, cancer still be present in the abdominal cavity. Her medical oncologist has taken the liberty of ordering her preoperative admission tests that include a CT scan of the abdomen and pelvis with contrast. The only remarkable study on her serum chemistry reveals a creatinine of 1.2. The next most appropriate step would be:

A. have the patient complete the studies and schedule her for an exploratory laparotomy

B. discontinue the order for the CT scan and order a pelvic ultrasonography instead

C. obtain a radio-labeled *lasix* renal scan to estimate the creatinine clearance in each kidney

D. order a magnetic resonance imaging study of the abdomen and pelvis

E. cancel the CT scan and schedule the patient for an exploratory laparotomy

28. Which of the following is not an independent risk factor for postoperative myocardial infarction?

A. significant aortic valvular stenosis

B. hypertension

C. evidence of congestive heart failure (S_3 gallop or jugular venous distension)

D. more than 5 PVCs per minute preoperatively

E. myocardial infarction within the last six months

Answers

1. D

While the process of obtaining preoperative "informed consent" includes the establishment of a relationship with the patient, and a clarification of the goals and specifics of the proposed operation, the principal purpose (from a legal standpoint) is to document that you have informed the patient regarding the risks, benefits, and alternatives to the operation.
Reference: Pages 545–547

2. B

Preoperative nutritional status is an important correlate of postoperative outcome. While no single test accurately predicts the outcome in malnourished surgical patients, those whose weight is 12% or more below their ideal body weight are at higher risk for complications.
Reference: Pages 547–548

3. B

The body adjusts to higher and lower volumes of intake by changes in plasma tonicity. However, the typical intake that a patient without significant insensible losses is about 2 to 3 liters per day. Patients with high fever can have increased pulmonary and skin loss of free water, sometimes in excess of 2 to 3 liters per day. In patients with bowel obstruction, 1 to 3 liters per day of fluid can be sequestered in the gastrointestinal tract.
Reference: Page 551

4. C

The most common problem seen in patients is iatrogenic, i.e., too much fluid given. The fluid excess can occur with normal or decreased sodium because large amounts of isotonic fluids will remain in the extracellular space. Simple fluid restriction will correct the problem. When necessary, diuretics can be used to increase urinary water excretion.

Reference: Page 555

5. B (see Table 19.3)

Alkalosis is usually of no clinical significance and resolves spontaneously. The most common etiologic factors are hyperventilation associated with pain; posttraumatic transient hyperaldosteronism, which results in a decrease in bicarbonate excretion; nasogastric suction, which removes hydrogen ions; infusion of bicarbonate with transfusions; and the use of diuretics. Alkalosis can usually be promptly reversed by removing the inciting cause.

Reference: Pages 556–558

6. D

The best way to control pain in the immediate postoperative period after major abdominal surgery is probably the PCA, because a relative steady state of drug can be maintained above the MEAC threshold. In this manner, peaks and valleys above and

Table 19.3   Acid-Base Disorders and Their Treatment

Primary Disorder	Defect	Common Causes	Compensation	Treatment
Respiratory acidosis	Carbon dioxide (hypoventilation)	Central nervous system depression Airway and lung impairment	Renal excretion of acid salts Bicarbonate retention Chloride shift into red cells	Restoration ventilation Control of excess dioxide production
Respiratory alkalosis	Hyperventilation	Central nervous excitation system Excess ventilator support	Renal excretion of sodium, potassium bicarbonate Absorption of hydrogen and chloride ions Lactate release from red cells	Correction hyperventilation
Metabolic acidosis	Excess loss of base Increased nonvolatile acids	Excess chloride versus sodium Increased bicarbonate loss Lactic, ketoacidosis Uremia Dilutation acidosis	Respiratory alkalosis Renal excretion of hydrogen and chloride ions Resorption of potassium bicarbonate	Increase sodium load Waste give bicarbonate for pH <7.2 Restore buffers, protein, hemoglobin
Metabolic acidosis	Excess loss of chloride and potassium Increased bicarbonate	Gastrointestinal losses of chloride Excess intake of bicarbonate Diuretics Hypokalemia Extracellular fluid volume contraction	Respiratory acidosis May be hypoxia Renal excretion of bicarbonate and potassium Absorption of hydrogen and chloride ions	Increased chloride content Potassium replacement Acetazolamide (Diamox) to waste bicarbonate Vigorous volume replacement Occasional 0.1 N HCl as needed

below this threshold can be minimized. This approach produces the best pain relief. Guidelines for the use of IV analgesics are presented in Table 19.4.
Reference: Pages 558–559

7. D

The benefit of prophylactic antibiotics in vaginal hysterectomy has been clearly established. However, the benefit in abdominal hysterectomy is controversial. Some data do indicate a benefit in the latter case, especially in obese women, the presence of malignancy, surgery that lasts longer than two hours, and low socioeconomic status.
Reference: Page 562

8. A

This definition has now been well accepted. Within 24 hours, higher temperatures often occur and the correlation with infection is low. If the fever is set higher than 38 degrees Celcius as a cut-off, significant morbidity is missed, especially in elderly patients who are less likely to mount a febrile response to infection.
Reference: Pages 563–564

9. A

The urinary tract has been the most common site of infection in surgical patients. However, this risk is substantially reduced in gynecologic patients who have received prophy-

Table 19.4   Guidelines for Front-Loading IV Analgesics* for Relief of Perioperative Pain

Drug	Total Front-Loaded Dose	Increments	Cautions
Morphine	0.08–0.12 mg/kg	0.03 mg/kg q 10 h	Histaminergic effects; nausea; biliary colic; reduce dose for elderly
Meperidine	1.0–1.5 mg/kg	0.30 mg/kg/q 10 h	Reduce dose or change drug for impaired renal function
Codeine	0.5–1.0 mg/kg	1/3 total q 15 h	Nausea
Methadone	0.08–0.12 mg/kg	0.03 mg/kg q 15 h	Do not administer maintenance dose after analgesia
Levorphanol	10.02 mg/kg	50–75 ug/kg q 15 h	Similar to *methadone*
Hydromorphone sulfate	0.02 mg/kg	25–50 ug/kg q 10 h	Similar to *morphine*
Pentazocine	0.5–1.0 mg/kg	1/2 total q 15 h	Psychomimetic effects; may cause withdrawal in narcotic-dependent patients
Nalbuphine	0.08–0.15 mg/kg	0.03 mg/kg q 10 h	Less psychomimetic effect than *pentazocine;* sedation
Butorphanol	0.01–0.04 mg/kg	0.01 mg/kg q 10 h	Sedation; psychomimetic effects like *nalbuphine*
Buprenorphine	Up to 0.2 mg/kg	1/4 total q 10 h	Long-acting like *methadone, levorphanol;* may precipitate withdrawal in narcotic-dependent patients; safe to give subcutaneous maintenance after analgesia—different from *methadone*

*A scheme for front-loading the opioids most commonly used in postoperative pain treatment.

156

lactic antibiotics. Recent literature has indicated a urinary tract infection rate as low as 4% in those women who have received prophylactic therapy. Most urinary tract infections occur in the lower urinary tract, and very few patients develop serious pyelonephritis.
Reference: Pages 564–565

10. A

One should minimize the shaving of the incision site, because shaving, particularly when it is done hours prior to the surgery instead of immediately before the incision, increases the rate of wound infection. All of the other parameters are associated with lower infection rates.
Reference: Pages 566–567

11. A

While *hemolytic streptococcus* is responsible for many of these cases, it is not the only organism. Furthermore, this infection may predispose to other infections and a polymicrobial infection often exists. Other organisms, including other Gram-positive organisms, coliforms, and anaerobes are often cultured in addition to the *hemolytic streptococcus*. Bacterial enzymes such as hyaluronidase and lipase are released in the subcutaneous space and destroy the fascia and fatty tissues producing a liquefactive necrosis.
Reference: Page 568

12. C

The principal reason for the performance of a "bowel prep" is to reduce the incidence of postoperative infectious morbidity. The rate of infection associated with intestinal resection in unprepared bowel is as high as 40%, whereas it is 5 to 10% after a preparation. When resection of the colon is a possibility, the intestinal preparation should include both mechanical and antibiotic preparation (see Table 19.7).
Reference: Page 570

13. C

Although the mechanism of ileus is somewhat unclear, there is a disruption in normal intestinal motility that is associated with peritoneal infection, various surgical procedures performed in the abdomen, and electrolyte disturbances. The primary therapy is

Table 19.7   Bowel Preparation Regimens to Begin Day Prior to Surgery

Time	*Mechanical Prep*	*Antibiotic Prep*
Preoperative day 2 *pm*	Clear liquid diet	
Preoperative day 1 *Noon*	Clear liquid diet *Magnesium citrate* (240 cc po), or *GoLYTELY* (4 l po over 3 hrs)	
1 pm		*Erythromycin* base 500 mg po, plus *Neomycin* 1 gm po *Metronidazole* 500mg po may be substituted
2 pm		Repeat po antibiotics
8 pm	Enemas until clear IV D5/0.5 NS + 20 mEq KCL at 125 cc/hr (optional)	
11 pm		Repeat po antibiotics
Operative day *12 midnight* *am*	Nothing by mouth Surgery	Prophylactic IV antibiotics

decompression of the bowel, typically with a nasogastric tube, and careful administration of fluids and electrolytes. Pharmacological and radiological stimulate are of limited value. Surgery should be performed if the condition does not resolve over several days and a true mechanical obstruction is suspected.
Reference: Pages 571–572

14. C

With complete colonic obstruction (typically be a gynecologic neoplasm), the colon can rapidly dilate and perforate. A normal lower colon may dilate to 4 to 5 centimeters, but when it reaches 10 to 12 centimeters, the colon is dangerously dilated. Immediate management with colostomy or colectomy is warranted.
Reference: Pages 572–573

15. D

The use of external pneumatic compression results in a reduction of postoperative venous thromboembolic complications by nearly threefold. This reduction is similar to that seen with low-dose *heparin* and has the advantage of not increasing the likelihood of bleeding complications.
Reference: Pages 574–575

16. B

A randomized trial of a 5-day versus a 10-day regimen of *heparin* showed that the 5-day regimen was equally effective and it had a lower risk of complications.
Reference: Page 578

17. D

The preoperative variable that most likely predisposes to a postoperative myocardial infarction is the presence of jugular venous distention or an S_3 gallop (indicating congestive heart failure) and the occurrence of a myocardial infarction in the preceding six months (Table 19.8). Therefore, in women who have had a recent MI, elective surgery should be postponed at least for six months.
Reference: Page 583

Table 19.8   Risk Factors for Postoperative Myocardial Infarction

Independent Risk Factors	Points
1. Jugular venous distension or S_3 gallop immediately preoperatively	11
2. Myocardial infarction in preceding 6 months	10
3. Presence of premature atrial contractions on preoperative ECG or any rhythm other than sinus	7
4. More than 5 premature ventricular contractions per minute preoperatively	7
5. Evidence of significant aortic valvular stenosis	3
6. Age older than 70 years	5
7. Emergency operation	4
8. Intraperitoneal operation	3
9. Poor general medical condition PO$_2$ <60 or PCO$_2$ 50 mm Hg K<3.0 or HCO$_3$ <20 mEq/l BUN >50 or creatinine >3.0 mg/dl Liver disease or debilitated patient	3

ECG, electrocardiogram.

18. C

Otherwise known as the "wedge pressure," the measurement of the pulmonary capillary wedge pressure (PCWP) reflects the LVEDP and is most useful in the management of fluid replacement in the perioperative period.
Reference: Pages 587, 590–591

19. A

The American Heart Association recommends this regimen for antibiotic valvular prophylaxis (Table 19.12). The use of *vancomycin/gentamicin* is for *penicillin*-allergic patients. Oral *amoxicillin* is recommended for low-risk patients for minor procedures only.
Reference: Page 589

20. D

With extensive blood loss, the most likely requirement for transfusion relates to the consumption of clotting factors and platelets. Therefore, intraoperative determinations of the platelet count and the partial thromboplastin time are useful to help assess whether platelet or fresh-frozen plasma should be transfused.
Reference: Pages 594–595

21. D

Chronic bronchitis and emphysema are diseases that often occur in tandem. Cigarette smoking is involved in the pathogenesis of both. Preoperative treatment with bronchodilators, antibiotics, respiratory therapy, and cessation of smoking are important to decrease the risk of postoperative pulmonary complications.
Reference: Pages 598–599

22. A

Atelectasis accounts for 90% of all pulmonary complications. The most important maneuvers for prevention and therapy are those that promote maximal inspiratory pressure. These include the use of incentive spirometry, deep breathing exercises, coughing, and in some cases, the use of positive-end expiratory pressure with a mask. Oversedation should be avoided and early ambulation should be encouraged.
Reference: Page 599

23. D

Otherwise known as noncardiogenic pulmonary edema, ARDS is a condition requiring aggressive pulmonary resuscitation and treatment of the underlying cause. In gynecologic patients, the underlying cause is usually septicemia, and thus, the use of broad-spectrum antibiotics in addition to the specific treatment of respiratory failure, which typically involves ventilator support and shock management, is employed.
Reference: Page 600

Table 19.12   Recommendations for Prophylaxis of Bacterial Endocarditis

Standard Regimen:	
Ampicillin	2 g, 30 minutes to 1 hour bid, and
Gentamicin	1.5 mg/kg IM or IV, 30 minutes to 1 hour before.
Penicillin-Allergic Patients:	
Vancomycin	1 g IV slowly over 1 hour, and
Gentamicin	1.5 mg/kg IM or IV 1 hour before; may be repeated once in 12 hours.
Oral Regimen for Minor Procedures in Low-Risk Patients:	
Amoxicillin	3 g po, 1 hour before and 1.5 q 6 hours later.

IM, intramuscularly; IV, intravenously.

24. D

Immediate treatment of postoperative deep-vein thrombosis is aimed at preventing propagation of deep thrombosis and prevention of pulmonary embolism. Long-term treatment should aim at prevention of rethrombosis while at the same time minimize the risks of bleeding complications. *Streptokinase* is contraindicated in the postoperative surgical patient except under the most life-threatening conditions. The risks of postoperative hemorrhage are extremely high with this therapy. The most widely evaluated and recognized method of deep-vein thrombosis treatment is the use of intravenous *heparin* therapy with the goal of achieving an activated partial thromboplastin time (APPT) of approximately 1.5 to 2.0 times the control value. This is usually accomplished with immediate intravenous bolus of *heparin* followed by continuous infusion.

The duration of *heparin* therapy has been evaluated in randomized prospective studies comparing what had been "traditional" therapy of 10 days of *heparin* versus a shorter infusion of 5 days of *heparin*. Both *heparin* regimens were then followed with three months of oral *Coumadin* administration achieving an INR of approximately 2.0 times control value. Five days of *heparin* therapy were found to be equally effective in preventing rethrombosis and, at the same time, shortened the hospital stay by approximately five days.
Reference: Page 577–579

25. D

An elderly patient undergoing surgery for gynecologic cancer is at very high risk to develop postoperative venous thrombolic complications. Prophylactic methods are clearly warranted, and prospective studies have identified that both low-dose *heparin* and intermittent pneumatic leg compression are effective in this patient group. However, the intensity of prophylaxis is critical. Randomized trials have shown that *heparin* given every 12 hours (answer A) and short duration (24 hours) of pneumatic compression (answer C) are not effective in patients with gynecologic cancers while they are effective in lower risk groups of patients. Low-dose *heparin* given at an eight-hour regimen or pneumatic compression continued for five days postoperatively have both been found to be effective in preventing venous thrombolic complications in this high-risk group of patients. Because of the decreased risks of bleeding complications, intermittent pneumatic leg compression was considered to be the most cost- effective regimen available.
Reference: Pages 574–576

26. D

Necrotizing fasciitis is an uncommon infectious disorder with approximately 1000 cases occuring annually in the United States. It is characterized by a rapidly progressive bacterial infection that involves the subcutaneous tissues and fascia and characteristically spares underlying muscle. Systemic toxicity is a frequent feature of the disease. The pathogenesis of necrotizing fasciitis involves a polymicrobial infection with common organisms including hemolytic streptococcus as well as other organisms, including gram-positive organisms and anaerobes. Enzymes released by bacteria into the subcutaneous space destroy the fascia, adipose tissue, and induce a liquefactive necrosis. In addition, noninflammatory and intravascular coagulation and thrombosis frequently will occur in the small vessels in the subcutaneous tissues, resulting in ischemia and necrosis of the subcutaneous tissues. Late in the course of infection, destruction of the superficial nerves can produce anesthesia in the involved skin. Release of bacteria and toxins into the systemic circulation can cause septic shock, acid base abnormalities, and multi-organ impairment.

Predisposing risk factors for necrotizing fasciitis include diabetes mellitus, trauma, alcoholism, an immuno-compromised state, hypertension, peripheral vascular disease, intravenous drug abuse, and obesity. The mortality rate of the disease is high. However, early diagnosis and aggressive management has led to improved survival rates. Clinical and laboratory findings can include a disproportionally greater amount of pain than expected from the clinical findings; temperature abnormalities—both hypothermia and hyperthermia; tenderness; erythema and warmth of the involved skin; edema and erythema spread diffusely, invading into normal skin. Most patients have a leukocytosis and develop acid-based abnormalities. Successful management involves early recognition of the problem and immediate initiation of resuscitative measures, including correction of fluid and acid-base electrolyte abnormalities, and hematologic abnormalities. Aggressive surgical debridement and re-debridement need to be performed, and broad-spectrum antibiotic therapy should be initiated. An incision should be made through the infected tissue, down to the fascia. An ability to undermine the skin and subcutaneous tissues with digital palpation often will confirm the diagnosis. Multiple incisions can be made sequentially toward the periphery of the infected tissue until well-vascularized healthy tissue is reached at all margins. Many patients have benefited from central venous monitoring as well as from high caloric and nutritional support. In addition, in one study, the use of hyperbaric oxygen therapy after surgical debridement was associated with an improvement in overall mortality. Once the infection has resolved and granulation has begun, skin flaps can be mobilized to help cover open wounds.

Reference: Pages 568–569

27. E

Further imaging studies are not likely to change the surgeon's approach to this patient. If she has a solid mass compressing her sigmoid colon, which was present before the chemotherapy, it is probable that this is related to the malignancy and probably represents her ovary. An ultrasound and MRI, and a CT scan will not change the management or the surgical approach in this patient. A CT scan of the abdomen and pelvis with contrast to identify the anatomy of the pelvic ureter is not only unnecessary but would likely result in acute tubular necrosis in a patient with a history of insulin-dependent diabetes and a prior history of *cisplatin*. It should be noted that the patient already has a component of nephropathy (of creatinine of 1.2), which may be due either to the long-standing hypertension, diabetes, and/or the *cisplatin* treatments. Intravenous contrast agents are associated with approximately a 70% incidence of acute tubular necrosis. Therefore, the right answer would be to proceed with an exploratory laparotomy and then debulk the pelvic mass. Since the patient initially presented with a stage IV lesion, additional debulking should be limited only to those areas in which the colon or small intestine were in jeopardy of obstruction, as it would probably not change her overall survival.

Reference: Pages 1174–1181 (see Chapter 33)

28. B

Because of the high mortality and morbidity associated with perioperative myocardial infarction, much effort has been made to predict perioperative cardiac risk. A prospec-

Table 19.9   Risk Classes for Postoperative Myocardial Infarction

Total Class	Score	Patients	Patients with life-threatening Complications* or Death
I	0–5	537	5 (1%)
II	6–12	316	21 (7%)
III	13–25	130	18 (14%)
IV	>26	18	14 (78%)

Modified from **Goldman L.** Multifactorial index of cardiac risk in noncardiac surgical procedures. *N Engl J Med* 1977;297:845–50.
*Life-threatening complications are documented intraoperative or postoperative myocardial infarction, pulmonary edema, or ventricular tachycardia without progression to cardiac death.

tive evaluation of preoperative cardiac risk factors using a multivariate analysis identified independent cardiac risk factors, as presented in Table 19.8. Using these factors, a *cardiac risk index* has been created that places a patient in one of four risk classes (Table 19.9). Unstable angina, probably because it is relatively uncommon, did not appear as a risk factor, although many believe that patients with unstable angina should be considered at extremely high risk of perioperative cardiac mortality and should undergo coronary artery revascularization prior to any elective gynecologic surgery.
Reference: Page 583–584

20 Incontinence, Prolapse, and Disorders of the Pelvic Floor

Felipe L.G. Videla
L. Lewis Wall

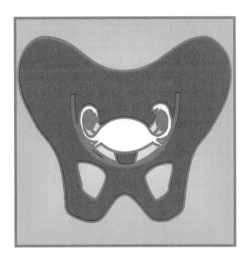

Learning Objective

1. Describe the functional anatomy of the pelvic floor and its relationship to urinary and fecal continence and incontinence.

2. Understand normal continence mechanisms of the lower urinary tract and colorectal system.

3. Outline the principles of investigation used in the evaluation of patients with incontinence and/or prolapse.

4. Understand clinical urodynamic testing and its application in the evaluation of urinary incontinence.

5. Describe the causes of urinary incontinence and the appropriate means for diagnosing them.

6. Understand the terminology used to describe pelvic relaxation and incontinence.

7. Understand the basic principles involved in nonsurgical management of urinary incontinence.

8. Understand the surgical procedures used for treating urinary incontinence and prolapse, and understand which procedures are useful for which type of incontinence.

9. Describe the evaluation and treatment of patients with colorectal dysfunction.

Questions

Multiple Choice

1. Intrinsic factors that contribute to the integrity of the urethral sphincteric mechanism include:

    A. The smooth muscle of the urethral wall
    B. Urethral elasticity
    C. Coaptation of the epithelial folds of the urethra
    D. Vascular congestion of the submucosal urethral venous plexus
    E. All of the above

2. The initial evaluation of most patients with urinary incontinence should include all of the following **except:**

    A. Urinalysis, with culture and cytology as appropriate
    B. Pressure/flow voiding studies
    C. Frequency/volume bladder chart
    D. Medication history
    E. Measurement of residual urine after voiding

3. The functional capacity of the bladder is defined most accurately by using which of the following studies?

    A. Frequency/volume bladder chart
    B. Bladder filling test
    C. Urethral pressure profile
    D. Subtracted cystometry
    E. Leak-point pressure test

4. Which of the following is *not* true concerning sling procedures for stress incontinence?

    A. They are only needed in about 10 to 15% of patients with stress urinary incontinence
    B. They are the procedures of choice in patients with high leak-point pressures
    C. Slings can be made from autologous, heterologous, or synthetic materials
    D. Slings can cause urinary outflow obstruction
    E. None of the above

5. Which of the following is *not* associated with the syndrome of interstitial cystitis:

    A. Frequency
    B. Urgency
    C. Painful voiding
    D. Bladder pain
    E. Small bladder capacity

6. Which of the following factors is *not* associated with rectal prolapse:

    A. Chronic constipation
    B. Female sex
    C. Cesarean delivery
    D. Redundant rectosigmoid colon
    E. Deep cul-de-sac of Douglas

Matching

7–10. Match the following points of attachment of the endopelvic fascia to the appropriate procedures:

—— **7.** Marshall-Marchetti-Krantz retropubic urethropexy
—— **8.** Burch colposuspension
—— **9.** Paravaginal defect repair
—— **10.** Turner-Warwick vagino-obturator shelf procedure

A. Arcus tendineus fascia pelvis
B. Periosteum of the pubic symphysis
C. Iliopectineal ligament (Cooper's ligament)
D. Obturator internus fascia
E. Rectus abdominis fascia

True or False

11. The major support for the pelvic organs is provided by their ligamentous attachments to the bony pelvis.

12. When the pubovisceral muscle contracts, it pulls the rectum, vagina, and urethra anteriorly toward the pubic bone. In doing this, it constricts the lumens of these organs, thereby helping to maintain continence.

13. Connective tissue abnormalities can be significant factors that contribute to prolapse and related conditions.

14. Active control of bladder contraction leading to complete bladder emptying is under the primary control of the sympathetic nervous system.

15. Urinary incontinence is defined as involuntary loss of urine that can be demonstrated objectively by a clinician.

16. Stress urinary incontinence is the most common form of transurethral incontinence in women.

17. Urinary urge incontinence refers to urine loss that occurs with an accompanying strong desire to void.

18. Detrusor overactivity is often initially managed best through a combination of drug therapy and behavior modification.

19. The mainstay of therapy for women with chronic urinary retention is clean intermittent self- catheterization.

20. Examining a patient with genital prolapse in the standing position is difficult and generally does not provide clinically useful information.

Answers

Multiple Choice

1. E

Normal urethral closure is maintained by a combination of intrinsic and extrinsic factors working together. Factors intrinsic to the urethra that contribute to normal closure include the smooth muscle of the urethral wall, urethral elasticity, coaptation of the epithelial folds within the urethral lumen, and vascular congestion of the submucosal venous plexus of the urethra. It is important to understand that urethral support by itself does not maintain urinary continence; rather, a complex interplay exists between intrinsic urethral factors and external urethral support.
Reference: Pages 636–638

2. B (see Figures 20.7 and 20.8)

The initial evaluation of the incontinent patient is straightforward and well within the capabilities of the general clinician. A systematic approach to the investigation of incontinence usually will yield an appropriate diagnosis, or clarify the need for more sophisticated urodynamic testing. The initial steps in investigating urinary incontinence include taking a complete medical and surgical history with a detailed review of specific urinary tract symptoms; performing a thorough physical examination; obtaining a complete urinalysis (with culture and cytology, if indicated); measuring the urine that remains after normal voiding; and having the patient keep a frequency/volume bladder chart. Simple uroflowmetry and pressure/flow voiding studies are more sophisticated tests that can be used to look at bladder emptying as part of a complete urodynamic evaluation of a patient.
Reference: Page 629

Figure 20.7 Subtracted filling cystometry. Pressure catheters are in place in the bladder and rectum. An additional filling catheter has been placed in the bladder. Volume infused, total bladder pressure, rectal (abdominal) pressure, and subtracted detrusor pressure (intrinsic bladder pressure) are recorded. (Reproduced with permission from **Wall LL, Addison WA.** Basic cystometry in gynecologic practice. *Postgrad Obstet Gynecol* **1988;26(2):3.)**

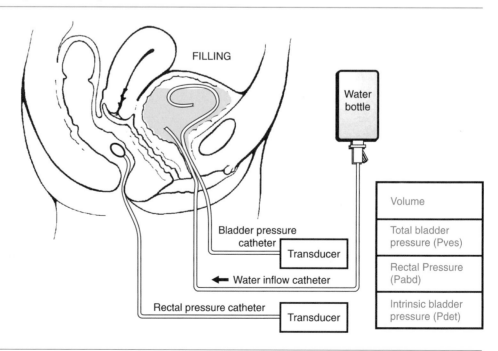

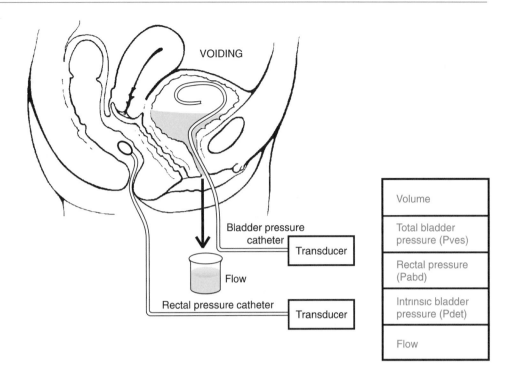

Figure 20.8 Pressure-flow voiding study. The filling catheter has been removed. Volume voided, urine flow rate, total bladder pressure, rectal (abdominal) pressure, and subtracted detrusor pressure are recorded. (Reproduced with permission from **Wall LL, Addison WA.** Basic cystometry in gynecologic practice. *Postgrad Obstet Gynecol* 1988;26(2):3.)

3. A (see Figure 20.6)

The frequency/volume bladder chart is an invaluable (and often-neglected) aid in diagnosing many types of urinary dysfunction. To keep a bladder chart, the patient records the time of each void and measures the amount of urine that she passes for several days, along with any symptoms or incontinent episodes. The resulting record provides accurate information about urinary frequency, the average voided volume, and total urinary output. The functional bladder capacity is the largest voided volume recorded on a bladder chart that has been kept for several days. This represents the largest volume that a patient is likely to keep in her bladder during the course of normal daily activities. Obtaining this information before performing urodynamic studies is particularly important, because it helps delineate the volumes at which the patient has symptoms. It also provides a useful target volume to aim at during filling cystometry, since there is no reason to believe that a patient should hold a greater bladder volume during urodynamic studies than she does in normal life, and if the bladder is overfilled, artifactual information may be obtained that is not relevant to the patient's complaint. In addition, obtaining the total urinary output in 24 hours will let the clinician pick out those patients with abnormally high (or abnormally low) urine production in a simple and reliable fashion. High urine output (as in uncontrolled diabetes) is particularly relevant to treating incontinence, since reducing the volume that the bladder must contend with may, by itself, restore continence in some patients.
Reference: Page 632

4. B

Sling procedures are used primarily for patients with complicated or recurrent stress incontinence, particularly patients with intrinsic sphincter deficiency (sometimes called "Type III incontinence"). Patients with intrinsic sphincter deficiency lose urine with

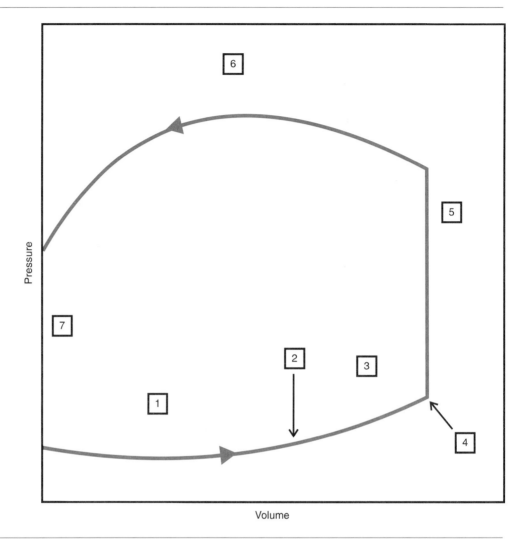

Figure 20.6   Pressure/volume relationship of the micturition cycle. 1) The normal bladder accommodates increasing urine volumes without a significant increase in pressure. 2) At around 200 ml, the first sensation of bladder fullness is appreciated. 3) The micturition reflex can be suppressed until a socially acceptable time and place for urination presents itself. 4) At this time, a voluntary detrusor contraction is initiated, in conjunction with pelvic floor relaxation. 5) There is a brief isometric pressure rise before the bladder neck is open and flow starts. 6) Normal voiding is accomplished by a sustained detrusor contraction until bladder emptying is complete. 7) The detrusor muscle then relaxes and the process of filling begins anew. (Reproduced with permission from **Wall LL, Addison WA.** Basic cystometry in gynecologic practice. *Postgrad Obstet Gynecol* 1988;26(2):2.)

relatively little effort; thus, they have low leak-point pressures. High leak-point pressures are indicative of a strong urethral sphincter mechanism. Slings can be made from a variety of materials including autologous grafts of rectus fascia or fascia lata taken from the patient herself, banked cadaveric tissues such as fascia lata, or heterologous materials from other species such as ox dura mater or porcine dermis. A variety of synthetic materials (such as Gore-Tex, Marlex, or Mersiline) have been used in performing sling operations, but these materials seem to be more prone to infection or erosion than organic materials. One of the most common problems occurring after a sling procedure is the development of obstructed voiding as the result of a sling that is too tight, often necessitating long-term clean intermittent self-catheterization.

Reference: Pages 649–650

5. C

The classic syndrome associated with interstitial cystitis (sometimes also called "painful bladder syndrome") includes urgency, frequency, and bladder pain in the presence of a small-capacity bladder. Bladder pain tends to increase with bladder filling and is relieved with voiding. The etiology of interstitial cystitis is unknown; most probably, a variety of disorders with a common clinical presentation are lumped together because the underlying pathophysiology is unknown. The diagnosis is often made by the exclusion of other etiologies in patients with painful bladder symptoms.
Reference: Page 656

6. C (see Table 20.8)

Rectal prolapse is a condition in which the rectum slips through the levator hiatus, intussuscepts, and finally protrudes through the anus. Factors that predispose to the development of this condition include chronic straining at stool, neurologic disease, female sex, nulliparity, redundant rectosigmoid, a deep cul-de- sac of Douglas, patulous anus, diastasis of the levator ani muscle, intussusception, and prior operative procedures (e.g., hemorrhoidectomy, fistulectomy).
Reference: Pages 665–666

Matching

7. B

The Marshall-Marchetti-Krantz retropubic urethropexy was first described in 1949 and has served as a starting point for the development of a number of subsequent retropubic bladder neck suspension procedures. The original MMK operation involves attaching the periurethral endopelvic fascia to the periosteum of the pubic symphysis. In some cases, this can lead to the development of osteitis pubis, an inflammatory condition of the pubic bone, which is both debilitating and difficult to treat.
Reference: Pages 645–646

8. C

The Burch colposuspension began originally as a modification of the MMK procedure. As originally described by Dr. John Burch, the operation involves placing sutures from the endopelvic fascia at the level of the bladder neck to the iliopectineal ligament

---

Table 20.8 Factors Associated With Or Predisposing To Rectal Prolapse

Poor bowel habits (especially constipation)

Neurologic disease (e.g. congenital anomaly, cauda equina lesion, spinal cord injury, senility)

Female sex

Nulliparity

Redundant rectosigmoid

Deep Douglas' pouch

Patulous anus (weak internal sphincter)

Diastasis of levator ani muscle (defect in pelvic floor)

Lack of fixation of rectum to sacrum

Intussusception (also secondary to colonic lesions)

Operative procedure (e.g., hemorrhoidectomy, fistulectomy, abdominoanal pull-through)

Reproduced with permission from **Corman ML.** Rectal prolapse. In: *Colon and Rectal Surgery.* 2nd ed. Philadelphia: JB Lippincott, 1989:209–47.

(Cooper's ligament). This procedure eliminated the risk of osteitis pubis seen with the MMK operation, and provided a more secure point of attachment for sutures, but it is not without its complications. Because the procedure elevates the bladder neck to a high retropubic position, the Burch operation is associated with a fairly high rate of postoperative prolapse (rectocele, enterocele), and the development of obstructed voiding, conditions which are also common after an MMK procedure.
Reference: Pages 645–646

9. A

The paravaginal defect repair operation can be performed either vaginally or abdominally. The abdominal route is easier for most surgeons. When a lateral detachment of the endopelvic fascia from the arcus tendineus fascia pelvis is present and results in urethral hypermobility, the associated stress incontinence can usually be cured by reattaching the endopelvic fascia laterally along the pelvic sidewall where it has become separated.
Reference: Pages 645–646

10. D

The vagino-obturator shelf procedure (originally described by the British urologic surgeon Richard Turner-Warwick) is similar philosophically to the paravaginal defect repair operation. In this procedure, either the vagina or the endopelvic fascia at the level of the bladder neck is sutured laterally to the fascia overlying the obturator internus muscle. This operation, like the paravaginal defect repair, is associated with less symptoms of obstructed voiding than is either the MMK or the Burch procedure.
Reference: Pages 645–646

True or False

11. False (see Table 20.1)

The majority of support to the pelvic organs is provided by tonic contraction of the muscles of the pelvic floor. The ligamentous attachments of the pelvic organs are only of secondary importance. The belief that the ligaments provide most of the support for pelvic organs such as the uterus is common, but erroneous, and is derived mainly from the fact that the "ligaments" are used in the surgical repair of prolapse and related conditions. In fact, ligaments are not well suited to provide support because they tend to stretch when subjected to constant tension over time.
Reference: Pages 619, 621

12. True

One of the most important continence mechanisms of the pelvic floor is the tonic contraction of the pubovisceral muscle (more commonly, but less descriptively, known as the puborectalis or pubococcygeus muscle). The pubovisceral muscle forms a sling around the genital hiatus; when contracted, this muscle pulls the rectum, vagina, and urethra anteriorly toward the pubic bone. In doing this, it closes the hiatus and constricts the lumens of the pelvic organs, helping to maintain both urinary and fecal continence as well as decreasing the opportunity for pelvic organ prolapse. The sling effect created by this muscle is aided by its medial attachments to the endopelvic fascia of the vagina, its lateral attachments to the arcus tendineus fascia pelvis, and its attachments to the pubic bone superiorly.
Reference: Page 621

13. True

The fascia that covers muscles and tendons, allowing them to attach to other structures, is composed mainly of collagen. Women with collagen abnormalities appear to have an increased incidence and prevalence of genital prolapse and associated disorders.
Reference: Pages 622–623

Table 20.1   Classification and Definition of Lower Urinary Symptoms In Women

I. Abnormal Storage

Incontinence: Involuntary urine loss that is a social or hygienic problem.
Stress incontinence: Incontinence occurring under conditions of increased intra-abdominal pressure.
Urge incontinence: Incontinence accompanied by a strong desire to void.
Mixed incontinence: Stress and urge incontinence occurring together.
Unconscious incontinence: Incontinence occurring without urgency and without conscious recognition of leakage.
Frequency: The number of voids per day, from waking in the morning until falling asleep at night.
Nocturia: The number of times the patient is awakened from sleep to void at night.
Nocturnal enuresis: Urinary incontinence during sleep.

II. Abnormal Emptying

Hesitancy: Trouble initiating voiding.
Straining to void: Voiding accompanied by abdominal straining.
Poor stream: Decreased force of flow of the urinary stream.
Intermittent stream: A "stop-and-start" pattern of urination.
Incomplete emptying: A persistent feeling of bladder fullness after voiding.
Postmicturition dribble: Urine loss occurring just after normal voiding has been completed.
Acute urinary retention: Sudden inability to void resulting in painful bladder overdistention and the need for catheterization to obtain relief.

III. Abnormal Sensation

Urgency: A strong desire to void.
Dysuria: Burning pain with urination.
Bladder pain: Conscious, hurting, suprapubic pain in the bladder.
Flank pain: Pain between the lower rib cage and the ilial crest.
Pressure: A feeling of heaviness or constant force being exerted in the bladder or lower pelvis.
Loss of bladder sensation: Decreased sensation in the bladder.

IV. Abnormal Bladder Contents

Abnormal color
Abnormal smell
Hematuria
Pneumaturia
Stones
Foreign bodies

14. False

Control of the lower urinary tract is maintained by a complex interaction between the sympathetic and parasympathetic nervous systems and the somatic nervous system. Motor control of the bladder (initiation and maintenance of a sustained vesical contraction) is controlled primarily by the parasympathetic nervous system, which arises in the sacral segments (S_2–S_4) of the spinal cord. Acetylcholine is the main neurotransmitter in both the preganglionic and postganglionic synapses of the parasympathetic nervous system. For this reason, nearly all medications used to control detrusor overactivity have anticholinergic properties.
Reference: Pages 625–626

15. False (see Table 20.2)

The International Continence Society defines urinary incontinence as loss of urine that is objectively demonstrable *and is a social or hygienic problem for the patient or her caregivers.* Many women leak small amounts of urine occasionally. Subclinical urine loss of this kind may even be seen during a routine pelvic examination; however, *occasional* loss of urine is not the same as clinical urinary incontinence. It is only when the frequency, duration, and amount of urine lost become socially problematic that clinical urinary in-

---

Table 20.2   Differential Diagnosis Of Urinary Incontinence

I. Extraurethral incontinence

   A. Congenital
      1. Ectopic ureter
      2. Bladder exstrophy
      3. Other
   B. Acquired (fistulas)
      1. Ureteric
      2. Vesical
      3. Urethral
      4. Complex combinations

II. Transurethral incontinence

   A. Genuine stress incontinence
      1. Bladder neck displacement (anatomic hypermobility)
      2. Intrinsic sphincteric dysfunction
      3. Combined
   B. Detrusor overactivity
      1. Idiopathic detrusor instability
      2. Neuropathic detrusor hyperreflexia
   C. Mixed incontinence
   D. Urinary retention with bladder distention and overflow
      1. Genuine stress incontinence
      2. Detrusor hyperactivity with impaired contractility
      3. Combinations
   E. Urethral diverticulum
   F. Congenital urethral abnormalities (e.g., epispadias)
   G. Uninhibited urethral relaxation ("urethral instability")
   H. Functional and transient incontinence

---

continence begins. The threshold at which this occurs is different for individual women. While it is important to demonstrate urine loss objectively before undertaking surgical treatment, when stress leakage of urine is seen, the patient should always be asked if what has been demonstrated bothers her and if it is the problem for which she is seeking help.
Reference: Page 628

16. **True (see Figure 20.10 and Table 20.4)**

Stress incontinence—the loss of urine occurring coincidentally with sudden increases in intra-abdominal pressure—is the leading cause of urinary incontinence in women. "Genuine stress urinary incontinence" is a specific term that refers to loss of urine occurring during an increase in intravesical pressure caused by elevated abdominal pressure, in the absence of a detrusor contraction. The term "genuine stress incontinence" therefore implies that stress incontinence has been demonstrated in the urodynamics laboratory under conditions in which pressure measurement of this type has been carried out. The term should be used to refer only to patients who have had multichannel urodynamic studies performed with appropriate findings.
Reference: Pages 639–640

17. **True**

Urge incontinence is the loss of urine associated with the strong desire to void. The presence of this symptom can be discovered by taking a careful history of the circumstances surrounding episodes of incontinence. When urge incontinence is demonstrated during a cystometrogram and is associated with a concurrent detrusor contraction, it is called "motor urge incontinence." "Detrusor overactivity" refers to the presence of involuntary detrusor contractions during cystometry, which produce symptoms in the patient (irrespective of the amplitude of those contractions). Detrusor overactivity can be due to a known, relevant, neurological condition (such as multiple sclerosis, a cerebrovascular accident, Parkinsonism, etc.); in these cases it is referred to as "detrusor hyperreflexia." In cases where a known,

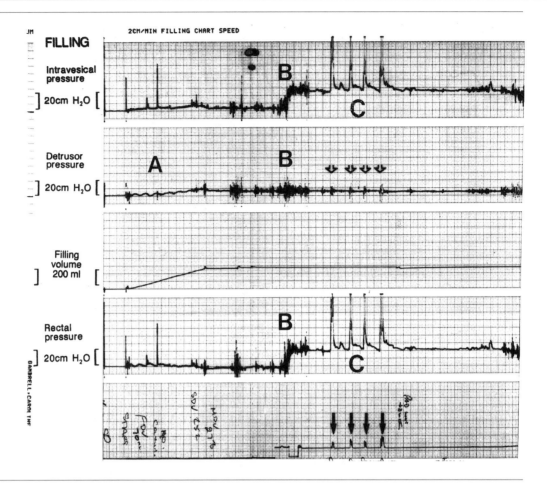

Figure 20.10   Subtracted cystometrogram showing a stable bladder with genuine stress incontinence. During the filling phase (*A*), there is no rise in detrusor pressure. When the patient stands (*B*), there is a rise in intravesical and rectal pressure as the position of the intra-abdominal contents changes, but the subtracted detrusor pressure remains stable. When the patient coughs in the standing position, the detrusor remains stable. Coughs appear as sharp, isolated pressure spikes (*C*) on the intravesical and rectal pressure tracings, but there are no spikes on the subtracted detrusor tracing. The presence of leakage occurring simultaneously with each cough (*arrows*) confirms that the patient has genuine stress incontinence caused by ineffective urethral closure rather than incontinence from detrusor overactivity.

Table 20.4   Pharmacologic Agents Useful in the Treatment of Stress Incontinence

Drug	Dose*
Imipramine	10–25 mg p.o. b.i.d./t.i.d.
Phenylpropanolamine	50–75 mg p.o. b.i.d.
Pseudoephedrine	30–60 mg p.o. t.i.d./q.i.d.
Ephedrine	15–30 mg p.o. b.i.d./t.i.d.
Norephedrine	100 mg p.o. b.i.d.

*p.o., by mouth; b.i.d., two times per day; t.i.d., three times per day; q.i.d., four times per day.

relevant, neurological condition is not present, detrusor overactivity is called "idiopathic detrusor instability." Patients may have urine loss due to detrusor overactivity during a cystometrogram without the forewarning symptom of urgency. Conversely, some patients with complaints of urge incontinence may have a stable tracing when they undergo subtracted urodynamic studies. In these cases, it is important for the clinician to realize that the patient being examined has a stable *cystometrogram,* but not necessarily a stable *bladder,* since conventional urodynamic studies provide a window of only 20 minutes into bladder activity. Some patients may well have urge incontinence due to detrusor contractions at other times and under other circumstances than those in the laboratory.
Reference: Page 650

18. True (see Figure 20.17 and Table 20.5)

Detrusor overactivity, particularly idiopathic detrusor instability, represents the bladder's escape from previously established cortical control, with the development of a

Figure 20.17   Subtracted cystometrogram showing detrusor overactivity. Notice that the rectal pressure stays relatively constant throughout bladder filling in the supine position, whereas there are phasic changes in intravesical pressure and subtracted detrusor pressure. These changes are diagnostic of uninhibited contractions of the detrusor muscle. In this patient, these contractions produced a large amount of urine loss. Note that the rise in rectal pressure that occurs when the patient stands (S) provokes an additional detrusor contraction.

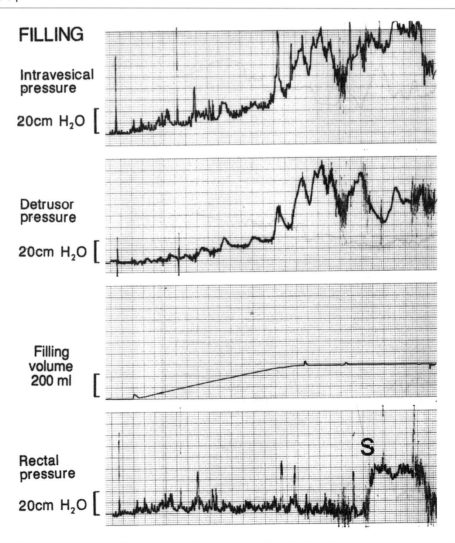

Table 20.5   Drugs Useful In Treating Detrusor Overactivity

Drug	Dose*
Propantheline bromide	15–30 mg p.o. q.i.d.
Hyoscyamine sulfate	0.125–0.25 mg p.o. q. 4–6 hours
Hyoscyamine sulfate, extended release	0.375 mg p.o. b.i.d.
Oxybutynin chloride	5–10 mg p.o. t.i.d./q.i.d.
Dicyclomine hydrochloride	20 mg p.o. q.i.d.

*p.o., by mouth; b.i.d., two times per day; t.i.d., three times per day; q.i.d., four times per day.

syndrome of increasing frequency, urgency, and urge incontinence. This syndrome can be treated successfully by behavior modification programs that "re-train" the bladder, replacing the cycle of increasingly frequent voids and episodes of incontinence with a more structured and gradually less frequent pattern of urination. Regaining detrusor control often can be facilitated by the use of drugs with anticholinergic effects that help relax bladder smooth muscle; however, most of these medications have unpleasant side effects. Even if such drugs are effective in suppressing unwanted detrusor contractions, most patients will not take them for prolonged periods of time. The best long-term therapy for detrusor instability is a program of behavior modification that is adhered to conscientiously. Establishment of the process if often helped by the use of anticholinergic preparations, which can be weaned down to a minimal dosage or stopped all together as bladder control is regained. Patients with detrusor hyperreflexia due to neurologic disease do not respond as well to behavior modification (since their incontinence is rooted in neuropathy), and most of them will require prolonged use of drug therapy to control detrusor activity.
Reference: Pages 652–653

19. **True**

Chronic urinary retention in women is less common than is incontinence; however, it can be associated with serious adverse sequelae. Voiding dysfunction in women is due to either failure of the detrusor muscle to contract appropriately or failure of the pelvic floor to relax during voiding. True outlet obstruction (low urinary flow in the presence of high detrusor voiding pressure) is quite rare in women unless they have had bladder neck surgery (such as a needle suspension, Burch procedure, or sling for stress incontinence). The treatment of incomplete bladder emptying has been revolutionized by the introduction of clean intermittent self-catheterization, which avoids the chronic use of indwelling catheters.
Reference: Pages 654–655

20. **False**

Understanding the particular defects in pelvic support that are present is crucial in planning appropriate therapy for any given patient. Although examination of a patient in the traditional dorsal lithotomy position permits some evaluation of the severity of pelvic organ prolapse, the full extent of the prolapse often cannot be assessed without examining the patient in the erect position. In evaluating any patient with complaints of prolapse, the examiner should always take care to see the prolapse developed to its maximum extent, and should confirm with the patient that this has been done. More subtle defects, such as an occult enterocele, are often uncovered only when the patient is examined while standing.
Reference: Page 659

21 Gynecologic Endoscopy

Malcolm G. Munro

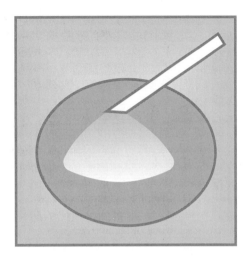

Learning Objectives

1. Understand the role of endoscopy in the diagnosis and treatment of gynecologic conditions.

2. Acquire a technical understanding of the equipment and supplies necessary for performing endoscopic and laparoscopic procedures.

3. Be able to effectively counsel patients who may be candidates for endoscopic gynecologic procedures.

4. Understand the complications associated with gynecologic endoscopic procedures.

Questions

1. Avoiding injury to the deep inferior epigastric vessels is facilitated by a thorough understanding of their location. These vessels are best identified by:

    A. Transillumination of the anterior abdominal wall using the laparoscope as a light source

    B. Laparoscopically identifying their origin from the external iliac arteries and tracing their course cephalad and lateral to the medial umbilical ligament

    C. Positioning any lower quadrant trocars within 3 centimeters of the medial umbilical ligaments, thereby avoiding injury to the inferior epigastric vessels, which invariably course cephalad and more laterally

2. The risk of capacitive coupling associated with monopolar laparoscopic surgery may be minimized by all of the following **except:**

    A. Use of all-metal cannula systems

    B. Use of all-plastic cannula systems

    C. Using "cutting" current

    D. Use of coagulation current

    E. All of the above

    F. None of the above

3. Which of the following circumstances are most likely to result in electrosurgical bowel injuries secondary to direct coupling?

    A. Using a monopolar grasping forceps to desiccate a vessel which is being held by a noninsulated laparoscopic needle driver

    B. The use of monopolar "coagulation" to fulgurate oozing vessels through a metal laparoscopic cannula held by a plastic sleeve anchor

    C. The use of bipolar electrosurgical forceps passed through the instrument channel of an operating laparoscope to desiccate the oviducts for purposes of sterilization

4. Which of the following best describes the type of electrical current used for performing electrosurgery?

    A. Low-voltage, direct current

    B. High-wattage, low-frequency, alternating current

    C. Variable-voltage, radio-frequency current

5. Which of the following is considered an acceptable site for placement of an insufflation needle in a woman undergoing laparoscopy with a history of two previous laparotomies for pelvic disease?

    A. Suprapubic

    B. Left upper quadrant

    C. Right upper quadrant

    D. McBurney's point

    E. None of the above

6. Which of the following findings is suggestive of extraperitoneal positioning of the insufflation needle?

    A. An early insufflation pressure of 12 mm mercury

    B. Persistence of dullness to percussion under the right costal margin after 500 cc insufflation CO_2

    C. The absence of measured negative pressure following elevation of the anterior abdominal wall, prior to insufflation

    D. All of the above

    E. None of the above

7. Which of the following would *not* be considered an appropriate method for securing the infundibulopelvic ligament when performing laparoscopic oophorectomy?

   A. Suture ligature with extracorporeal tie
   B. Endoscopic stapling device
   C. Bipolar technique using "cutting" current
   D. Unipolar technique using coagulation current
   E. All are equally appropriate

8. Which of the following may be a complication associated with the performance of laparoscopy for prolonged periods of time with the intraperitoneal pressure exceeding 20mm of mercury?

   A. Carbon dioxide embolus
   B. Hypercarbia
   C. Hypotension
   D. All of the above

9. Avoidance of injury to the great vessels secondary to insertion of a laparoscopic trocar in the umbilicus can be reduced by:

   A. Ensuring that the angle of incidences is always between 45° and 90° to horizontal
   B. By utilizing disposable instrumentation incorporated with safety shields
   C. By maintaining the trocar in the saggital plane
   D. All of the above

10. Which of the following is true regarding diagnostic hysteroscopy?

    A. It should be part of the work-up for all infertile patients.
    B. It is generally difficult to perform in an office setting because of patient discomfort.
    C. Comparative studies have demonstrated it superior to D&C and radiological hysterography for the identification of structural anomalies of the uterus.
    D. All of the above
    E. None of the above

11. Which of the following is untrue regarding 1.5% glycine when used as a distention medium for operative hysteroscopy?

    A. Patients may suffer from hyperglycemia with high infused volumes.
    B. Significant and, occasionally, rapid systemic absorption may result in hypo-osmolar encepalopathy.
    C. Hypernatremia is an occasional complication.
    D. None of the above

12. Which of the following causes loss of uterine distention at the time of hysteroscopy?

    A. Uterine perforation
    B. An overdilated cervix
    C. An open outflow valve
    D. All of the above
    E. None of the above

13. Which of the following steps may reduce the incidence and severity of systemic absorption of uterine distention media?

    A. Frequent, accurate measurement of total inflow and outflow in the uterine cavity
    B. Main retaining intra-uterine pressure above mean arterial pressure
    C. Use of an in-line pump
    D. Adding suction to the outflow collecting system

179

14. Which of the following is true regarding laparoscopic hysterectomy?

A. It is a procedure that involves complete laparoscopically directed section of the bladder and all vascular and ligament peddles.

B. It has been demonstrated to be a more cost-effective procedure in both vaginal and abdominal hysterectomy.

C. Postoperative morbidity has been demonstrated to be less than a vaginal hysterectomy.

D. All of the above

E. None of the above

Answers

1. B (see Figure 21.3)

The deep inferior epigastric vessels can rarely, if ever, be seen by a transillumination because they lie deep to the anterior rectus sheath and often inferior to the rectus muscle itself. While the *superficial* inferior epigastrics may frequently be identified using transillumination, these vessels do not align with the larger deep inferior epigastric vessels.

Lower quadrant trocars should be passed *lateral* to, not within, 3 centimeters of the medial umbilical fold (ligaments) for the deep inferior epigastric vessels generally course in this area.

The deep inferior epigastric vessels are usually seen shortly distal to their origin from the external iliac arteries where the artery begins its intraperitoneal course between the internal inguinal ring (marked by the round ligament) and the most distal visible attachment of the medial umbilical ligament.
Reference: Pages 684, 690

Figure 21.3   Vascular anatomy of the anterior abdominal wall. Location of the vessels that can be traumatized when inserting trocars into the anterior abdominal wall.

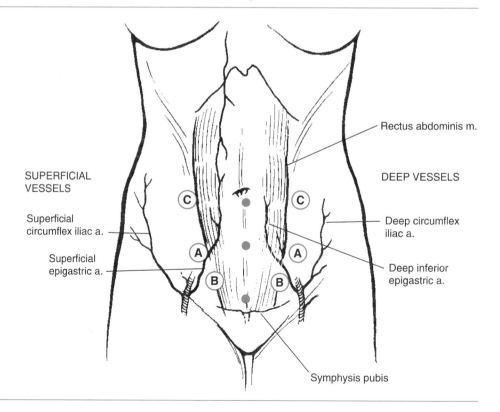

2. D (see Figure 21.16)

All-metal cannula systems generally prevent capacitance by allowing current to be widely dispersed via the relatively large area of the abdominal wall in contact with the conductive surface. All-plastic systems reduce the chance of capacitance to adjacent bowel because of the nonconductive nature of all of the system's materials.

High-voltage currents predispose to the formation of a capacitor. "Cutting" current is of relatively low voltage and is appropriately used for desiccation, vaporization, and the creation of incisions. It is far less likely to result in capacitive coupling than "coagulation" current, which has relatively high voltage.
Reference: Page 700

3. A (see Figure 21.15)

Monopolar grasping forceps are invariably insulated while laparoscopic needle drivers are not. If an uninsulated hand instrument is utilized to grasp tissue undergoing unipolar desiccation, the entire shaft becomes a conductor and, therefore, has the potential to directly couple to the bowel. Monopolar fulguration through a metal laparoscopic cannula held by a plastic sleeve anchor is more likely to result in capacitive, not direct, coupling (see Figure 21.16C). Bipolar forceps may safely be passed through the instrument channel of an "operating" laparoscope without concern. However, when monopolar instruments are inserted through the instrument channel, it causes an increased risk of capacitive coupling to the metal jacket of the laparoscope.
Reference: Page 700

4. C

The electrosurgical generators convert low-frequency wall current (60 Hz in North America) to a frequency similar to that used in AM radio broadcasts (around 500 Hz).
Reference: Pages 698–700

5. B (see Figure 21.6)

In the presence of known or suspected adhesions under the umbilicus, the left upper quadrant is an ideal site for primary entry, provided it has not been exposed to previous potentially adhesiogenic procedures such as splenectomy or abdominal radiation therapy. Prior to such an entry, the stomach is routinely decompressed with an orogastric or nasogastric tube. Use of a small caliber (< 3mm) "scout" laparoscope via an insufflation needle will minimize postoperative pain and cosmetic concerns, and is usually adequate to allow assessment of the underside of the umbilicus and, if necessary, to direct required adhesiolysis.

The suprapubic area is inappropriate because of risks of adhesions, at least in this patient. Blind insertion at McBurney's point is immediately above the right iliac vessels and should not be performed. Right upper quadrant insertion places the patient at risk for injury to the liver, the gallbladder, the great hepatic vessels, and the bilary collecting system. Some have suggested that open laparoscopy reduces the risk of bowel injury but there are no data supporting such a contention.
Reference: Pages 687, 689, 705

6. D

Insufflation pressure that exceeds 10 millimeters of mercury early in the insufflation process is suggestive of extraperitoneal positioning or of the needle tip being located within the posterior abdominal wall, or the lumen of a vessel or abdominal viscera. Gas dispersing to the left upper quadrant separates the costal margin from the liver resulting in a tympana to percussion—a distinct change from the preexisting dullness to percussion prior to insufflation. Failure of this tympanitic change by 500 cc of insufflation gas may be an early sign of inappropriate needle placement.

If the insufflation needle is in the peritoneal cavity, the negative intraperitoneal pressure created by lifting the abdominal wall may be demonstrated with the aspiration of

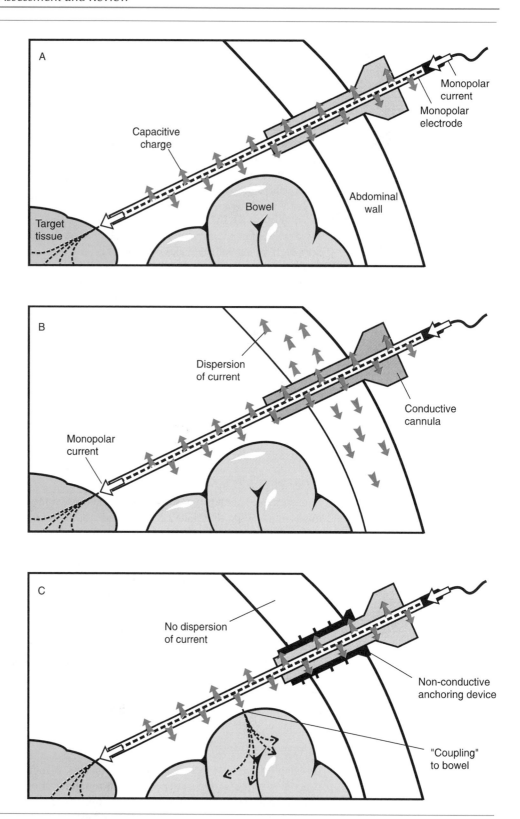

Figure 21.16   Capacitative coupling. *A,* All activated monopolar electrodes emit a surrounding charge, proportional to the voltage of the current. This makes the electrode a potential capacitor. *B,* Generally, as long as the charge is allowed to disperse through the abdominal wall, no sequelae result. However, if the "return" to the dispersive electrode is blocked by insulation, such as a plastic anchor (*C*), the current can couple to a conductive cannula or directly to bowel.

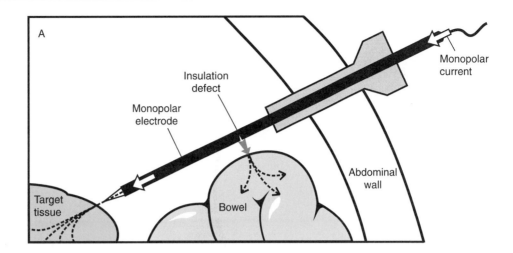

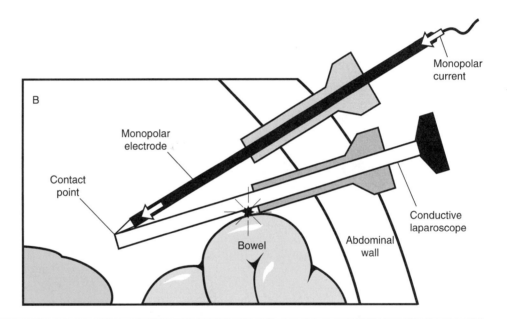

Figure 21.15 Direct coupling. Direct coupling is a potential complication of monopolar electrosurgery and may occur secondary to defects in the insulation (*A*) or, classically, to contract with a conductive instrument that in turn touches other intraperitoneal structures. In the example depicted (*B*), the active electrode is touching the laparoscope, and current is transferred to bowel via a small enough contact point that thermal injury results. Another common target of such coupling is to noninsulated hand instruments.

a drop of fluid placed at the proximal opening of the needle. This negative pressure gradient is perhaps more accurately demonstrated by attaching the needle to the insulator using insufflation tubing and reading the pressure meter as the abdominal wall is sharply lifted.

Reference: Page 686

7. D

"Cutting current" of appropriate output results in even desiccation of the tissue interposed between the jaws of the unipolar or bipolar grasping instrument. "Coagulation current" is interrupted and of relatively high voltage resulting in uneven areas of des-

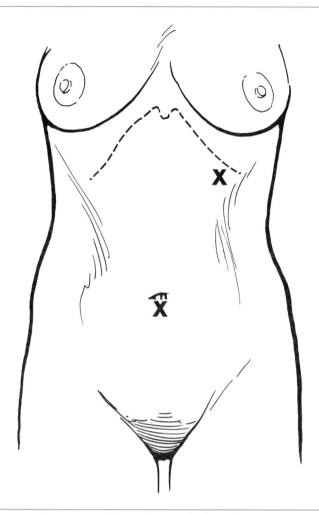

Figure 21.6 Insufflation needle and cannula insertion sites. In most instances, both the insufflation needle, if used, and the primary cannula are inserted through the umbilicus. When subumbilical adhesions are known or suspected, the insufflation needle may be placed through the pouch of Douglas or in the left upper quadrant following evacuation of the gastric contents with an orogastric tube.

iccation. These focally desiccated areas of tissue can impede conduction of current throughout the rest of the tissue, potentially leaving parts of the lumen intact. In the case of a fallopian tube, the result could be pregnancy; for blood vessels, the result could be hemorrhage.
Reference: Page 695

8. D

Carbon dioxide embolus may be facilitated by a number of aspects of laparoscopic surgery including extensive dissection under high intraperitoneal pressures (> 20mm Hg) . The risk of hypercarbia has been demonstrated to increase gradually, with time, even between 12 to 15 mm Hg.

High intraperitoneal pressure may compress the great veins of the pelvis as well as the Venn cave, thereby reducing end diastolic flow to the right atrium, reducing cardiac output.
Reference: Pages 686, 696–697

9. C (see Figure 21.4)

For most patients of normal weight, the incision angle should be approximately 45° to the plane of the operating table. With increasing body habitués, the location of the umbilicus tends to fall below the bifurcation of the great vessels, thereby allowing for a more vertical insertion of the trocar. The "safety shields" integrated into the design of many disposable laparoscopic canals have never been demonstrated to reduce the rate of injury to great vessels.

The surgeon should *always* maintain the trocar-cannula in the saggital plane when inserting at the umbilicus to prevent injury to the common and external iliac vessels.
Reference: Pages 686, 687–689

10. C

Many infertile patients receive adequate primary evaluation of the endometrial cavity with the hysterosalpingogram for it is able to provide information regarding patency of the fallopian tubes. Hysteroscopy is generally performed with ease in an office setting, providing the diameter of the hysteroscope is small, or with one or a combination of conscious sedation and an effective intracervical block using local anesthetic. Diagnostic hysteroscopy is clearly superior to both D&C and hysterosalpingogram in detecting structural abnormalities of the uterus.
Reference: Page 708

11. D

Sorbitol is a sugar solution which, if absorbed in sufficient amounts, can contribute to hyperglycemia, a problem not experienced with glycine. Large amounts of absorbed electrolyte-free distention media of any type may result in an hypo-osmolar state and potentially result in encepalopathy. Hyponatremia is a complication associated with glycine and other electrolyte-free distention media. Of the "low-viscosity" electrolyte-free media, only 5% mannitol is iso-osmolar.
Reference: Page 719

12. D

Uterine perforation will invariably result in loss of distention of the endometrial cavity. Overdilation of the cervix may also prevent generation of adequate intracavitary pressure. In such instances, the problem usually can be overcome by using an additional

Figure 21.4 Vascular anatomy. Location of the great vessels and their changing relationship to the umbilicus with increasing patient weight (from left to right).

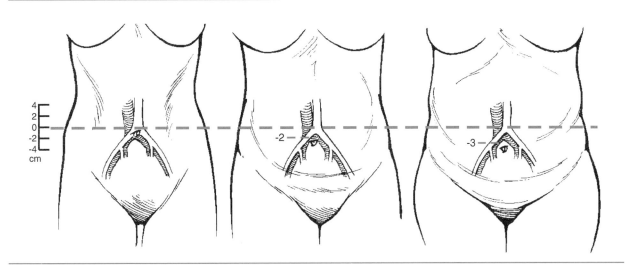

tenaculum or other clamp to more tightly secure the cervix around the hysteroscope. If a gravity-flow system is used, the surgeon should always check to ensure that the outflow valve is set appropriately to maintain some degree of intrauterine pressure.
Reference: Page 718

13. A

The incidence and severity of absorption of uterine distention media is decreased when the surgeon operates at pressures that are *below* mean arterial pressure. An in-line pump can result in increasing intracavitary pressure and systemic absorption unless there is a pressure threshold above which the pump shuts off. Regardless, frequent and accurate measurement of total inflow and outflow must take place at least every 15 minutes during a case.
Reference: Page 719

14. E

Laparoscopic hysterectomy (LH) is a spectrum of procedures that vary depending upon the relative amount of dissection performed vaginally and laparoscopically. A number of classification systems exist that allow for various "types" of LH to be defined.

While LH *may* be more cost effective for many women who would otherwise undergo abdominal hysterectomy, neither morbidity or cost is saved when compared to vaginal hysterectomy.
Reference: Page 680

22 Hysterectomy

Jonathan S. Berek

Learning Objectives

1. Know the indications for hysterectomy.

2. Understand the different methods for performing hysterectomy, their advantages, and their disadvantages.

3. Know concurrent surgical procedures that are performed with hysterectomy.

4. Be able to articulate the perioperative complications of hysterectomy.

5. Understand the psychosomatic effects of hysterectomy.

Questions

1. The most common indication for hysterectomy in North America is:

   A. malignancy
   B. benign uterine tumors
   C. benign uterine bleeding
   D. pelvic pain
   E. pelvic infection

2. A 46-year-old woman who has had two prior full-term pregnancies needs to undergo a hysterectomy because of severe menorrhagia unresponsive to medication. She wishes to preserve her ovaries. In counseling the patient regarding the pros and cons of a vaginal versus an abdominal hysterectomy, an important issue for the discussion is the difference of the two procedures on outcome for which of the following variables:

   A. sexual function
   B. ovarian function
   C. complications
   D. cancer prophylaxis

3. A 40-year-old women is to undergo a hysterectomy for symptomatic uterine leiomyomata. She has no personal or family history of ovarian or breast disease. She asks you whether or not she should undergo bilateral oophorectomy. The principal reason for ovarian preservation is:

   A. the risk of malignancy is low and compliance with estrogen replacement therapy is low
   B. the risk of malignancy is unknown and the morbidity of prophylactic oophorectomy is significant
   C. the psychological effects of oophorectomy are unknown
   D. the pelvic support structures are more likely to be retained

4. During the performance of an abdominal hysterectomy, the best way to identify the ureter is:

   A. observe the course of the ureter transperitoneally
   B. palpate the ureter at the pelvic brim
   C. enter the retroperitoneum and visualize the ureter
   D. the ureter need not be identified if proper clamping techniques are used

5. During the performance of an abdominal hysterectomy for uterine leiomyomata, an inadvertent cystotomy is created in the dome of the bladder. The management of the cystotomy is:

   A. postoperative bladder drainage with an indwelling Foley catheter for 14 days
   B. resection of the bladder dome with three-layered closure
   C. one- or two-layered closure with absorbable suture
   D. no repair is necessary

6. An inadvertent enterotomy is created in the ileum during the performance of a lysis of adhesions prior to a planned abdominal hysterectomy. The defect is 1 centimeter. The repair should be:

   A. closed in two layers in a direction perpendicular to the intestinal lumen
   B. closed in two layers in a direction parallel to the intestinal lumen
   C. a small bowel resection 2 cm proximal and distal to the defect with an end-to-end reanastamosis
   D. a small bowel resection and diverting colostomy

7. After the performance of a hysterectomy for benign disease, the best predictor of post-operative sexual functioning is:

A. the results of psychological testing
B. the patient's preoperative sexual satisfaction
C. whether the cervix has been preserved
D. whether the ovaries have been preserved
E. vaginal length

Answers

1. B

The most common indication listed for the performance of a hysterectomy is uterine leiomyomata. However, available data strongly suggest that hysterectomy for leiomyomata should only be considered in symptomatic patients who do not desire future fertility.
Reference: Pages 728–729

2. C

The risk of one or more complications after abdominal hysterectomy is 1.7 times the risk after vaginal hysterectomy. The two major categories of complications are febrile morbidity and hemorrhage requiring transfusion. The risk of febrile morbidity is 2.1

Figure 22.4   Identification of the ureter in the retroperitoneal space on the medial leaf of the broad ligament. (From Mann WA, Stovall TG. *Gynecologic Surgery.* New York: Churchill Livingstone, 1996.)

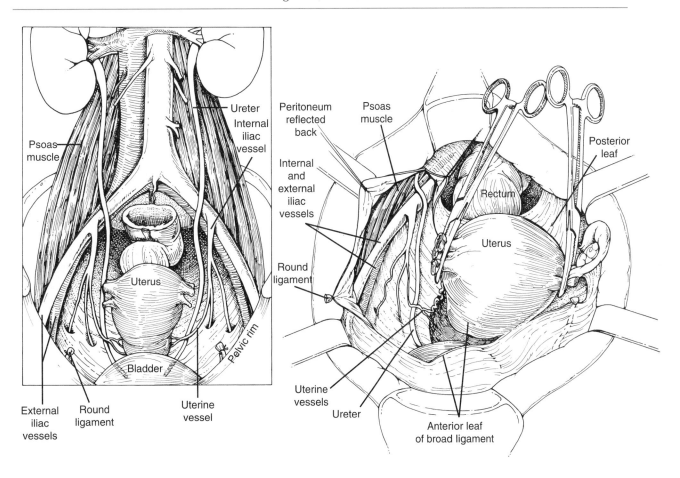

times higher for abdominal hysterectomy than vaginal hysterectomy, and the risk of transfusion is 1.9 times higher.
Reference: Page 731

3. A

The risk of developing ovarian cancer after a hysterectomy performed in women for benign conditions is low. If there is no significant family history of ovarian cancer or a past history of ovarian pathology, the risk of subsequent malignancy may be as low as 0.14%. A 40-year-old woman is more than 10 years younger than her anticipated menopause. Long-term compliance with post-hysterectomy estrogen replacement therapy is about 20 to 40% at five years. The optimal duration of replacement therapy is unknown.
Reference: Page 733

4. C (see Figure 22.4 in Appendix)

The most consistent means of identification of the ureter is by entering the retroperitoneal space. This is accomplished by extending the incision made into the broad ligament in a cephalad direction on the medial leaf of the broad ligament. The ureter is identified crossing the common iliac artery.
Reference: Pages 736, 742–743 (see also 118–119)

5. C

Uncomplicated cystotomy should be repaired in the manner described. Postoperative drainage for two to three days should be sufficient. Defects near the trigone are more involved and often require passage of retrograde ureteral catheters and, occasionally, ureteral reimplantation.
Reference: Pages 743–744

6. A

When a small inadvertent enterotomy occurs, it should be repaired in this manner to minimize the risk of lumenal stenosis. Resection or diversion of the intestine is unnecessary.
Reference: Pages 744–745

7. B

The literature supports that hysterectomy does not cause psychiatric sequelae or diminished sexual functioning in most patients.
Reference: Pages 761–762

REPRODUCTIVE ENDOCRINOLOGY

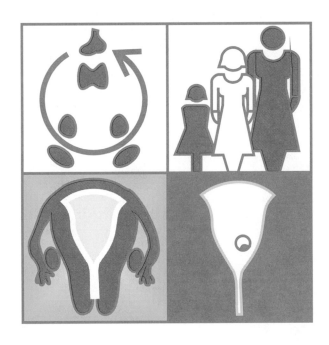

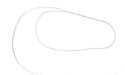

23 Puberty

Robert W. Rebar

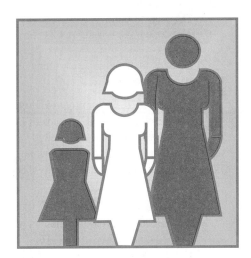

Learning Objectives

1. Be able to describe the physical and hormonal changes that occur during normal pubertal development.

2. Be capable of developing a classification for the possible disorders of pubertal development.

3. Be able to outline the evaluation of delayed and precocious puberty.

4. Understand the evaluation of the newborn infant with genital ambiguity.

Questions

1. The usual sequence of events in normal pubertal development from first to last is:

   A. Peak growth velocity, appearance of pubic hair, breast budding, menarche
   B. Breast budding, appearance of pubic hair, peak growth velocity, menarche
   C. Appearance of pubic hair, peak growth velocity, breast budding, menarche
   D. Breast budding, menarche, appearance of pubic hair, peak growth velocity
   E. Appearance of pubic hair, breast budding, menarche, peak growth velocity

2. Each of the following hormonal changes occurs early in normal pubertal development in girls **except:**

   A. Increased circulating estradiol
   B. Sleep-entrained increases in LH and FSH
   C. Increased circulating dehydroepiandrosterone sulfate
   D. Decreased circulating estrone
   E. Increased circulating dehydroepiandrosterone

3. Each of the following statements about Turner's syndrome is true **except:**

   A. Affected individuals may have a variety of karyotypes, including 45X, 45X/46XY, and 45X/46XX.
   B. 45X is the most common chromosomal disorder in humans.
   C. Associated abnormalities include multiple pigmented nevi, lymphedema at birth, hyperconvex nails, coarctation of the aorta, and abnormalities of the kidneys.
   D. Most individuals have below average intelligence.
   E. Diabetes mellitus and thyroid disorders are common.

4. Genital ambiguity at birth may be caused by maternal ingestion of which of the following steroids?

   A. *Ethinyl estradiol*
   B. *Prednisolone*
   C. *Danazol*
   D. *Medroxyprogesterone*
   E. *17α-hydroxyprogesterone*

5. Causes of precocious puberty may include each of the following **except:**

   A. McCune-Albright syndrome
   B. 11β-hydroxylase deficiency
   C. Prader-Labhardt-Willi syndrome
   D. Granulosa-theca cell tumors
   E. Hypothalamic hamartomas

6. The initial change in the hypothalamic-pituitary-gonadal axis with puberty in girls is:

   A. Decreased sensitivity to inhibitory effects of the low levels of sex steroids
   B. Maturation of the positive feedback response to estrogen
   C. Reversal of the estrogen/estradiol ratio with concomitant follicular development
   D. Reversal of the LH/FSH ratio in response to changing GnRH pulse frequency

7. Treatment of Turner's syndrome begins with:

   A. *Congested estrogen* 0.625 mg daily plus *medroxyprogesterone* 5 mg daily
   B. *Conjugated estrogen* 1.25 mg daily plus *medroxyprogesterone* 10 mg for 14 days each month
   C. *Conjugated estrogen* 0.625 mg daily
   D. *Medroxyprogesterone* 10 mg daily

8. The most common cause of delayed puberty is:

   A. Isolated gonadotropin deficiency
   B. Cuanio pharyngioma
   C. Constitutional delay
   D. Anorexia nervosa
   E. Primary hypothyroidism

9. A six-year-old girl is brought to your office with Tanner III breast and pubic hair development. Gonadotropin levels are low, but serum estradiol is 60 pg/ml. Which of the following diagnoses is consistent with these findings?

   A. Constitutional precocious puberty
   B. McCune-Albright syndrome
   C. Hypothalamic hamartoma
   D. Hydrocephalus
   E. Septo-optic dysplasia

10. A young girl presents with what you believe is heterosexual precocious puberty and hyperandrogenism. Investigation reveals elevated levels of 17-hydroxypregnenolone and DHEA; 17-hydroxyprogesterone is low. The most likely diagnosis is:

    A. 21-hydroxylase deficiency
    B. 11-hydroxylase deficiency
    C. 17-hydroxylase deficiency
    D. 3-β-hydroxysteroid dehydrogenase deficiency
    E. 17, 20-desmolase deficiency

Answers

1. B

In girls, pubertal development typically requires 4.5 years in all (see Figure 23.2). Although the first sign of puberty is generally accelerated growth, breast budding is usually the first recognized pubertal change, followed by the appearance of pubic hair, peak growth velocity, and, later, menarche. The stages initially described by Marshall and Tanner are commonly used to describe breast and pubic hair development.
Reference: Page 772

2. D

Several of the hormonal changes associated with pubertal development begin even before any of the physical changes are obvious. Early in puberty there is increased sensitivity of LH to GnRH. Sleep-entrained increases in both LH and FSH can be documented early in puberty. In boys, the nocturnal increases in gonadotropins are accompanied by simultaneous increases in circulating testosterone levels. In girls, in contrast, the nighttime increases in circulating gonadotropin levels are followed by increased secretion of estradiol the next day. This delay in estradiol secretion is believed to be due to the additional synthetic steps required in the aromatization of estrogens from androgens. Basal levels of both FSH and LH increase through puberty, with the patterns differing in boys and girls and with LH levels, in terms of milli-international units per milliliter, eventually becoming greater than FSH. Although it now appears that gonadotropins are always secreted in an episodic or pulsatile fashion, even before puberty, the pulsatile secretion of gonadotropins is more easily documented as puberty progresses and basal levels increase.

Increased adrenal androgen secretion is important in stimulating adrenarche—the appearance of pubic and axillary hair—in both boys and girls. (Pubarche specifically refers to the appearance of pubic hair.) Progressive increases in circulating levels of the

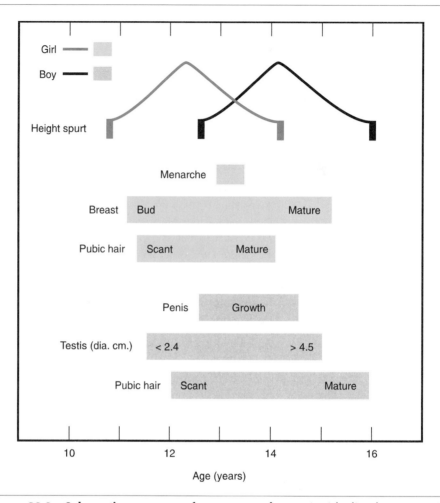

Figure 23.2   Schematic sequence of events at puberty. An idealized average girl (upper panel) and an idealized average boy (lower panel) are represented. (Reproduced with permission from **Rebar RW.** Practical evaluation of hormonal status. In: **Yen SSC, Jaffe RB,** eds. *Reproductive Endocrinology: Physiology, Pathophysiology and Clinical Management.* 3rd ed. Philadelphia: WB Saunders, 1991:830. Based on data from **Marshall WA, Tanner JM.** Variations in patterns of pubertal changes in girls. *Arch Dis Child* 1969;44:291–303; and **Marshall WA, Tanner JM.** Variation in the pattern of pubertal changes in boys. *Arch Dis Child* 1970;45:13–23.)

major adrenal androgens, dehydroepiandrosterone (DHEA) and its sulfate (DHEAS), begin as early as 2 years of age, accelerate at 7 to 8 years of age, and continue until 13 to 15 years of age. The accelerated increases in adrenal androgens begin about 2 years before the increases in gonadotropin and gonadal sex steroid secretion when the hypothalamic-pituitary-gonadal is still functioning at a low prepubertal level.

In girls, estradiol, secreted predominantly by the ovaries, increases during puberty. Although, as noted, increases in estradiol first appear during the daytime hours, basal levels increase during both the day and night. Estrone, which is secreted in part by the ovaries and arises in part from extraglandular conversion of estradiol and androstenedione, also increases early in puberty but plateaus by midpuberty. Thus, the ratio of estrone to estradiol decreases throughout puberty, indicating that ovarian production of estradiol becomes increasingly important and peripheral conversion of androgens to estrone less important during maturation.

Reference: Pages 777–779

3. D

Most affected individuals have a 45X karyotype and Turner's syndrome; still others have mosaic karyotypes (45X/46XX; 45X/46XY; etc.) and may present with the Turner's phenotype as well. These patients generally grow slowly beginning in the second or third year of life. They typically have many of the associated stigmata, including lymphedema at birth; a webbed neck; multiple pigmented nevi; disorders of the heart, kidneys (horseshoe), and great vessels (most commonly coarctation of the aorta); and small hyperconvex fingernails. Diabetes mellitus, thyroid disorders, essential hypertension, and other autoimmune disorders are often present in individuals with 45X karyotypes. Most 45X patients have normal intelligence, but many affected individuals have an unusual cognitive defect characterized by an inability to appreciate the shapes and relations of objects with respect to one another (i.e., space-form blindness). Affected children typically become shorter compared to their peers as they get older. Although they do not develop breasts at puberty, some pubic or axillary hair may develop because of appropriate adrenarche with failure of thelarche (i.e., breast development). Although less severe short stature and some adolescent development may occur with chromosomal mosaicism, the tenet that any short, slowly growing, sexually infantile girl has Turner's syndrome until proved otherwise is reasonable because this disorder is so prevalent (approximately 1 in 2500 newborn phenotypic females). In fact, the 45X karyotype is the single most frequent chromosomal disorder in humans, but most affected fetuses are aborted spontaneously early in pregnancy.
Reference: Pages 783–784

4. C

It is important to recognize that ambiguous genitalia can result from the maternal ingestion of various teratogens, most of which are synthetic steroids (Table 23.3). Exposure to the teratogen must occur early in pregnancy during genital organogenesis. Moreover, not all exposed fetuses manifest the same anomalies or even the presence of any anomalies.

In principle, most synthetic steroids with androgenic properties, including weakly androgenic progestins, can affect female genital differentiation. However, the doses required to produce genital ambiguity are generally so great that the concern is only theoretical. The one agent that clearly can lead to genital ambiguity when ingested in clinically used quantities is *danazol*. There is no evidence that inadvertent ingestion of oral contraceptives, which contain relatively low doses of either *mestranol* or *estradiol* and a 19-nor-steroid, results in virilization.
Reference: Pages 803–804

Table 23.3 Androgens and Progestogens Potentially Capable of Producing Genital Ambiguity*

Proved	*No Effect*	*Insufficient Data*
Testosterone enanthate	Progesterone	Ethynodiol diacetate
Testosterone propionate	17α-hydroxyprogesterone	Dimethisterone
Methylandrostenediol	Medroxyprogesterone	Norgestrel
6α-methyltestosterone	Norethynodrel	Desogestrel
Ethisterone		Gestodene
Norethindrone		Norgestimate
Danazol		

*Those agents proved to cause genital ambiguity do so only when administered in relatively high doses. Insufficient data exist regarding effects of *dimethisterone* and *norgestrel*. In low doses (e.g., as in oral contraceptives), progestins, even including *norethindrone,* seem unlikely to virilize a female fetus.

197

5. C (see Table 23.1)

Precocious puberty is pubertal development beginning before the age of eight years. Precocious pubertal development is characterized in several ways. In iso-sexual precocious puberty, the early changes are common to the phenotypic sex of the individual. In heterosexual precocious puberty, the development is characteristic of the opposite sex. Precocious puberty is sometimes termed "true" when it is of central origin with activation of the hypothalamic-pituitary unit. In precocious pseudopuberty, also known as precocious puberty of peripheral origin, secretion of hormones in the periphery (commonly by neoplasms) stimulates pubertal development.
Reference: Pages 781–782

6. A

The mechanisms responsible for the numerous hormonal changes occurring during puberty are poorly understood, although it is recognized that a "CNS program" must be responsible for initiating puberty. It appears that the hypothalamic-pituitary-gonadal axis in girls develops in two distinct stages during puberty. First, sensitivity to the negative or inhibitory effects of the low levels of circulating sex steroids present in childhood decreases early in puberty. Second, late in puberty, there is maturation of the positive or stimulatory feedback response to estrogen, which is responsible for the ovulatory mid-cycle surge of LH.

Current evidence suggests that the central nervous system inhibits the onset of puberty until the appropriate time. Based on this theory, the neuroendocrine control of puberty is mediated by GnRH-secreting neurons in the medial basal hypothalamus, which act together as an endogenous pulse generator. At puberty, the GnRH pulse generator is reactivated (i.e., disinhibited), leading to increased amplitude and frequency of GnRH pulses. In turn, the increased GnRH secretion results in increased gonadotropin and then gonadal steroid secretion. What causes this "disinhibition" of GnRH release is unknown.
Reference: Pages 779–780

7. C

In order to increase final adult height, treatment strategies utilizing exogenous growth hormone (GH) are commonly accepted. It is not yet known what dose of GH is optimal or if an anabolic steroid such as oxandrolone will provide additional growth. However, GH in doses 25% greater than those recommended for GH deficiency are proving safe and effective, with a net increase in height of 8.1 cm over the average height of approximately 146 cm in untreated individuals.

The treatment of patients with Turner's syndrome is as follows:

1. To promote sexual maturation, therapy with exogenous estrogen should be initiated when the patient is psychologically ready, at approximately 12 to 13 years of age, and after GH therapy is completed.
2. Because the intent is to mimic normal pubertal development, low-dose estrogen alone (such as 0.3 to 0.625 mg *conjugated estrogens* orally each day) should be initiated.
3. Progestins (5 to 10 mg *medroxyprogesterone acetate* given orally for 12 to 14 days every 1 to 2 months) can be added to prevent endometrial hyperplasia after the patient first experiences vaginal bleeding or after 6 months of unopposed estrogen use if the patient has not yet had any bleeding.
4. The dose of estrogen is increased slowly over 1 to 2 years until the patient is taking about twice as much estrogen as is administered to postmenopausal women.
5. Girls with gonadal dysgenesis must be monitored carefully for the development of hypertension with estrogen therapy.
6. The patients and their parents should be counseled regarding the emotional and physical changes that will occur with therapy.

Reference: Pages 785–786

Table 23.1   Aberrations of Pubertal Development

I. Delayed or interrupted puberty
   A. Anatomic abnormalties of the genital outflow tract
   1. Müllerian dysgenesis (*Rokitansky-Küster-Hauser syndrome*)
   2. Distal genital tract obstruction
      a. Imperforate hymen
      b. Transverse vaginal septum
   B. Hypergonadotropic (follicle-stimulating hormone >30 mIU/ml) hypogonadism (gonadal "failure")
   1. Gonadal dysgenesis with stigmata of *Turner's syndrome*
   2. Pure gonadal dysgenesis
      a. 46XX
      b. 46XY
   3. Early gonadal "failure" with apparent normal ovarian development
   C. Hypogonadotropic (LH and FSH <10 mIU/ml) hypogonadism
   1. Constitutional delay
   2. Isolated gonadotropin deficiency
      a. Associated with midline defects (*Kallmann's syndrome*)
      b. Independent of associated disorders
      c. Prader-Labhardt-Willi syndrome
      d. Laurence-Moon-Bardet-Biedl syndrome
      e. Many other rare syndromes
   3. Associated with multiple hormone deficiencies
   4. Neoplasms of the hypothalamic-pituitary area
      a. Craniopharyngiomas
      b. Pituitary adenomas
      c. Other
   5. Infiltrative processes (Langerhans-cell type histiocytosis)
   6. After irradiation of the central nervous system
   7. Severe chronic illnesses with malnutrition
   8. Anorexia nervosa and related disorders
   9. Severe hypothalamic amenorrhea (rare)
   10. Antidopaminergic and gonadotropin-releasing hormone inhibiting drugs (especially psychotropic agents, opiates)
   11. Primary hypothyroidism
   12. *Cushing's syndrome*

II. Asynchronous pubertal development
   A. Complete androgen insensitivity syndrome (testicular feminization)
   B. Incomplete androgen insensitivity syndrome

III.Precocious puberty
   A. Central (true) precocious puberty
   1. Constitutional (idiopathic) precocious puberty
   2. Hypothalamic neoplasms (most commonly hamartomas)
   3. Congenital malformations
   4. Infiltrative processes (Langerhans-cell-type histiocytosis)
   5. After irradiation
   6. Trauma
   7. Infection
   B. Precocious puberty of peripheral origin (precocious pseudopuberty)
   1. Gonadotropin-secreting neoplasms
      a. Human chorionic gonadotropin-secreting
         i. Ectopic germinomas (pinealomas)
         ii. Choriocarcinomas
         iii. Teratomas
         iv. Hepatoblastomas
      b. Luteinizing hormone-secreting (pituitary adenomas)
   2. Gonadal neoplasms
      a. Estrogen-secreting
         i. Granulosa-theca cell tumors
         ii. Gonadal sex-cord tumors
      b. Androgen-secreting
         i. Arrhenoblastomas
         ii. Teratomas
   3. Congenital adrenal hyperplasia
      a. 21-Hydroxylase (P450c21) deficiency

Table 23.1—*continued*

III. Precocious puberty
        b. 11 β-Hydroxylase (P450c11) deficiency
        c. 3 β-Hydroxysteroid dehydrogenase deficiency
    4. Adrenal neoplasms
        a. Adenomas
        b. Carcinomas
    5. Autonomous gonadal hypersecretion
        a. Cysts
        b. *McCune-Albright syndrome*
    6. Iatrogenic ingestion/absorption of estrogens or androgens

IV. Heterosexual puberty
   A. Polycystic ovarian syndrome
   B. Nonclassic forms of congenital adrenal hyperplasia
   C. Idiopathic hirsutism
   D. Mixed gonadal dysgenesis
   E. Rare forms of male pseudohermaphroditism (*Reifenstein syndrome,* 5α-reductase
        deficiency)
   F. *Cushing's syndrome* (rare)
   G. Androgen-secreting neoplasms (rare)

8. C

Hypothalamic-pituitary disturbances are usually associated with low levels of circulating gonadotropins (with both LH and FSH <10 mIU/ml). There are both sporadic and familial causes of hypogonadotropic hypogonadism, and the differential diagnosis is extensive. It is important to remember, however, that low levels of LH and FSH are normally present in the prepubertal years; thus, girls with constitutionally delayed puberty may be mistakenly presumed to have hypogonadotropic hypogonadism. In fact, constitutional delay is the most common cause of delayed puberty. Constitutional delayed growth and adolescence can be diagnosed only after careful evaluation excludes other causes of delayed puberty and longitudinal follow-up documents normal sexual development. The farther below the third percentile for height that the young girl is, the less likely it is that constitutional explanations are correct.
Reference: Pages 787–788

9. B

In central precocious puberty, GnRH prematurely stimulates increased gonadotropin secretion. Central precocious puberty may occur in children in whom no structural abnormality exists, in which case it is termed *constitutional* or *idiopathic.* Alternatively, central precocious puberty may result from a tumor, infection, congenital abnormality, or traumatic injury affecting the hypothalamus. Tumors of the hypothalamus include hamartomas and, less frequently, neurogliomas and pinealomas. It appears that harmartomas produce GnRH in a pulsatile manner and thus stimulate gonadotropin secretion. A number of congenital malformations, including hydrocephalus, craniostenosis, arachnoid cysts, and septo-optic dysplasia, can also be associated with precocious puberty (as well as with sexual infantilism).

In gonadotropin-independent precocious puberty, production of estrogens or androgens from the ovaries, adrenals, or rare steroid-secreting neoplasms leads to early pubertal development. Small functional ovarian cysts, typically asymptomatic, are common in children and may cause transient sexual precocity. Simple cysts (with a benign ultrasonographic appearance) can be observed and usually resolve over time. Of the various ovarian neoplasms that can secrete estrogens, granulosa-theca cell tumors occur most frequently but are still rare. Although such tumors may grow rapidly, more than two-thirds are benign.

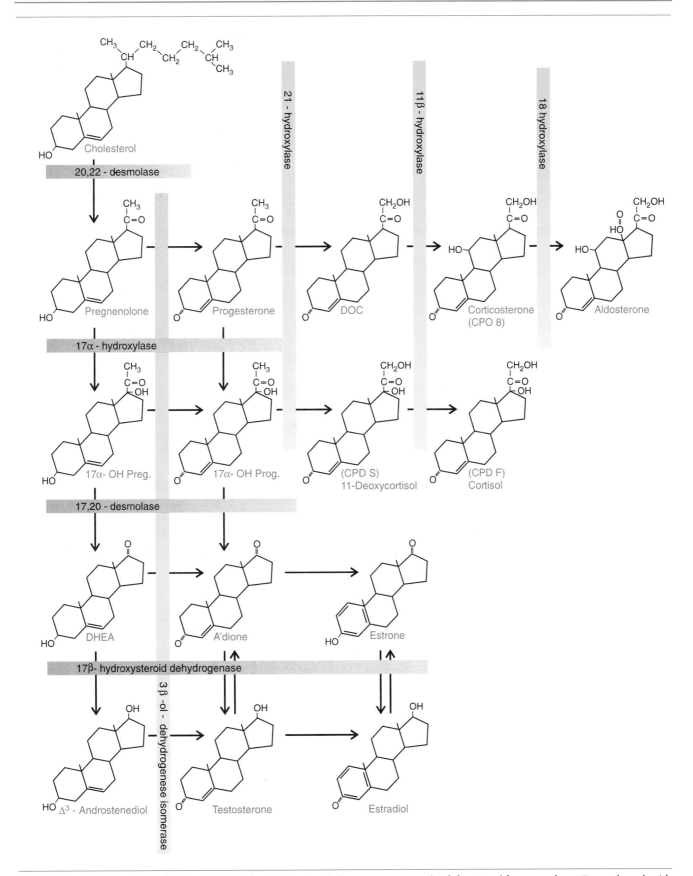

Figure 23.19 Gonadal and adrenal steroid pathways and the enzymes required for steroid conversion. (Reproduced with permission from **Rebar RW, Kenigsberg D, Hodgen GD.** The normal menstrual cycle and the control of ovulation. In: **Becker KL,** ed. *Principles and Practice of Endocrinology and Metabolism.* 2nd ed. Philadelphia: JB Lippincott, 1995:868–80.)

The *McCune-Albright syndrome* is characterized by polyostotic fibrous dysplasia of bone, irregular *café au lait* spots on the skin, and hyperfunctioning endocrinopathies. Girls develop sexual precocity as a result of functioning ovarian cysts. Other endocrinopathies may include hyperthyroidism, hypercortisolism, hyperprolactinemia, and acromegaly. It is now known that mutations of the $G_{S\alpha}$ subunit of the G protein, which couples extracellular hormonal signals to the activation of adenylate cyclase, are responsible for the autonomous hyperfunction of the endocrine glands and, presumably, for the other defects present in this disorder. Exposure to exogenous estrogens can mimic gonadotropin-independent precocious puberty. Ingestion of oral contraceptives, other estrogen-containing pharmaceutical agents, and estrogen-contaminated foods and the topical use of estrogens have been implicated in cases of precocious development in infants and children. Severe primary hypothyroidism has also been associated with sexual precocity; associated hyperprolactinemia may result in galactorrhea in affected individuals.
Reference: Pages 795–796

10. D

Heterosexual precocious puberty is always of peripheral origin and is most often caused by CAH. Three adrenal enzyme defects—21-hydroxylase deficiency, 11β-hydroxylase deficiency, and 3β-hydroxysteroid dehydrogenase deficiency—can lead not only to heterosexual precocity but also to virilization of the external genitalia because of increased androgen production beginning *in utero*.

Deficiency of 3β-hydroxysteroid dehydrogenase (3β-HSD) affects the synthesis of glucocorticoids, mineralocorticoids, and sex steroids. Typically, levels of 17-hydroxypregnenolone and DHEA are elevated (see Figure 23.19). The classic form of the disorder, detectable at birth, is quite rare, and affected girls may be masculinized only slightly. In severe cases, salt-wasting may also be present.

A nonclassic form of this disorder may be associated with heterosexual precocious pubertal development (as in the classic form if untreated), but postpubertal hyperandrogenism occurs more often. The androgen excess in individuals with nonclassic 3β-HSD deficiency appears to result from androgens derived from the peripheral conversion of increased serum concentrations of DHEA. This disorder is inherited in autosomal recessive fashion, with allelism at the 3β-HSD gene on chromosome 1 believed to be responsible for the varying degrees of enzyme deficiency.
Reference: Pages 796–798

24 Amenorrhea

Wendy J. Scherzer
Howard D. McClamrock

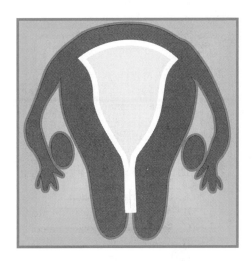

Learning Objectives

1. Understand organ system abnormalities that may cause amenorrhea.

2. Understand the relationship of amenorrhea to anovulation and luteal phase defect.

3. Be able to present a strategy for the workup of the patient with amenorrhea.

4. Be able to determine the appropriate treatment for the patient with amenorrhea according to medical needs and personal desires.

Questions

1. The underlying etiology of premature ovarian failure may be any of the following **except:**

    A. Turner's syndrome
    B. Autoimmune dysfunction
    C. Hyperandrogenism
    D. Galactosemia
    E. Radiation exposure

2. The following are all associated with Kallmann's syndrome, **except:**

    A. XX karyotype
    B. Insufficient pulsatile secretion of GnRH
    C. Blind vaginal pouch
    D. Anosmia
    E. Normal height for age

3. The following are associated with congenital androgen insensitivity, **except:**

    A. Blind vaginal pouch
    B. Absence of uterus and fallopian tubes
    C. Serum total testosterone concentrations in the normal male range
    D. Anosmia
    E. Breast development at puberty

4. Asherman's syndrome is most commonly seen with which one of the following:

    A. Curettage, especially postpartum
    B. Imperforate hymen
    C. Transverse vaginal septum
    D. Congenitally absent endometrium
    E. Use of intrauterine device

5. A luteal phase defect is caused by:

    A. Abnormal pulsatility of gonadotropin-releasing hormone
    B. Absence of oocytes in the ovary
    C. Absence of nerve cells which secrete gonadotropin-releasing hormone
    D. Uterine scarring
    E. Chromosomal abnormalities

6. Patients with the following conditions may present initially with amenorrhea, anovulation, or luteal phase defects, **except:**

    A. Hyperprolactinemia
    B. Hypothyroidism
    C. Anorexia nervosa
    D. Polycystic ovarian syndrome
    E. Müllerian agenesis

7. The following conditions may be associated with ovulation in the presence of amenorrhea, **except:**

    A. Asherman's syndrome
    B. Mayer-Rokitansky-Küster-Hauser syndrome
    C. Imperforate hymen
    D. Congenitally absent endometrium
    E. Androgen insensitivity

8. The following condition may be associated with anovulation and amenorrhea, because of abnormalities of GnRH production or release, **except:**

   A. Asherman's syndrome
   B. Exercise-induced amenorrhea
   C. Kallmann's syndrome
   D. Stress-induced amenorrhea
   E. Physiologic delay of puberty

9. The initial workup for a patient with secondary sexual characteristics and amenorrhea usually includes all of the following **except:**

   A. Pregnancy test
   B. Pelvic ultrasound
   C. Prolactin level
   D. TSH level
   E. Assessment of estrogen status

10. The following disorder is associated with absent secondary sexual characteristics, lack of an anatomic cause for amenorrhea demonstrable on physical exam, and an elevation in FSH:

    A. Physiological delay of puberty
    B. Kallmann's syndrome
    C. Pure gonadal dysgenesis
    D. Disorders of low-estrogen status occurring before puberty
    E. Central nervous system tumors

11. The following condition has an anatomic defect demonstrable on physical exam that is associated with amenorrhea:

    A. Pure gonadal genesis
    B. Savage syndrome
    C. Congenital adrenal hyperplasia
    D. Androgen insensitivity
    E. Hypothalamic dysfunction

12. All of the following conditions are treated surgically **except:**

    A. Asherman's syndrome
    B. Imperforate hymen
    C. Transverse septum of the vagina
    D. Absent endometrium
    E. Androgen insensitivity

13. Estrogen replacement therapy is generally needed in the following conditions, **except:**

    A. Turner's syndrome (45X)
    B. Eugonadotropic chronic anovulation
    C. Hypothalamic hypogonadism
    D. Savage syndrome
    E. Premature ovarian failure

14. Clomiphene citrate is generally ineffective in inducing ovulation in the following conditions, **except:**

    A. Hypogonadotropic hypogonadism
    B. Hypergonadotropic hypogonadism
    C. Anorexia nervosa
    D. Savage syndrome
    E. Eugonadotropic chronic anovulation

15. All of the following statements regarding treatment options are correct, **except:**

A. *Clomiphene citrate* is generally the first agent used when attempting to induce ovulation in a patient with polycystic ovarian syndrome.

B. Injectable human menopausal gonadotropins or pulsatile GnRH therapy may be used to induce ovulation in patients with hypogonadotropic hypogonadism.

C. Oral contraceptives may be effective in treating hirsutism by decreasing ovarian androgen production and by decreasing circulating levels of sex-hormone binding globulin.

D. *Spironolactone* may be effective in treating hirsutism by decreasing androgen production and by competing with androgens for the androgen receptor.

E. Patients with Turner's syndrome may become pregnant using donated oocytes through *in vitro* fertilization.

Answers

1. C (see Table 24.3)

Premature ovarian failure occurs due to decreased follicular endowment or accelerated follicular atresia. It occurs in approximately 1% of the population. Once this condition has been diagnosed, the underlying etiology should be explored. Genetic abnormalities such as Turner's syndrome, iatrogenic causes such as radiation exposure, metabolic dysfunction such as galactosemia and autoimmune disorders all cause accelerated follicular atresia. Hyperandrogenism causes abnormalities in gonadotropic secretions and the local environment that a follicle is exposed to but it does not cause accelerated atresia of the follicles.
Reference: Pages 811–813, 820–822

2. C

Kallmann's syndrome was originally described as a triad of hypogonadism, anosmia, and color blindness in men. While it is more common in men, women may be affected as well. It is also known as isolated gonadotropin deficiency and occurs as a result of an absence of GnRH neurons in the hypothalamus and olfactory bulbs and, consequently, hypogonadotropic hypogonadism and anosmia. Cleft lip and palate may also be associated with the syndrome. Patients with Kallmann's syndrome traditionally have normal height for age, in contrast to patients with physiologic delay of puberty, who generally are short for their chronologic age, but of normal height for their bone age. Kallmann's syndrome is not associated with anatomical defects, therefore, it is not associated with a blind vaginal pouch.
Reference: Pages 813–814

**Table 24.3   Causes of Ovarian Failure After
Development of Secondary Sexual Characteristics**

Chromosomal etiology
Iatrogenic causes
   Radiation
   Chemotherapy
   Surgical alteration of ovarian blood supply

Infections

Autoimmune disorders

Galactosemia (mild form or heterozygote)

Savage syndrome

Cigarette smoking

Idiopathic

3. D

Androgen insensitivity (previously known as testicular feminization) occurs in individuals with an XY karyotype, but a defect in androgen receptor function which leads to development of the female phenotype. Anti-müllerian hormone is present and functions normally in these patients, therefore, internal female (müllerian) structures such as a uterus, vagina, and fallopian tubes are absent. The gonads are testes rather than ovaries and occur in the abdomen or inguinal hernias where they secrete testosterone leading to circulating testosterone concentrations in the normal male range. Testosterone does not function during development to suppress formation of breast tissues, and at puberty, the conversion of androgens to estrogens stimulates breast growth, often leading to well-developed breasts. Due to the defect in androgen receptor function, external genitalia are phenotypically female and a blind vaginal pouch is characteristic of the disorder. There is no association with anosmia or midline facial defects.
Reference: Pages 817–820

4. A (see Figure 24.1 and Table 24.2)

Imperforate hymen, transverse vaginal septum, and congenitally absent endometrium are all causes of amenorrhea associated with normal secondary sexual characteristics. Asherman's syndrome is not associated with imperforate hymen or transverse vaginal septum because there is no history of uterine instrumentation in those individuals. Congenitally absent endometrium is a very rare condition and is basically a diagnosis of exclusion. Asherman's syndrome may be seen in patients after infections related to the use of an intrauterine device, however, it is much more common after a pregnancy-related uterine curettage. It has been reported to occur in 39% of patients undergoing hysterosalpingography who have previously undergone postpartum curettage.
Reference: Page 817

5. A

In the luteal phase of the cycle, progesterone is secreted from the corpus luteum. This promotes development of the endometrial lining to support implantation of an embryo. Abnormalities in the luteal phase are caused by abnormal stimulation of the follicle development in the follicular phase leading to inadequate development of the corpus luteum. GnRH secreted in a pulsatile manner stimulates FSH to be secreted from the pituitary, which in turn stimulates estrogen production by granulosa cells in the ovarian follicle. Both FSH and estrogen stimulate the granulosa cells to multiply and differentiate. Estrogen through positive feedback causes the midcycle surge of LH, which leads to ovulation and luteinization of follicular cells (formation of the corpus luteum). Luteinized cells secrete progesterone. If the frequency of the GnRH pulses is altered, ovulation may occur but the corpus luteum formation may not be adequate. Patients with uterine scarring are not considered to have luteal phase defects because the defect is not related to hormonal abnormalities. Patients with absent oocytes cannot ovulate and, therefore, do not have any luteal phase. Likewise, patients who have no cells that secrete GnRH cannot stimulate follicles to ovulate and, therefore, cannot have a luteal phase defect. Chromosomal abnormalities cause rapid loss of oocytes.
Reference: Pages 809, 823

6. E

Any condition that effects gonadotropin pulsatility leads to disruption of the hormonal signals which control the normal reproductive cycle. Gonadotropins need to be released in pulses in order to stimulate follicular growth and estrogen production in the ovary, which leads to ovulation and adequate corpus luteum development. Gonadotropin secretion is directly stimulated by the pulsatile release of gonadotropin releasing hormone (GnRH) from the hypothalamus. GnRH release is influenced by a variety of neurotransmitters and hormones. Prolactin, thyroid hormone, and androgens all can cause abnormal secretion of GnRH.

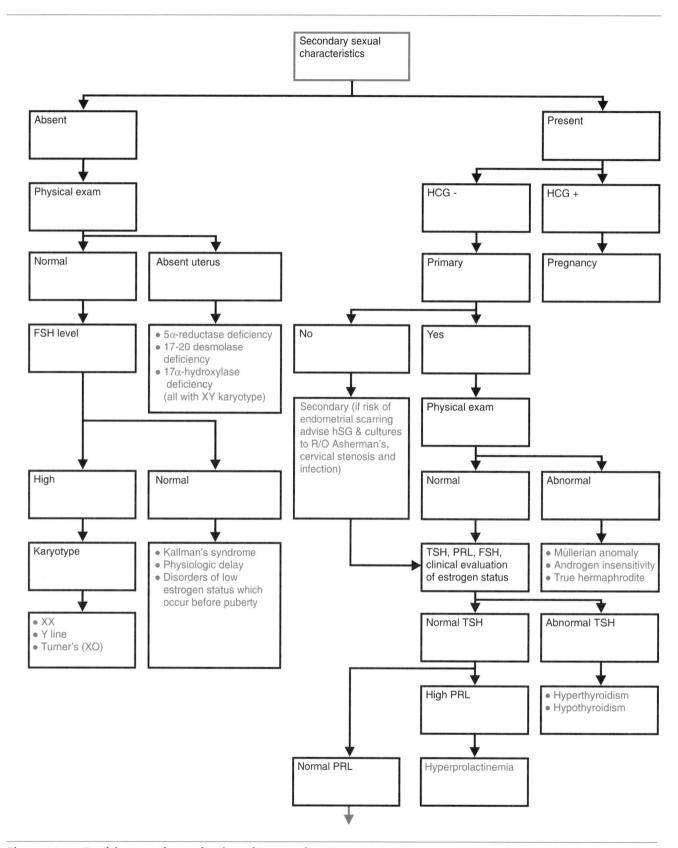

Figure 24.1   Decision tree for evaluation of amenorrhea.

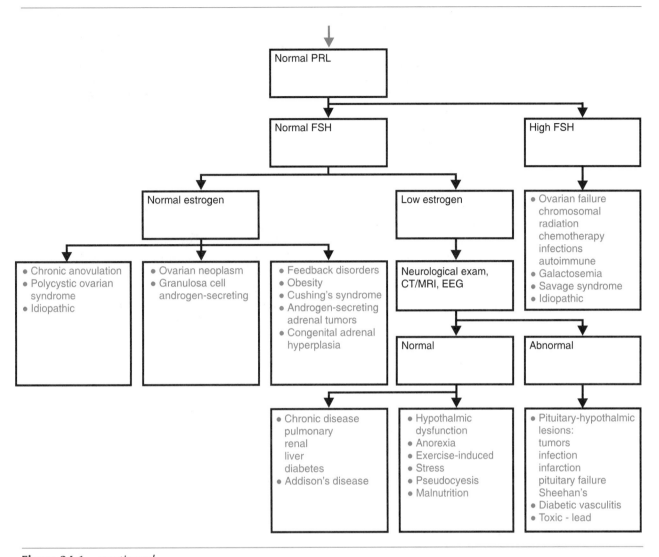

Figure 24.1—*continued*

Table 24.2   Anatomic Causes of Amenorrhea

Absent Secondary Sexual Characteristics

Müllerian anomalies
   Imperforate hymen
   Transverse vaginal septum
   Mayer-Rokitansky-Küster-Hauser syndrome
Androgen insensitivity
True hermaphrodites
Absent endometrium
Asherman's syndrome
   Secondary to prior uterine or cervical surgery
      Currettage, especially postpartum
      Cone biopsy
      Loop electroexcision procedure
   Secondary to infections
      Pelvic inflammatory disease
      IUD-related
      Tuberculosis
      Schistosomiasis

Anorexia nervosa, malnutrition, and chronic diseases can also disrupt the normal secretion of GnRH. If the normal GnRH pulsatile secretion is severely disrupted, amenorrhea will result. Less severe abnormalities in GnRH secretion cause the patient to develop oligomenorrhea. Minor disruptions in the secretion of GnRH lead to luteal phase defect where ovulation occurs, but the corpus luteum is not able to secrete enough progesterone to allow for normal development of the endometrial lining to support implantation. Müllerian agenesis is an anatomic defect that presents as amenorrhea and is frequently associated with cyclic pain.
Reference: Pages 809–830

7. E (see Tables 24.4 and 24.5)

Asherman's syndrome results in amenorrhea due to intrauterine scarring, often as a result of pregnancy-related uterine curettage. Ovulation is not effected. Mayer-Rokitansky-Küster-Hauser syndrome is a congenital absence of the uterus, cervix, and/or vagina, with the ovaries intact, which leads to normal ovulation. Imperforate hymen results in amenorrhea because of outflow obstruction but, again, ovulation is not effected. Amenorrhea in patients with a congenitally absent endometrium is a result of the inability of the endometrium to develop despite normal circulating hormone levels in association with ovulation. Ovulation does not occur in androgen insensitivity, because the gonads are testes rather than ovaries and the individuals are genotypically male.
Reference: Pages 816–820

8. A

Kallmann's syndrome is also known as isolated gonadotropin deficiency due to an absence GnRH neurons in the hypothalamus and olfactory bulbs. Amenorrhea induced by exercise or stress occurs as a result of hypogonadotropic hypogonadism and the resulting abnormalities of GnRH production. Physiologic delay of puberty results in amenorrhea because of a delayed reactivation of the hypothalamic pulse generator. Asherman's syndrome occurs as a result of intrauterine scarring and is not associated with any abnormalities of GnRH production.
Reference: Pages 813–814

9. B

Any patient of reproductive age with amenorrhea should be tested for pregnancy. History and physical, including a pelvic exam, are always necessary when evaluating a

---

Table 24.4   Pituitary/Hypothalamic Lesions

Pituitary/Hypothalamic

Craniopharyngioma
Germinoma
Tubercular granuloma
Sarcoid granuloma
Dermoid cyst

Pituitary

Nonfunctioning adenomas
Hormone-secreting ademonas
    Prolactinoma
    Cushing's disease
    Acromegaly
    Primary hyperthyroidism
Infarction
Lymphocytic hypophysitis
Surgical or radiological ablations
Sheehan's syndrome
Diabetic vasculitis

Table 24.5   Abnormalities Affecting Release of Gonadotropin-Releasing Hormone

Variable Estrogen Status*

Anorexia nervosa
Exercise-induced
Stress-induced
Pseudocyesis
Malnutrition
Chronic diseases
   Diabetes mellitus
   Renal disorders
   Pulmonary disorders
   Liver disease
   Chronic infections
   Addison's disease
Hyperprolactinemia
Thyroid dysfunction

Euestrogenic States

Obesity
Hyperandrogenism
   Polycystic ovarian syndrome
   Cushing's syndrome
   Congenital adrenal hyperplasia
   Androgen-secreting adrenal tumors
   Androgen-secreting ovarian tumors
Granulosa cell tumor
Idiopathic

*Severity of the condition determines estrogen status—the more severe, the more likely to manifest as hypoestrogenism.

patient with secondary sexual characteristics and amenorrhea. Unless the diagnosis is made by the physical exam, one needs to determine if thyroid, prolactin, and estrogen are normally secreted. Serum levels for prolactin and thyroid-stimulating hormone should be obtained. In order for secondary sexual characteristics to develop, estrogen secretion had to be adequate at some point in development. However, evaluation of estrogen status needs to be obtained, usually by a progesterone withdrawal test but physical exam and estradiol level may also be helpful. A pelvic ultrasound is not usually part of the initial workup but could be considered if an anatomic defect is found on physical exam.
Reference: Pages 818–819, 825–827

10. **C**

Physiologic delay of puberty and Kallmann's syndrome are both associated with an absence of secondary sexual characteristics and the lack of an anatomic cause for amenorrhea demonstrable on physical exam. Physiologic delay of puberty is due to a delayed reactivation of the hypothalamic pulse generator; therefore, FSH levels remain low. Kallmann's syndrome is associated with extremely low FSH levels due to absence of GnRH neurons in the hypothalamus. Disorders of low estrogen status occurring before puberty and central nervous system tumors may also be associated with lack of sexual characteristics if these occur prior to the development of sexual characteristics. Again, patients lack demonstrable anatomic causes for amenorrhea on physical exam, and FSH levels remain low to normal because the ovaries remain normal and these patients have a normal complement of oocytes. FSH elevation implies gonadal failure and the resultant lack of oocytes. In the selections given for this question, only gonadal genesis is associated with ovarian failure.
Reference: Pages 811–813

11. D (see Table 24.1)

Pure gonadal genesis is a genetic disorder resulting in ovarian failure. There is no anatomic abnormality that is necessary to make this diagnosis. In Savage syndrome, amenorrhea again results from anovulation due to ovarian resistance. Despite the fact that oocytes are present in the ovary, they do not respond with follicular development and ovulation in response to gonadotropin stimulation. There is no anatomic defect associated with Savage syndrome. Congenital adrenal hyperplasia results in increased circulating androgen levels, which in turn interferes with feedback mechanisms leading to amenorrhea in some individuals. Patients with congenital adrenal hyperplasia are anatomically normal. Any of the many conditions associated with hypothalamic dysfunction result in amenorrhea due to abnormalities in the pulsatile release of GnRH. These individuals are generally anatomically normal. Androgen insensitivity is associated with a blind vaginal pouch that is demonstrable on physical exam. Despite circulating testosterone levels in the normal male range, external genitalia remain female in phenotype due to receptor defects. The uterus, cervix, fallopian tubes, and upper vagina are absent, however, due to normal function of anti-müllerian hormone.
Reference: Pages 816–819

12. D

There is no surgical treatment for an absent endometrium. An imperforate hymen and a transverse septum need to be removed surgically to allow for the release of menstrual flow. Asherman's syndrome (uterine scarring) can be treated surgically to improve menstrual flow and pregnancy outcome. A patient with androgen sensitivity has intra-abdominal testes that can develop malignancies. Therefore, the testes should be removed surgically after puberty to prevent tumor development.
Reference: Pages 819–820

13. B

Estrogen replacement therapy is needed in conditions where circulating estrogen levels are low (hypoestrogenism). Hypoestrogenism may be a result of ovarian failure or a result of hypothalamic dysfunction leading to insufficient ovarian stimulation and estrogen production. Turner's syndrome and premature ovarian failure are both associated with hypoestrogenism as a result of ovarian failure and the associated lack of oocytes. Savage syndrome is associated with oocytes in the ovary, but these oocytes do

---

Table 24.1   Amenorrhea Associated with a Lack of Secondary Sexual Characteristics

Abnormal Physical Examination

    5α-reductase deficiency in XY individual
    17–20 desmolase deficiency in XY individual
    17α-hydroxylase deficiency in XY individual

Hypergonadotropic Hypogonadism

    Gonadal dysgenesis
    Pure gonadal dysgenesis
    Partial deletion of X chromosome
    Sex chromosome mosaicism
    Environmental and therapeutic ovarian toxins
    17α-hydroxylase deficiency in XX individual
    Galactosemia
    Other

Hypogonadotropic Hypogonadism

    Physiological delay
    Kallman's syndrome
    Central nervous system tumors
    Hypothalamic/pituitary dysfunction

not respond to gonadotropin stimulation resulting in hypoestrogenism. Hypoestrogenism also results in hypothalamic hypogonadism because of inappropriate GnRH production. This leads to insufficient gonadotropin levels for ovarian stimulation of folliculogenesis and a resulting hypoestrogenism. Eugonadotropic chronic anovulation is not associated with hypoestrogenism. In some cases, the patient may be in a state of chronic unopposed estrogen. Androgen levels may be elevated, which in turn may be converted to estrogens. These patients do not need estrogen replacement, but may need cyclic progestin therapy to combat the unopposed estrogen state and to lead to withdrawal bleeding.

Reference: Pages 815–816, 828

14. E

Clomiphene citrate is primarily indicated in patients with adequate levels of estrogen and normal levels of FSH and prolactin. It is generally ineffective in patients with a poor estrogen supply. This includes patients with hypogonadotropic hypogonadism and patients with hypergonadotropic hypogonadism resulting from a decreased supply of oocytes. It may be ineffective in anorexia nervosa because these patients are also hypoestrogenic. Patients with Savage syndrome may have oocytes demonstrable by biopsy, but these oocytes do not respond to stimulation with either clomiphene or human menopausal gonadotropins. *Clomiphene citrate* is generally effective in eugonadotropic chronic anovulation and up to 80% of well-selected patients can be expected to ovulate after therapy with clomiphene citrate.

Reference: Page 829

15. C

Clomiphene citrate is generally the first agent used for ovulation induction as long as the patient is not hypoestrogenic. Patients with polycystic ovarian syndrome are not hypoestrogenic and may respond to *clomiphene citrate,* however, rates of ovulation in patients with polycystic ovarian syndrome are lower than in patients with other forms of chronic anovulation. In patients with hypogonadotropic hypogonadism, *clomiphene citrate* is generally ineffective. These patients will respond to either injectable human menopausal gonadotropins or pulsatology GnRH therapy. *Spironolactone* is one of several agents that may be used in treating hirsutism. This mechanism acts by decreasing the androgen production and by competing with androgens for the androgen receptor.

Patients with Turner's syndrome or other forms of ovarian failure may become pregnant using donated oocytes through *in vitro* fertilization. Oocytes obtained from donors may be fertilized with sperm from the recipient's husband and transferred into the recipient's uterus after the endometrium has been appropriately prepared with hormonal regimens. Estrogen and progestins are used to prepare the endometrium for implantation of the transferred embryos. Patients with Turner's syndrome, other forms of ovarian failure, or natural menopause may all carry pregnancies derived from oocyte donation. Pregnancy rates from anonymous oocyte donation are very high and average over 50% per transfer in better programs.

Oral contraceptives may be effective in treating hirsutism in some patients. The mechanism acts by decreasing ovarian androgen production and by increasing circulating levels of sex-hormone binding globulin (SHBG). Oral contraceptives have a net estrogenic effect leading to increases in SHBG. The increases in SHBG are associated with the increased androgen binding, which therefore leaves less free androgen available.

Reference: Pages 815–816, 819–820, 827–830

25 Endocrine Disorders

David L. Olive

Learning Objectives

1. Understand the evaluation and treatment of the hirsute patient.

2. Be able to explain the pathophysiology and treatment of polycystic ovarian disease.

3. Be aware of the causes of Cushing's Syndrome.

4. Understand the different types of congenital adrenal hyperplasia, including the genetics, time of onset, manifestations, and diagnosis.

5. Recognize the many causes of hyperprolactinemia, including their diagnoses and treatment.

6. Realize the prevalence increase of thyroid disease in women.

Questions

1. The presence of hair in androgen-dependent sites in which hair does not normally appear in women is called:

   A. Hirsutism
   B. Hypertrichosis
   C. Virilization

2. The initial laboratory tests for hirsutism should consist of:

   A. Free testosterone and TSH
   B. Total testosterone, DHEAS, and 17-hydroxyprogesterone
   C. Total testosterone only
   D. Free testosterone only
   E. Androstanediol glucuronide

3. The hyperinsulinemia seen in polycystic ovarian disease is a result of:

   A. Obesity
   B. Acanthosis nigricans
   C. Insulin resistance
   D. Excessive isolated insulin secretory activity

4. In the hirsute patient, the only permanent means of hair removal is:

   A. *Finasteride*
   B. *Spironolactone*
   C. Electrolysis
   D. *Cyproterone acetate*
   E. Depilatory creams

5. The most common cause of ACTH-independent Cushing's Syndrome is:

   A. Ectopic ACT-secreting tumor
   B. Ectopic CRH-secreting tumor
   C. Adrenal adenoma
   D. Adrenal cancer
   E. Iatrogenic

6. Which of the following is *true* regarding prenatal diagnosis and treatment of 21-hydroxylase deficiency?

   A. Diagnosis and treatment only occur when a female fetus has been identified.
   B. Diagnosis and treatment must be performed in the second trimester.
   C. Diagnosis is performed by HLA determination, and treatment is carried out only in males.
   D. Diagnosis is performed by PCR, and treatment is initiated in all fetuses at risk.

7. In the patient with hyperprolactinemia who desires future fertility, the imaging technique of choice is:

   A. None
   B. Coned down x-ray of the sella turcica
   C. CT scan
   D. Tomograms
   E. MRI

8. Which of the following statements is *true* regarding pituitary adenomas in pregnancy?

    A. *Bromocriptine* does not work to reduce symptoms.
    B. Prolactin levels are followed to determine clinical course.
    C. Breastfeeding is contraindicated.
    D. These tumors rarely create complications during pregnancy.

9. The laboratory test that represents the best single screen for thyroid function is:

    A. Free T_4 index
    B. Total serum T_4
    C. T_3 resin uptake
    D. Free T_3 index
    E. TSH

10. The most common clinical state associated with autoimmune thyroid disease is :

    A. Hypothyroidism
    B. Hyperthyroidism
    C. Euthyroidism

Answers

1. A

Hirsutism, which is the most frequent manifestation of androgen excess in women, is preceded by acne, chronic anovulation, and virilization. Hirsutism is defined as the presence of hair in androgen-dependent sites in which hair does not normally appear in women. This refers particularly to "midline hair," sideburns, mustache, beard, chest or intermammary hair, and inner thigh and midline lower back hair entering the intergluteal area.

Two features should be distinguished from hirsutism. *Hypertrichosis* is the term reserved for androgen-independent growth of hair that is prominent in nonsexual areas such as the trunk and extremities. This may be an autosomal-dominant congenital disorder or may be caused by metabolic disorders (anorexia nervosa, hyperthyroidism, porphyria, cutanea tarda) or medications (phenytoin, minoxidil, cyclosporine, diazoxide). *Virilization* is characterized by male-pattern baldness (vertex most of the time and temples occasionally), coarsening of the voice, decrease in breast size, increase in muscle mass, loss of female body contour (obesity particularly of the upper segment, and waist-to-hip ratio) and enlargement of the clitoris (the mean transverse diameter of the gland is 3.4 + 1 mm and the longitudinal diameter is 5.1 + 1.4 mm).
Reference: Pages 833–834

2. B (see Table 25.1)

Initial laboratory testing for the assessment of hirsutism should include total testosterone, DHEAS, and 178-hydroxyprogesterone (17-HP) measurements. If a patient is oligomenorrheic, LH, FSH, prolactin, and thyroid-stimulating hormone (TSH) values

Table 25.1   **Normal Values for Serum Androgens***

Serum Androgens	Value
Testosterone	20–80 ng/dl
Free testosterone	0.3–1.9 ng/dl
Androstenedione	20–250 ng/dl
Dehydroepiandrosterone sulfate	100–350 μg/dl
17-hydroxprogesterone (follicular phase)	30–200 ng/dl

*May vary among different laboratories.

may be useful in the initial evaluation. In cases in which Cushing's syndrome is suspected, patients should undergo screening with a 24-hour urinary cortisol (most sensitive) assessment or an overnight *dexamethasone* suppression test. For this test, the patient takes 1 mg of *dexamethasone* at 11:00 PM, and a blood cortisol assessment is performed at 8:00 AM the next day. Cortisol levels of 2 μg/ml or higher require a further workup for Cushing's syndrome.

Many hirsute women manifest testosterone levels above normal [(20–80 ng/dl) (0.723 nmol/l)]. There is no direct correlation between the level of hirsutism and the total testosterone concentration, because hirsutism is caused by the action of the testosterone metabolite, dihydrotestosterone, which in turn is related to the concentration of SHBG. Low SHBG levels, which frequently occur in the presence of elevated androgen and insulin levels, increase free testosterone levels. The result is hirsutism in the absence of an increase in total testosterone. A testosterone level in the male range (>200 ng/dl) is a marker of neoplasms, which are mostly ovarian but occasionally adrenal.

In the past, testing for androgen conjugates (e.g., 3-α-androstenediol G [3-α-diol G] and androsterone G [AOG] as markers for 5-α-reductase activity in the skin) was advocated. However, routine determination of conjugates to assess hirsute patients is not recommended, because hirsutism itself is an excellent bioassay of free testosterone action on the hair follicle and because documentation identifies that these androgen conjugates arise from adrenal precursors and are likely markers of adrenal steroid production.

The upper limit of a DHEAS level is 350 μg/dl (9.5 nmol/liter) in most laboratories. A random sample is sufficient because the level variation is minimized as a result of the long-life of the sulfated form. The presence of normal levels essentially rules out adrenal disease, and moderate elevations are a common finding in the presence of PCOS. As a rule, a DHEAS level >700 μg/dl (20 nmol/l) is indicative of an adrenal tumor. Occasionally, ovarian tumors are associated with high DHEAS levels.

Because the 17-HP level varies significantly in the cycle, standardized testing requires evaluation in the morning during the follicular phase. A baseline follicular phase 17-HP level should be less than 200 ng/dl (6 nmol/liter). When levels >200 ng/dl but <800 ng/dl (24 nmol), ACTH testing should be performed. Levels >800 ng/dl (24 nmol) also warrant ACTH testing but are virtually diagnostic of 21 hydroxylase deficiency. Reference:Pages 836–837

3. **C**

Patients with PCOS are at risk for hyperinsulinemia and insulin resistance. The most common cause of insulin resistance and compensatory hyperinsulinemia is obesity. The insulin resistance seen in PCOS seems to be independent of the expected insulin resistance that occurs with obesity alone. The following observations provide evidence that the insulin resistance associated with PCOS is not the result of hyperandrogenism:

1. Hyperinsulinemia is not a characteristic of hyperandrogenism in general but is uniquely associated with PCOS.
2. In obese women with PCOS, 20% have glucose intolerance or frank diabetes mellitus, whereas ovulatory hyperandrogenic women have normal insulin levels and glucose tolerance. It seems that the negative effects of PCOS and obesity on the action of insulin are synergistic.
3. Treatment with long-acting GnRH analogs does not change insulin levels or insulin resistance.
4. Oophorectomy in patients with hyperthecosis accompanied by hyperinsulinemia and hyperandrogenemia does not change insulin resistance, despite a decrease in androgen levels.

Acanthosis nigricans is considered a marker for insulin resistance in hirsute women. This thickened, pigmented, velvety skin is most often found in the vulva and may be present on the axilla, on the nape of the neck, below the breast, and on the inner thigh.

Women with severe insulin resistance develop *hair-AN syndrome,* consisting of hyperandrogenism, insulin resistance, and acanthosis nigricans. These patients usually have high testosterone levels ($>$1.5 ng/ml), fasting insulin levels of more than 25 μg/ml (normal 20 μg/ml), and maximal serum insulin responses to glucose load exceeding 300 μg/ml (normal is $<$150 μg/ml).

Insulin alters ovarian steroidogenesis independent of gonadotropin secretion in PCOS. Insulin and insulin-like growth factor 1 receptors are present in the ovarian stromal cell. A specific defect in the early steps of insulin receptor-mediated signaling (diminished autophosphorylation) has been identified in 50% of women with PCOS.

Clinically, it is important to realize that patients with PCOS are at increased risk for glucose intolerance or frank diabetes mellitus early in life. Therefore, it is appropriate to screen obese women with PCOS for glucose intolerance on a regular basis once or twice a year. Abnormal glucose metabolism may be improved with weight reduction, which may also reduce hyperandrogenism and restore ovulatory function. In obese, insulin-resistant women, caloric restriction that results in weight reduction will reduce the severity of insulin resistance (a 40% decrease in insulin level with a 10-kilogram weight loss). This decrease in insulin levels should result in a marked decrease in androgen production (a 35% decrease in testosterone levels with a 10-kilogram weight loss). Reference: Pages 839–840

4. C

Spironolactone is a specific antagonist of aldosterone, which competitively binds to the aldosterone receptors in the distal tubular region of the kidney. Therefore, it is an effective potassium-sparing diuretic, which was originally marketed for treatment of hypertension. At least a modest improvement in hirsutism can be anticipated in 70 to 80% of women using at least 100 mg of *spironolactone* per day for 6 months. Most authors agree that *spironolactone* reduces the daily linear growth rate of sexual hair, hair shaft diameters, and daily volume production. The most common doses are 25 to 100 mg twice daily.

Women treated with *spironolactone* 200 mg/day show a greater reduction in hair shaft diameter than women receiving 100 mg/day.

Maximal effect on hair growth is between 3 and 6 months but continues for 12 months. Electrolysis can be recommended thereafter for permanent hair removal.

The most common side effects of *spironolactone* is menstrual irregularity (usually metrorrhagia), which may occur in up to 68% of patients with a dose of 200 mg/day. Normal menses may resume with reduction of the dosage. Infrequently, other side effects such as urticaria, mastodynia, or scalp hair loss occur. Nausea and fatigue can occur with high doses. Because *spironolactone* can raise serum potassium levels, its use is not recommended in patients with renal insufficiency or hyperkalemia. Periodic monitoring of potassium and creatinine levels is required.

Return of normal menses in amenorrheic patients is reported in up to 60% of cases. Patients must be counseled to use contraception with *spironolactone,* because it theoretically can feminize a male fetus.

Cyproterone acetate is a synthetic progestin derived from 17-HP with potent antiandrogenic properties. The primary mechanism of *cyproterone acetate* is competitive inhibition of testosterone and dihydrotestosterone at the level of androgen receptors. This agent also induces hepatic enzymes and may increase the metabolic clearance rate of plasma androgens.

The combination of ethinyl estradiol with *cyproterone acetate,* which was commonly used in Europe for many years, significantly reduces plasma testosterone and androstenedione levels, suppresses gonadotropins, and increases SHBG. *Cyproterone acetate* also shows mild glucocorticoid activity and may reduce DHEAS levels. Administered in a reverse sequential regimen (*cyproterone acetate,* 100 mg/day on days 5 to 15, and *ethinyl estradiol,* 30 to 50 µg/day on cycle days 5 to 26), this cyclic schedule allows regular menstrual bleeding, provides excellent contraception, and is effective in the treatment of even hirsutism and acne. When a desired clinical response is achieved, the dose of *cyproterone acetate* may be tapered gradually at 3- to 6-month intervals.

Side effects of *cyproterone acetate* include fatigue, weight gain, decreased libido, irregular bleeding, nausea, and headaches. These symptoms occur less often when *ethinyl estradiol* is added. *Cyproterone acetate* administration has been associated with liver tumors in beagles and is not approved by the Food and Drug Administration for use in the United States.

Finasteride is a specific inhibitor of 5-α-reductase enzyme activity (5-α-RA) that has been approved in the United States for the treatment of benign prostatic hyperplasia. In a study in which *finasteride* (5 mg daily) was compared with *spironolactone* (100 mg daily), both drugs resulted in similar significant improvement in hirsutism despite differing effects on androgen levels. Further studies are needed to clarify the role of this family of drugs in the treatment of hirsutism.

Depilatory creams remove hair only temporarily. They break down and dissolve hair by hydrolyzing disulfide bonds. Although depilatories can have a dramatic effect, many women cannot tolerate these irritative chemicals. The topical use of corticosteroid cream may prevent contact dermatitis.

Electrolysis is the only permanent means recommended for hair removal. Under magnification, a trained technician destroys each hair follicle individually. When a needle is inserted into a hair follicle, galvanic current and electrocautery alone or in combination ("the blend") destroy the hair follicle. After the needle is removed, forceps are used to remove the hair. Hair regrowth ranges from 15 to 50%. Problems with electrolysis include pain, scarring, pigmentation, and cost.
Reference: Pages 842–845

5. E

The six recognized causes of Cushing's syndrome can be either *ACTH-dependent* or *ACTH-independent.*

The ACTH-dependent causes can result form ACTH secreted by pituitary adenomas or from an ectopic source. Pituitary ACTH-secreting adenomas, or Cushing's disease, are the most common cause of Cushing's syndrome. These growths are usually microadenomas (<10 mm in diameter) that may be as small as 1 mm. They behave as if they are resistant, to a variable degree, to the "feedback" effect of cortisol. Like the normal gland, these tumors secrete ACTH in a pulsatile fashion; unlike the normal gland, the diurnal pattern of cortisol secretion is lost. *Ectopic ACTH syndrome* is most often caused by malignant tumors. About one-half of these tumors are small-cell carcinomas of the lung. Other tumors include bronchial and thymic carcinomas, carcinoid tumor of the pancreas, and medullary carcinoma of the thyroid.

Ectopic cortical-releasing hormone (CRH) tumors are rare and include such tumors as bronchial carcinoids, medullary thyroid carcinoma, and metastatic prostatic carcinoma.

The presence of an ectopic CRH-secreting tumor should be suspected in patients who react biochemically similar to those with pituitary ACTH-dependent disease but who have rapid disease progression and very high plasma ACTH levels.

The hallmark of ACTH-dependent forms of Cushing's syndrome is the presence of normal or high plasma ACTH concentrations with increased cortisol levels. The adrenal glands are hyperplastic bilaterally.

The most common causes of ACTH-independent Cushing's syndrome are *exogenous* or *iatrogenic* (superphysiologic therapy with cortical steroids) or *factitious* (self-induced). Cortical steroids in pharmacologic quantities are used to treat a variety of diseases with an inflammatory component. Over time, this practice will result in Cushing's syndrome. When glucocorticoids are taken by the patient but not prescribed by a physician, the diagnosis may be especially challenging.
Reference: Pages 845–846

6. D

In families at risk for CAH, first-trimester prenatal screening is advocated. The previously used hormonal and HLA determinations have been replaced by polymerase chain reaction (PCR) amplification of the CYP 21 gene. An aggressive and still controversial approach involves the use of *dexamethasone* treatment for all pregnant women at risk of having a child with CAH. The dosage is 20 µg/kg in three divided doses administrated as soon as pregnancy is recognized and prior to performing chorionic villus sampling or amniocentesis. *Dexamethasone* crosses the placenta and suppresses ACTH in the fetus. If the fetus is a male, *dexamethasone* administration is stopped; if it is female, DNA analysis is performed to detect the 21-hydroxylase gene. *Dexamethasone* therapy is discontinued if the fetus is unaffected and continued if the fetus is affected. When *dexamethasone* is administrated before nine weeks of gestation and is continued to term, it effectively reduces genital ambiguity in genetic females. However, at least two-thirds of treated females still require surgical repair of the genitalia. Although prenatal treatment does reduce virilization in females, the efficacy and safety to both mother and baby have not been verified. The unnecessary treatment of seven out of every eight pregnancies poses serious ethical dilemmas.
Reference: Pages 850–851

7. E

Prolactin levels in patients with larger microadenomas and macroadenomas are usually higher than 100 ng/ml. However, levels may be lower with smaller microadenomas and other suprasellar tumors that may be missed on a "coned-down" view of the sella turcica. In patients with clearly identifiable drug-induced or physiologic etiology for hyperprolactinemia, scanning may not be necessary. Coned-down views of the pituitary are occasionally obtained as a screening technique to rule out a mass effect in the sella. The community standard of care, resources available, and expertise of the operator will influence the imaging technique: coned-down view of sella, CT scan, or MRI. An MRI is considered by neuroradiologists to be the optimal technique to evaluate the sella/suprasellar region. The cumulative radiation dose from multiple CT scans may cause cataracts, and the coned-down views or tomograms of the sella are very insensitive and likewise expose the patient to radiation. Even modest elevations of prolactin can be associated with microadenomas, nonlactotroph pituitary tumors, and other central nervous system abnormalities.

For patients with hyperprolactinemia who desire future fertility, MRI is indicated to differentiate a pituitary microadenoma from a macroadenoma as well as to identify other potential sellar-suprasellar masses. Although they are infrequent when pregnancy-related complications occur, sellar-suprasellar masses are associated with macroadenomas twice as often as with microadenomas, and patients should make informed decisions.
Reference: Page 860

8. D

Prolactin-secreting microadenomas rarely create complications during pregnancy. However, monitoring of patients with serial gross visual field examinations and fundoscopic examination is recommended. If persistent headaches, visual field deficits, or visual or fundoscopic changes occur, MRI scanning is advisable. Because serum prolactin levels are elevated throughout pregnancy, prolactin measurements are of no value.

Although not recommended, *bromocriptine* use during pregnancy in women with symptomatic (visual field defects, headaches) microadenoma enlargement has resulted in resolution of deficits and symptoms.

Women with previous transsphenoidal hypophysectomy and macroadenomas are monitored, as are those with microadenomas, with the addition of monthly Goldman perimetry visual field testing. Periodic MRI scanning may be necessary in women with symptoms or visual change. *Bromocriptine* has been used on a temporary basis to resolve symptoms and visual field deficits in symptomatic macroadenoma patients to allow completion of pregnancy before initiation of definitive therapy. Breastfeeding is not contraindicated in the presence of microadenomas or macroadenomas.
Reference: Page 864

9. E

Total serum T4 is measured by radioimmunoassay. Conditions that elevate the levels of thyroid-binding globulin (TBG) (pregnancy, oral contraceptive, estrogen replacement, hepatitis, and genetic abnormalities of TBG) necessitate measuring T3 resin uptake for clarification.

The T3 resin uptake determines the concentration of radiolabeled T3 bound to serum TBG and an artificial resin. The number of binding sites available in TBG is inversely proportional to the amount of labeled T3 bound to the artificial resin. Therefore, high TBG T3 receptor site availability results in a low T3 resin uptake.

The free T4 index (FTI) is obtained by multiplying the serum T4 concentration by the T3 resin uptake percentage, yielding an indirect measurement of free T4.
$$\% \text{ free T4} \times \text{T4 total} = \text{free T4}$$
Equilibrium dialysis may be used to determine the percentage of free T4. Free T4 and T3 may also be determined by radioimmunoassay.

The present TSH sandwich immunoassays are extremely sensitive and are capable of differentiating low-normal from pathological or iatrogenically subnormal values and elevations. Thus, TSH measurements provide the best single screen for thyroid dysfunction and accurately predict thyroid hormone dysfunction in about 80% of cases.
Reference: Page 865

10. A

Autoimmune thyroid disease is the predominant class of thyroid disorders; hypothyroidism is three times more common than hyperthyroidism. The most common thyroid abnormalities in women, autoimmune thyroid disorders, represent the combined effects of the multiple antibodies produced. The various antigen-antibody reactions result in the varied clinical spectrum of these disorders. The transmission of these immunoglobulins transplacentally also potentially complicates thyroid function in the fetus. The presence of autoimmune thyroid disorders, particularly Graves' disease, is associated with other autoimmune conditions. Other autoimmune conditions associated with Graves' disease are Hashimoto's thyroiditis, Addison's disease, ovarian failure, rheumatoid arthritis, Sjögren's syndrome, diabetes mellitus (type I), vitiligo, pernicious anemia, myasthenia, gravis, and idiopathic thrombocytopenic purpura.
Reference: Page 866

26 Endometriosis

David L. Olive

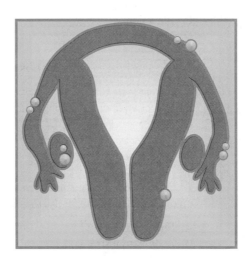

Learning Objectives

1. Be able to list the theories of etiology and histogenesis of endometriosis.

2. Know the options for diagnosing endometriosis, as well as the advantages and disadvantages of each method.

3. Be aware of the classification systems used for endometriosis.

4. Know the different types of treatment for endometriosis, including both medical and surgical approaches.

Questions

1. The theory for the etiologic mechanism of endometriosis that has the most experimental support and is the likely mechanism for most patients with the disease is:

   A. Transplantation
   B. Coelomic metaplasia
   C. Induction
   D. Müllerian rest

2. The diagnosis of endometriosis is best made by:

   A. Patient symptoms
   B. Objective findings on physical examination
   C. CA125 level
   D. Laparoscopic visualization
   E. Laparoscopic biopsy

3. To be defined as endometriosis, a lesion must be located outside the uterine cavity and myometrium. Histologically, the diagnosis is made by the presence of:

   A. Endometrial glands
   B. Endometrial stroma
   C. Endometrial glands and stroma
   D. Hemosiderin-laden macrophages
   E. Endometrial glands and hemosiderin-laden macrophages

4. The internationally accepted classification scheme for endometriosis is:

   A. The Acosta classification system
   B. The Buttram classification system
   C. The American Fertility Society classification system
   D. The revised American Fertility Society classification system
   E. The Kistner classification system

5. Which of the following treatments is effective in the treatment of endometriosis-associated pain?

   A. Oral contraceptives
   B. *Danazol*
   C. Progestins
   D. *Gestrinone*
   E. GnRH agonists
   F. All of the above

6. Which of the following medications has been shown to enhance fertility in patients with endometriosis-associated infertility?

   A. Oral contraceptives
   B. *Danazol*
   C. Progestins
   D. *Gestrinone*
   E. GnRH agonists
   F. None of the above

Answers

1. A (see Figure 26.1)

The transplantation theory, originally proposed by Sampson, is based on the assumption that endometriosis is caused by the seeding or implantation of endometrial cells by transtubal regurgitation during menstruation. Substantial clinical and experimental data support this hypothesis. Retrograde menstruation occurs in 70 to 90% of women, and it may be more common in women with endometriosis than in those without the disease. Also, endometriosis is most often found in dependent portions of the pelvis. Extrapelvic endometriosis can be explained by transplantation via lymphatics or by hematogenous spread. While other theories of endometriosis pathogenesis exist, they have little or no clinical and experimental support.

Reference: Pages 888–889

2. E

Endometriosis is frequently difficult to diagnose. Symptoms of pain or infertility are suggestive of the disease, but hardly diagnostic. The same is true for signs such as adnexal masses or cul-de-sac tenderness and nodularity. Laboratory tests such as CA125 lack sufficient sensitivity and specificity to be of much value. Laparoscopy remains the

Figure 26.1   Pelvic localization of endometriosis.

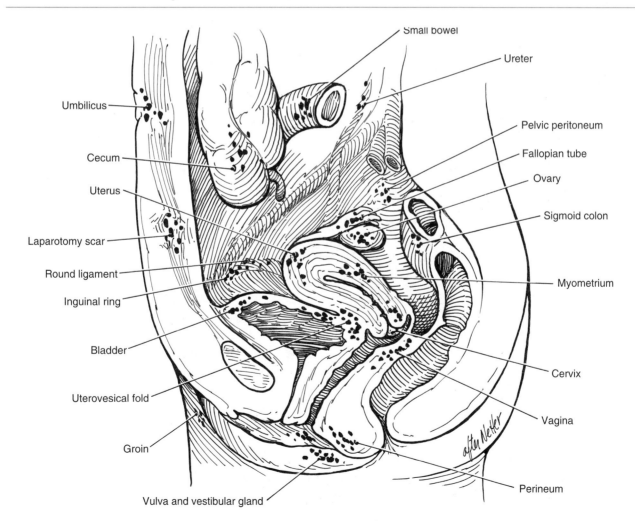

gold standard for diagnosis, but while simple visualization of lesions is highly suggestive, numerous other disorders can mimic the appearance of endometriosis. Thus, to maximize the chance of correctly determining the presence of disease, laparoscopy with biopsy of suspicious lesions is indicated.
Reference: Pages 890–898

3. C (see Figure 26.6)
Endometriosis is defined as the presence of ectopic endometrial glands and stroma, with or without the presence of hemosiderin-laden macrophages.
Reference: Page 893

Figure 26.6 Histological appearance of endometriosis: endometrial glandular epithelium, surrounded by stroma in (*A*) typical lesion and (*B*) clear vesicle.

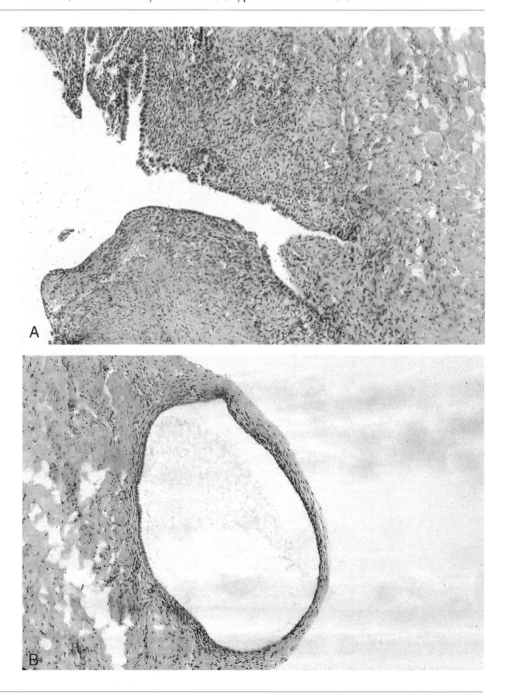

4. D (see Figure 26.5)

The current classification system of endometriosis is the revised American Fertility Society (AFS) system. It is based on appearance, size, and depth of peritoneal and ovarian implants; the presence, extent, and type of adnexal adhesions; and the degree of cul-de-sac obliteration. This system reflects the extent of endometriotic disease, but it is not based on the correlation of pain or infertility and it has considerable intraobserver and

Figure 26.5 Revised American Fertility Society Classification, 1985. (Reproduced with permission from **The America Fertility Society.** Revised American Fertility Society Classification of endometriosis. *Fertil Steril* 1985;43:351–2. Reproduced, with permission of the publisher, the American Society for Reproductive Medicine.)

Revised American Fertility Society Classification of Endometriosis: 1985

Patient's Name _____ Date _____

Stage I (Minimal) - 1-5
Stage II (Mild) - 6-15
Stage III (Moderate) - 16-40
Stage IV (Severe) - >40
Total _____

Laparoscopy _____ Laparotomy _____ Photography _____
Recommended Treatment _____
_____
Prognosis _____

PERITONEUM	ENDOMETRIOSIS	<1cm	1-3cm	>3cm
	Superficial	1	2	4
	Deep	2	4	6
OVARY	R Superficial	1	2	4
	Deep	4	16	20
	L Superficial	1	2	4
	Deep	4	16	20

	POSTERIOR CULDESAC OBLITERATION	Partial	Complete
		4	40

	ADHESIONS	<1/3 Enclosure	1/3-2/3 Enclosure	>2/3 Enclosure
OVARY	R Filmy	1	2	4
	Dense	4	8	16
	L Filmy	1	2	4
	Dense	4	8	16
TUBE	R Filmy	1	2	4
	Dense	4*	8*	16
	L Filmy	1	2	4
	Dense	4*	8*	16

*If the fimbriated end of the fallopian tube is completely enclosed, change the point assignment to 16.

Additional Endometriosis: _____

Associated Pathology: _____

To Be Used with Normal Tubes and Ovaries

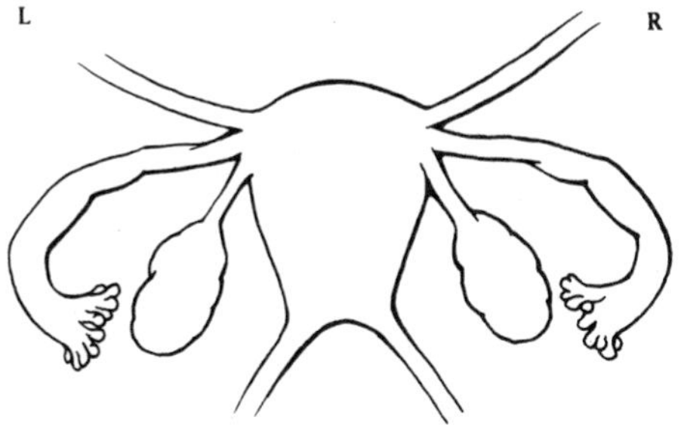

To Be Used with Abnormal Tubes and/or Ovaries

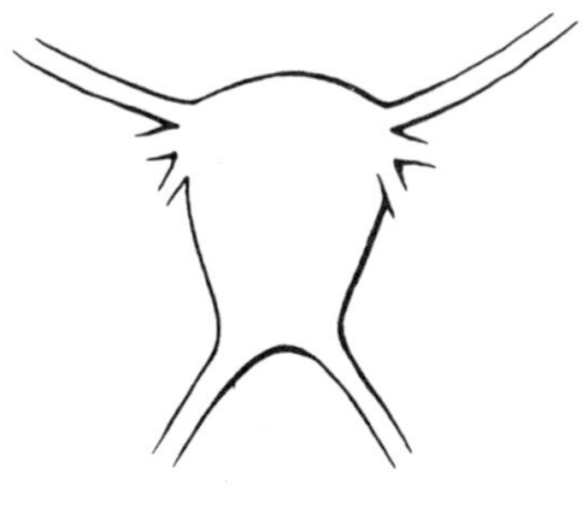

Table 26.1   Medical Treatment of Endometriosis-Associated Pain: Effective Regimens (Usual Duration: six months)

	Administration	Dose	Frequency
Progestogens			
Medroxyprogesterone acetate	PO	30 mg	daily
Megestrol acetate	PO	40 mg	daily
Lynestrenol	PO	10 mg	daily
Dydrogesterone	PO	20–30 mg	daily
Antiprogestins			
Gestrinone	PO	1.25 or 2.5 mg	twice weekly
Danazol	PO	400 (2 × 200) mg	daily
Gonodotropin-Releasing Hormone			
Leuprolide	SC	500 µg	daily
	IM	3.75 mg	monthly
Goserelin	SC	3.6 mg	monthly
Buserelin	IN	3 × 300 µg	daily
	SC	1 × 200 µg	daily
Nafarelin	IN	2 × 200 µg	daily
Tryptorelin	IM	3.75 mg	monthly

PO, oral; SC, subcutaneous; IM, intramuscular; IN, intranasal.

interobserver variability. However, the revised AFS classification of endometriosis is the only internationally accepted standard to evaluate spontaneous evolution and to compare therapeutic outcomes.
Reference: Pages 898–899

5. F (see Table 26.1)

Medical treatment with each of the above medications is effective in treating pain associated with endometriosis as shown in several prospective, randomized, placebo-controlled double-blind studies. Based on published studies, these drugs appear to have similar efficacy.
Reference: Pages 901–904

6. F

Numerous randomized trials have been carried out to assess fertility rates after medical therapy in women with endometriosis. To date, no study has been able to demonstrate an increase in fertility following medical treatment. In fact, since the patient cannot conceive while on these medications, they may actually have a detrimental effect upon fertility due to time lost during treatment.
Reference: Pages 901–904

27 Infertility

David L. Olive

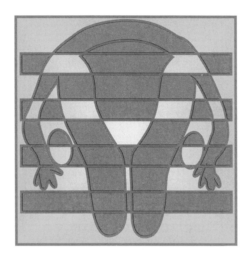

Learning Objectives

1. Understand the epidemiology of infertility.

2. Know the initial evaluation of the infertile couple.

3. Be able to articulate the different causes of infertility in the male and female.

4. Understand the treatments available to treat the infertile couple and their relative efficacies.

5. Know the different types of assisted reproduction.

Questions

1. The probability of achieving a live birth within a single cycle is termed:

   A. Fertility
   B. Fecundity
   C. Fecundability
   D. Fertilizability

2. The day 3 FSH level above which women show reduced pregnancy rates in IVF is:

   A. 5 mIU/ml
   B. 10 mIU/ml
   C. 15 mIU/ml
   D. 20 mIU/ml
   E. 25 mIU/ml

3. The most common cause of infertility is:

   A. Ovulatory dysfunction
   B. Male factor infertility
   C. Endometriosis
   D. Cervical factor infertility
   E. Pelvic adhesions

4. Which of the following chemicals can decrease sperm quality?

   A. *Penicillin*
   B. *Theophylline*
   C. DDT
   D. *Cimetidine*
   E. *Fluoxitene*

5. The most accurate method for documenting the day of ovulation is:

   A. Serum progesterone
   B. Basal body temperature
   C. LH monitoring kit
   D. Endometrial biopsy
   E. Ultrasound monitoring

6. The appropriate time to perform a postcoital test is:

   A. During menses
   B. 2 to 5 days after the cessation of menses
   C. 1 to 2 days before anticipated ovulation
   D. 1 day post-ovulation
   E. Midluteal phase

7. Poor prognostic factors for a successful pregnancy after neosalpingostomy includes each of the following **except:**

   A. Hydrosalpinx >30 mm diameter
   B. Absence of visible fimbriae
   C. Dense pelvic/adnexal adhesions
   D. Proximal and distal tubal disease
   E. Single fallopian tube

8. The most successful form of assisted reproductive technology is:

A. IVF
B. GIFT
C. ZIFT
D. Cryopreserved embryo transfer
E. Donor oocytes

Answers

1. B

Infertility is defined as one year of unprotected intercourse without pregnancy. This condition may be further classified as *primary infertility,* in which no previous pregnancies have occurred, and *secondary infertility,* in which a prior pregnancy, although not necessarily a live birth, has occurred. *Fecundability* is the probability of achieving pregnancy within a single menstrual cycle, and *fecundity* is the probability of achieving live birth within a single cycle. The fecundability of a normal couple has been estimated at 20 to 25%. On the basis of this estimate, approximately 90% of couples should conceive after 12 months.
Reference: Page 915

2. C

The age-related decline in fertility appears to be attributed to oocyte depletion. For women in their late thirties, a small increase in follicle-stimulating hormone (FSH) correlates with subtle changes in oocyte number and perhaps oocyte competence, translating into reduced fertility. As FSH levels rise and a women approaches menopause, the chances of successful pregnancy decline further. The data that correlate FSH levels with poor reproductive outcome show that women with FSH levels of >15 mIU/ml on cycle day 3 have reduced pregnancy rates in IVF, and women with higher FSH levels have even lower pregnancy rates. There is, however, a considerable variation in FSH assays, so the results depend on the method used.
Reference: Page 917

3. B

Abnormalities of the semen, or male factor infertility, probably represent the most common cause of infertility. Semen analysis is the basic laboratory study assessing such abnormalities. Because this test is inexpensive and noninvasive, it should be a part of every infertility workup. Assessment of semen parameters, however, is confounded by controversies regarding the proper range of normal values. Semen parameters in normal fertile men vary considerably over time and may even drop below established norms; this situation makes evaluation of the male patient more difficult. Before the value and interpretation of semen analysis and other tests for male infertility are considered, a brief review of male reproductive physiology is in order.
Reference: Pages 918–919

4. D

The mean sperm concentration and mean sperm volume in normal males have dropped substantially over the past 50 years. This decline in semen quality is suggested to be associated with increased levels of environmental toxins in the last half of the twentieth century. The nature of such toxins, however, remains speculative. Heavy marijuana and cocaine use can reduce sperm concentration. Certain drugs, such as anabolic steroids, chemotherapeutic agents, *cimetidine, erythromycin, nitrofurans, spironolactone, sulfasalazine,* and *tetracycline,* may reduce semen parameters. In addition, cigarette smoking and heavy coffee consumption diminish semen quality.
Reference: Page 923

5. E

The easiest and least expensive method of detecting ovulation is for the patient to record her temperature each morning on a basal body temperature (BBT) chart. The temperature should be determined orally before the patient arises, eats, or drinks. Smoking is forbidden. Use of a basal body thermometer is preferred because of its precision in the temperature range under consideration. The patient records her temperature daily and also records the times when coitus takes place. The principle of temperature charting is simple. Significant progesterone secretion by the ovary generally occurs only after ovulation. Progesterone is a thermogenic hormone; the secretion of progesterone leads to temperature increases of approximately 0.5°F over the base line temperature in the follicular phase, which is generally in the range of 97 to 98°F. The difference between the two phases of the cycle produces the characteristic biphasic pattern indicative of ovulation. Frequently, there is a nadir around the time of the LH surge, but this finding is inconsistent. The luteal phase is characterized by a temperature elevation lasting at least 10 days.

The BBT, although simple, has several drawbacks. Presumptive ovulation can be identified only retrospectively; i.e., the test merely confirms rather than predicts ovulation. Also, in a small percentage of patients, the BBT charts are monophasic despite the documentation of ovulation by other methods. The exact time of ovulation is difficult to predict, but in most instances, it is probably one day before temperature elevation. The unequivocal temperature rise generally occurs two days after the LH surge and correlates with serum progesterone levels of >4 ng/ml. The correlation between BBT rise and LH surge may be more reliable than correlations with progesterone levels.

Despite its limitations, BBT charting is a simple way to document ovulation. Unequivocal biphasic cycles are almost certainly ovulatory, but monophasic cycles require the confirmation of the patient's ovulatory status.

Elevations in serum levels of progesterone constitute indirect evidence of ovulation. The lower limit of progesterone levels in the luteal phase varies among laboratories, but a level of >3 ng/ml (10 nmol/l) confirms ovulation. The measurement should be made as progesterone secretion peaks in the midluteal phase (typically on days 21 to 23 of an ideal 28-day cycle). Typically, ovulatory levels are considerably higher than 3 ng/ml. Interpretation of a single measurement of the progesterone level is complicated by the pulsatile nature of the secretion of this hormone; therefore, low levels are not necessarily diagnostic of anovulation, but appropriate concentrations in the luteal phase confirm prior ovulation.

Numerous investigators have attempted to correlate elevated midluteal progesterone levels with adequate corpus luteum function. Others have tried to correlate progesterone levels with findings on endometrial biopsy. A single progesterone measurement is not a substitute for an endometrial biopsy in the assessment of adequacy in the luteal phase.

Luteinizing Hormone Monitoring. Documentation of the LH surge is a reproducible method of predicting ovulation. Ovulation occurs 34 to 36 hours after the onset of the LH surge and approximately 10 to 12 hours after the LH peak. Because LH is a pulsatile hormone, the detection of a true elevation may be difficult. A two- to threefold elevation of serum LH levels over base line, however, is sufficient to document an LH surge. A number of manufacturers have developed self-administered home kits to detect the LH surge in the urine. The kits are generally accurate, quick, convenient, and relatively inexpensive enzyme-linked immunoabsorbent assays. Unlike assays that measure serum LH levels, these tests detect urinary LH levels above a certain threshold.

Endometrial Biopsy. Another method of confirming ovulation is the endometrial biopsy; the finding of secretory endometrium confirms ovulation. Because this procedure is more invasive than other methods and may be somewhat uncomfortable for some patients, its major role in the infertility evaluation is not in documentation of ovulation but rather in diagnosis of luteal phase defects. Generally, the biopsy is performed 2 to 3 days before the expected onset of menses. The patient may be offered a sensitive serum pregnancy test prior to biopsy, but the risk that the biopsy will interrupt an early pregnancy is small. The biopsy is interpreted by dating of the endometrium according to the criteria of Noyes, Hertig, and Rock. Despite widespread agreement on the pathologic criteria, there may be significant variability in the dating of the specimen.

Ultrasound Monitoring. Ovulation can be documented by monitoring the development of the dominant follicle by ultrasound until ovulation takes place. Ovulation is characterized by a decrease in follicular size and the appearance of fluid in the cul-de-sac. Ovulation is reported to occur when follicular size reaches 21 to 23 mm, although it may occur with follicles as small as 17 mm or as large as 29 mm. Because of the inconvenience and expense of serial ultrasound measurements, use of this method for documenting ovulation is discouraged; instead, it is recommended that its use be confined to the monitoring of ovulation induction in ART patients. However, it stands as the most precise marker of ovulation.
Reference: Pages 923–924

6. C

The PCT should be performed just before ovulation because its proper interpretation requires the examination of cervical mucus at a time of sufficient estrogen exposure. Serum estrogen levels peak just before ovulation, providing optimal stimulation to the estrogen-sensitive, mucus-producing cervical glands. The PCT should be performed one or two days before the anticipated time of ovulation. The patient's urinary LH surge may be helpful in scheduling the test for patients with irregular cycles. One area of controversy concerns the timing of coitus preceding examination of the cervical mucus. Although an optimal interval may be less than two hours from intercourse to PCT, an adequate test can be performed within 24 hours of intercourse. Although the data are not definitive, intercourse after 2 days of abstinence, or approximately 2 to 12 hours before the PCT is performed, should yield adequate information. Couples should be reminded not to use lubricants that may contain spermicidal agents.
Reference: Pages 926–927

7. E

Treatment of distal tubal disease involves surgical correction via fimbrioplasty or neosalpingostomy. By definition, fimbrioplasty is the lysis of fimbrial adhesions or dilatation of fimbrial phimosis, whereas neosalpingostomy involves the creation of a new tubal opening in an occluded fallopian tube. Distal tubal disease can be treated with conventional microsurgical techniques, although laparoscopic management can be equally efficacious. The resurgence of the minilaparotomy in gynecologic surgery, however, has called this practice into question. Recent evidence suggests that neosalpingostomy can be performed via laparotomy with very brief postoperative hospital stays (less than 24 hours) and subsequent pregnancy rates equivalent to those obtained with laparoscopic management.

Regardless of the method used, the efficacy of neosalpingostomy or fimbrioplasty as treatment for distal tubal occlusion rests largely on the extent of tubal and peritubal disease, as assessed by hysterosalpingography and laparoscopy. The poor prognostic factors for a successful pregnancy after neosalpingostomy include hydrosalpinx >30 mm in diameter, absence of visible fimbriae, and dense pelvic or adnexal adhesions. The appearance of the tubal mucosa has added prognostic significance for the fertility outcome of laparoscopic tuboplasty for distal tubal occlusion. In one study, laparoscopic distal tuboplasty has produced an overall pregnancy rate of 27% and an ectopic pregnancy rate of 4.5% among 44 patients. Fimbrioplasty appeared to be more successful

Table 27.5 Comparison of Reported Outcomes for All ART Procedures

	IVF	GIFT	ZIFT	Donor*	Cryopreserved Embryo Transfers†
Cycles/procedures‡	29,404	5,767	1,993	1,802	5,354
Cancellation (%)	15.4	16.2	15.0	5.2	NA§
Retrievals	24,996	4,837	1,696	1,708	NA
Transfers	21,870	4,712	1,497	1,699	5,354
Transfers per retrieval (%)	87.5	97.4	88.3	99.4	NA
Pregnancies	5,279	1,621	488	625	820
Pregnancy loss (%)	20.0	16.9	21.1	14.9	23.8
Deliveries	4,206	1,273	386	534	619
Deliveries per retrieval (%)	16.8	26.7	22.8	31.3	NA
Singleton (%)	67.3	67.3	64.2	63.3	77.9
Ectopic pregnancy	272	61	20	14	32
Ectopic per transfer (%)	1.2	1.3	1.3	0.8	0.6
Birth defects per neonates delivered (%)	1.9	2.4	2.5	1.7	1.3

*Donor includes known or anonymous, but not surrogate.
†Cryopreserved embryo transfer cycles not done in combination with fresh Embryo Transfers and not with donor egg/embryo.
‡Includes all cycles, regardless of age or diagnosis.
§NA, not available.
||Birth defect reporting did not account for all neonatal outcomes.
Reproduced with permission from **American Fertility Society, Society for Assisted Reproductive Technology.** Assisted reproductive technology in the United States and Canada: 1992 results generated from the American Fertility Society/Society for Assisted Reproductive Technology Registry. *Fertil Steril* 1994;62:1121–8.

than neosalpingostomy; however, the choice of surgery may have been influenced by the extent of disease. Patients with both proximal and distal tubal disease represent the poorest candidates for surgical management of infertility. Studies of surgical treatment for these patients have had small numbers of patients but have universally yielded dismal results. This select group of patients should benefit from IVF.
Reference: Page 942

8. E (see Table 27.5)
The highest percentage of deliveries per retrieval is associated with donor oocytes, 31.3%.
Reference: Page 945

28 Recurrent Spontaneous Early Pregnancy Loss

Joseph A. Hill

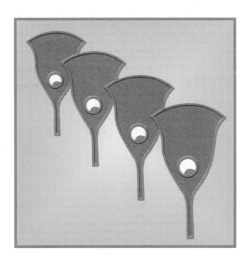

Learning Objectives

1. Understand the potential mechanisms involved in recurrent spontaneous abortion.

2. Be able to differentiate the diagnostic tests and therapies that are potentially useful and effective in treating recurrent spontaneous abortion from those that are not.

3. Be aware of the prognosis for viable birth following documentation of early fetal cardiac activity, as a function of the number of prior pregnancy losses (up to four), and in relation to the potential causes of loss.

4. Develop a caring, empathetic attitude toward the couple experiencing reproductive failure to ameliorate the emotional distress these couples often encounter and to facilitate a rational, cost-effective assessment leading to appropriate consultation and, ultimately, to therapy.

Questions

1. The potential causes of recurrent spontaneous abortion are all controversial **except:**

    A. Parental chromosomal abnormalities
    B. Müllerian anomalies
    C. Luteal phase insufficiency
    D. Antiphospholipid antibodies

2. The diagnostic tests potentially useful in the evaluation of the couple with recurrent spontaneous abortion include all of the following **except:**

    A. Parental peripheral blood karyotypes
    B. Structural study of the intrauterine cavity
    C. Luteal phase endometrial biopsy
    D. Parental HLA profiles and MLC reactivities

3. The following is/are potentially useful in treating women with recurrent spontaneous abortion:

    A. Operative hysteroscopy for an intrauterine filling abnormality
    B. Ovulation induction and/or progesterone supplementation for luteal phase insufficiency
    C. Aspirin and heparin for higher titer anticardiolipin antibody
    D. All of the above

4. The following should be given to treat recurrent spontaneous abortion of undetermined etiology:

    A. Progesterone
    B. *Aspirin* and *heparin*
    C. Intravenous immunoglobulin and/or leukocyte immunization
    D. None of the above

5. The most common single chromosomal abnormality in spontaneous abortion is:

    A. Trisomy 16
    B. 45X
    C. Trisomy 21
    D. Monosomy 3
    E. 47XXY

Answers

1. **A (see Table 28.1)**
Parental chromosomal abnormalities are the only undisputed cause of recurrent abortion. Such abnormalities occur in approximately 5% of couples who experience recurrent pregnancy loss. Other associations have been made with anatomic anomalies (12%), endocrinologic problems (17%), infections (5%), and immunologic factors (50%). Other miscellaneous factors have been implicated and account for 10% of cases. After a thorough evaluation, the potential cause in 60% of cases remains unexplained. Reference: Page 963

2. **D**
Laboratory assessment includes the following:

    1. Parental peripheral blood karyotyping with banding techniques.
    2. Assessment of the intrauterine cavity with either office hysteroscopy or hysterosalpingography, followed by operative hysteroscopy if a potential correctable anomaly is found.

Table 28.1 Proposed Etiologies for Recurrent Spontaneous Abortion

Etiology	Proposed Incidence
Genetic factors	5%
Chromosomal	
Multifactorial	
Anatomic factors	12%
1. Congenital	
a. Incomplete Müllerian fusion or septum reabsorption	
b. Diethylstilbestrol exposure	
c. Uterine artery anomalies	
d. Cervical incompetence	
2. Acquired	
a. Cervical incompetence	
b. Synechiae	
c. Leiomyomas	
d. Endometriosis, adenomyosis	
Endocrine factors	17%
1. Luteal phase insufficiency, including luteinizing hormone disorders	
2. Thyroid disorders	
3. Diabetes mellitus	
4. Androgen disorders	
5. Prolactin disorders	
Infectious factors	5%
1. Bacteria	
2. Viruses	
3. Parasites	
4. Zoonotic	
5. Fungal	
Immunologic factors	50%
1. Humoral Mechanisms	
a. Antiphospholipid antibodies	
b. Antisperm antibodies	
c. Antitrophoblast antibodies	
d. Blocking antibody deficiency	
2. Cellular Mechanisms	
a. TH1 cellular immune response to reproductive antigens (embryo/trophoblast–toxic factors/cytokines)	
b. TH2 cytokine, growth factor, and oncogene deficiency	
c. Supressor cell and factor deficiency	
d. Major histocompatibility antigen expression	
Miscellaneous factors	10%
1. Environmental	
2. Drugs	
3. Placental abnormalities	
a. Circumvallate	
b. Marginate	
4. Medical illnesses	
a. Cardiac	
b. Renal	
c. Hematological	
5. Male factors	
6. Dyssynchronous fertilization	
7. Coitus	
8. Exercise	

3. A well-timed luteal phase endometrial biopsy, ideally 10 days after the LH surge or after cycle day 24 of an idealized 28-day cycle. (If the cycle is abnormal by three or more days, the assessment should be repeated in a subsequent cycle; in out-of-phase biopsies, serum prolactin and androgen profile should be obtained.)

4. Thyroid-functioning testing, including thyroid-stimulating hormone and antithyroid antibodies. (Individuals with antithyroid antibodies may have an increased risk

of developing hypothyroidism in early pregnancy and are at increased risk of developing either postpartum or postabortal autoimmune thyroiditis).

5. Anticardiolipin and antiphosphatidylserine antibodies (IgG and IgM only) and a lupus anticoagulant (a PTT or Russell viper venom).
6. Platelet assessment.
7. Cervical cultures for mycoplasma, ureaplasma, and chlamydia should be considered.

There is no place in the clinical care of couples with recurrent abortion for testing of the following:

1. Antinuclear antibodies
2. Antipaternal cytotoxic antibodies
3. Parental HLA antibodies
4. MLC reactivities

Likewise, other immunologic tests are unnecessary unless they are performed, with informed consent, under a specific study protocol.
Reference: Page 969

3. D

Hysteroscopic resection of intrauterine filling defects represents state-of-the art therapy for submucous leiomyomas, intrauterine adhesions, and an intrauterine septum. Ultrasonographically guided transcervical metroplasty has also been reported to be safe and effective.

Stimulating folliculogenesis with ovulation induction or luteal phase support with progesterone should be considered for women with luteal phase insufficiency.

A combination of low-dose *aspirin* (80 mg/day) and subcutaneous *heparin* (5,000 to 10,000 units twice daily) has been advocated during pregnancy for women with antiphospholipid antibody syndrome. This therapy is not without potential risks, including gastric bleeding, osteopenia, and abruptio placenta. Prednisone has also been advocated but has not been found to offer any advantage over *aspirin* and *heparin*.
Reference: Pages 971–972

4. D

Recurrent spontaneous abortion is a frustrating problem for couples desiring children and often for their physicians. This frustration often renders the physician susceptible to being unsupportive or to recommending tests of little scientific validity and therapies of dubious efficacy. This results in significant emotional and financial costs to the couple who is experiencing recurrent abortion and to unnecessary increases in health care expenditures.

There is no definitive therapy of recurrent spontaneous abortion due to the fact that properly designed double-blind, randomized placebo-controlled trials have not been performed.

Epidemiological surveys indicate that the chance of a viable birth even after four prior losses may be as high as 60%. The live birth rate following documentation of fetal cardiac activity at six weeks of gestation in women with a history of two or more unexplained spontaneous abortions is as high as 77% (Table 28.3).

The ethical duty of every physician is to be sure that the tests and procedures he or she uses are worth the money, inconvenience, and risks involved.

Table 28.3 Prognosis for Viable Birth

Following:	
One abortion	76%
Two abortions	70%
Three abortions	65%
Four abortions	60%
With:	
Genetic factors	20–80%
Anatomic factors	60–90%
Endocrine factors	>90%
Infectious factors	70–90%
Antiphospholipid antibodies	70–90%
TH1 cellular immunity	70–87%
Unknown factors	40–90%
Following:	
Ultrasound detected fetal cardiac activity at 6 weeks of gestation	77%

Unfortunately, an entrepreneurial atmosphere has clouded the rationale care of many couples experiencing reproductive difficulty, resulting in a growing number of financially lucrative immunization clinics. However, no credible clinical or laboratory method exists to identify a specific individual who may benefit from such therapy.

The routine use of immunization therapy for recurrent abortion cannot be justified clinically. Intravenous immunoglobulin administration has been advocated to treat women with unexplained recurrent abortion, although in studies promoting this therapy, patients were neither prestratified by age nor number of prior losses before randomization, nor included in sufficient numbers to achieve meaningful results.

Progesterone has immunosuppressive effects in doses approaching 10^{-5} mmol/l, but has not been studied in properly designed trials to treat unexplained recurrent abortion.

Neither *aspirin* nor *heparin* has been studied in properly designed trials to treat unexplained recurrent abortion. The potential for adverse side effects further makes their empiric use unwarranted.

A caring, empathetic attitude is prerequisite to healing. The acknowledgment of the pain and suffering couples have experienced as a result of recurrent abortion can be a cathartic catalyst enabling them to incorporate their experience of loss into their lives rather than their lives into their experience of loss. Referral to support groups and counselors should be offered. Self-help measures, including meditation, yoga, exercise, and biofeedback, may also be helpful.
Reference: Pages 970–973

5. **B**

A description of all prior pregnancies and their sequence as well as whether histologic assessment and karyotype determinations were performed are important aspects of taking a history of the recurrent aborter. Approximately 60% of abortuses lost before eight weeks of gestation have been reported to be chromosomally abnormal; most of these pregnancies are affected by a type of trisomy, especially trisomy 16. The most common single chromosomal abnormality is monosome X (45X), especially in anembryonic conceptuses. Aneuploidy may be less likely in recurrent abortions when the couple is euploidic, although this hypothesis is controversial.
Reference: Pages 968–969

29 Menopause

William W. Hurd

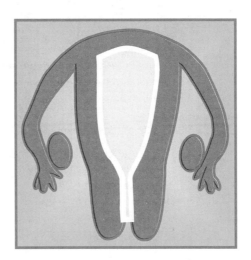

Learning Objectives

1. Understand the perimenopausal phases, including the most common presenting symptoms and health implications.

2. Be aware of the physiologic basis of the symptoms that occur in the perimenopausal period.

3. Understand the relative and absolute contraindications to estrogen replacement therapy.

4. Be aware of the common approaches to hormone replacement therapy.

Questions

1. The following statements are true about the perimenopause **except:**

   A. During the period that immediately precedes menopause, hormonal changes may lead to menstrual irregularity and/or subtle signs of relative estrogen deficiency.

   B. The menopause usually occurs at approximately 51 years of age as a result of a genetically determined depletion of ovarian follicles that are able to respond to gonadotropins.

   C. The menopause occurs earlier in smokers and women who have never had children.

   D. The loss of ovarian function results in absolute estrogen deficiency.

   E. Hormonal replacement therapy is one of the primary concerns of women's health after the menopause.

2. Which one of the following statements is *true* about perimenopausal symptoms:

   A. During the climacteric, the menopause, and the quiescence, the concerns that a woman has may be markedly different from the primarily medical concerns that gynecologists may have.

   B. Depression and irritability occurring in the perimenopausal period are almost always related to low estrogen levels.

   C. Irregular, heavy, or prolonged uterine bleeding are common but of little medical concern in the perimenopausal period.

   D. A decrease in libido is an extremely common symptom after surgical menopause.

   E. Skin changes seen during the quiescence are related solely to age rather than to hypoestrogenemia.

3. The following statements are *true* about estrogen replacement therapy contraindications **except:**

   A. In women with a history of breast cancer, estrogen replacement therapy should be used only with extreme caution.

   B. Estrogen replacement therapy should never be used in a patient with a history of endometrial cancer.

   C. Unopposed estrogen replacement therapy should be avoided in a patient who has undergone a hysterectomy for severe endometriosis.

   D. Estrogen replacement therapy is relatively safe in women with well-controlled hypertension.

   E. A history of thrombophlebitis is not a contraindication to estrogen replacement therapy.

4. Which one of the following statements is *true* about hormone replacement therapy:

   A. Oral estrogen is used only when the patient cannot tolerate the transdermal or vaginal route of administration.

   B. Medroxyprogesterone is by far superior to other available progestins.

   C. Unopposed estrogen is appropriate in a woman with a uterus in some cases.

   D. Androgen therapy should be considered whenever hormone replacement therapy is prescribed.

   E. Continuous low-dose progestin therapy is associated with a significant risk of endometrial hyperplasia.

Answers

1. D

A is correct. The period that precedes menopause is characterized by a varying degree of somatic and psychological changes that reflect alterations in the normal cyclic functioning of the ovary. Early recognition of symptoms and the use of appropriate screening tests can minimize the impact of this potentially disruptive period.

B and C are correct. The menopause occurs at a median age of approximately 51 years. The age of menopause appears to be determined genetically and does not seem to be affected by race or nutritional status. Menopause occurs earlier in cigarette smokers, in some women who have had hysterectomies, and in nulliparous women.

D is incorrect. The loss of ovarian function does not result in an absolute estrogen deficiency. Because of peripheral conversion of androgens of both ovarian and adrenal origin, some women are less affected by estrogen deficiency than others.

E is correct. Even though the long-term health impact of estrogen deficiency may be similar to that of thyroid or adrenal deficiencies, relatively little attention has been paid to this problem. This may be because the health problems associated with estrogen deficiency tend to be chronic rather than acute. For example, osteoporosis is usually not clinically apparent until decades after the menopause, when it is harder to treat. The impact of estrogen deficiency on cardiovascular disease is often confused with age-related changes. Reference: Pages 981–982

2. A

A is true. The loss of fertility and menstrual function that accompany natural and surgical menopause may have an impact on a woman's sense of well-being. The physician should be sensitive to the potentially significant emotional stress faced by these women and be prepared to offer psychological support.

B is false. Studies have failed to show a relationship between clinical depression and hormonal status, suggesting that many psychiatric symptoms that occur during this period may be more related to psychosocial events such as changes in relationships with children, marital status, and other life events. Many women report an increase in anxiety and irritability during the perimenopausal period; thus, these symptoms have become a prominent part of what is sometimes termed the "climacteric syndrome." It is commonly accepted by the lay public that anxiety and irritability are the result of estrogen deficiency. Despite this, multiple studies have found no evidence that most psychological symptoms experienced during the menopausal transition are related to estrogen deficiency or that they resolve with estrogen replacement therapy. The increased anxiety and irritability associated with the perimenopausal period is more clearly associated with psychosocial factors than with estrogen status. It is important to investigate and treat the hormonal status of women who complain of a constellation of symptoms that occur during the menopausal transition. Psychological intervention may be helpful in some women.

C is false. During the climacteric, it has been estimated that menstrual irregularity occurs in more that half of all women. In most cases, uterine bleeding is related to anovulatory cycles. However, pregnancy should also be considered in any menstruating woman, because pregnancies are still reported in the late forties. Of more concern is endometrial cancer, with an incidence of approximately 10% in women with abnormal uterine bleeding. This risk is increased at least fivefold in women with a history of unopposed estrogen use and decreased by more than two-thirds in women taking a combination of estrogen and progestin.

D is false. A major concern is a decrease in libido or a decrease in sexual satisfaction that may occur with natural or surgical menopause. However, sexual activity remains relatively stable in women before and after the menopause. Although only one-half of menopausal women report being sexually active, this may be related to the relative decrease in the number of men in the aging population.

E is false. Estrogen therapy after menopause has been shown to maintain skin thickness. Although mechanisms underlying this effect are ill-understood, a major factor may be the ability of estrogen to both prevent and restore age-related loss of skin collagen. Because changes in collagen may be the major determinant in skin aging, these effects of estrogen may be important.
Reference: Pages 985–987

3. B (see Table 29.2)

A is true. The limited data available suggest no increased risk of recurrent breast cancer among postmenopausal estrogen users. Until more long-term data are available, estrogen should be used with caution in women with a history of breast cancer. In a woman with nonmetastatic (node-negative) estrogen-receptor breast cancer—particularly if she has a strong family history of osteoporosis and heart disease—the benefits of estrogen may outweigh the low theoretic risk that the hormone will predispose her to the development of recurrent cancer.

B is false. Although, theoretically, estrogen and progestin therapy should not increase the risk of recurrent endometrial cancer, there are few data regarding estrogen and progestin therapy in women who have been treated for endometrial cancer. Progestins have been used to treat recurrent endometrial cancer. One study of women successfully treated for a Stage I endometrial cancer revealed that a combination of estrogen and progestin therapy does not increase the risk of recurrence. Because of the limited information available, any woman with a history of endometrial cancer should be informed of the unknown risk of recurrence with hormonal therapy.

C is true. Anecdotal reports do exist of recurrent endometriosis or malignant transformation of endometriosis in women with endometriosis who take estrogen replacement therapy following bilateral oophorectomy. Therefore, these women should be treated with continuous estrogen and a progestin. In women with severe endometriosis, especially when bowel, bladder, or ureter are involved, a hormone-free period for up to six months immediately after surgery may also be advisable prior to instituting combined estrogen and progestin therapy.

D is true. The dose of conjugated estrogens used for estrogen replacement therapy have little effect on blood pressure. Because chronic hypertension is a well-established risk factor for both myocardial infarctions and stroke, women with this disorder should be encouraged to maintain low blood pressure levels and to take advantage of the protective effect of estrogen replacement therapy for cardiovascular disease.

Table 29.2   Indications and Contraindications for Estrogen Replacement Therapy

Indications	*Contraindications*
Menopause	**Absolute**
Hot flashes	Pregnancy
Vaginal atrophy	Undiagnosed uterine bleeding
Urinary tract symptoms	Active thrombophlebitis
High risk for osteoporosis	Current gallbladder disease
Family history	Liver disease
Cigarette smoker	
Low body weight	**Relative**
Radiographic evidence	History of breast cancer
High risk for cardiovascular disease	History of recurrent thrombophlebitis
Previous myocardial infarction/angina	or thromboembolic disease
Hypertension	
Family history	
Cigarette smoker	

E is true. No increased risk of thrombophlebitis associated with estrogen replacement therapy appears to exist. However, no study has addressed the risk of recurrent thrombophlebitis of women taking estrogen. Therefore, women who have a history of thrombophlebitis should be offered estrogen therapy with the understanding that it is unlikely, but uncertain, that this therapy alters the risk of recurrent thrombophlebitis. Reference: Pages 997–999

4. C (Table 29.3)

A is false. In general, oral estrogens are used as the first line of therapy in most women. Transdermal estradiol patches have also been found to be an effective method for hormone administration. However, several potential drawbacks are possible with this approach. On a physiologic level, it is uncertain whether the same benefit is achieved in terms of reduction of cardiovascular disease risks, because changes in lipoprotein profiles do not occur as rapidly as with oral therapy. Transdermal patches are more expensive than oral preparations and result in some skin irritation at the site of placement in one-third of the users. For women in whom oral estrogen therapy does not alleviate symptoms, is poorly tolerated, or in whom oral preparations create a problem with hypertriglyceridemia, estrogen patches may offer some advantage.

B is false. The most common progestin used is *medroxyprogesterone* given orally. However, many progestin formulations have been evaluated for the treatment of irregular bleeding and found to be effective. No single progestin is clearly superior to another. If a woman has significant side effects with one progestin dose, a lower dose or a different progestin formulation should be given.

C is true. Some women requiring estrogen replacement therapy experience intolerable side effects from progestin therapy. If no dose or formulation of progestin can be found that has acceptable side effects for an individual woman, unopposed estrogens may be given. A reasonable approach is the use of the lowest effective dose of estrogen daily coupled with yearly surveillance of the endometrium, since administration of unopposed estrogen is associated with an increased incidence of endometrial hyperplasia and cancer (see Figure 29.2).

D is false. Studies of testosterone administration have shown mixed results in terms of libido improvement. A six-month study of the oral preparation showed an adverse

Table 29.3 Standard Dosages of Commonly Used Estrogens and Progestins

Estrogens	Dosage range
Oral	
Conjugated estrogens	0.625–1.25 mg daily
Ethinyl estradiol	5–10 μg daily
Piperazine estrone sulfate	1.0 mg daily
Micronized 17β-estradiol	0.5–2.0 mg daily
Parenteral	
Transdermal estradiol	0.05–0.10 mg patch twice weekly
Vaginal conjugated estrogens	0.2–0.625 mg, 2–7 times per week
Vaginal 17β-estradiol	1.0 mg, 1–3 times per week
Progestins (Oral)	
Medroxyprogesterone	2.5–5.0 mg daily, or 10 mg 12–14 days/month
Norethindrone	5 mg daily
Norethindrone acetate	1.25–5 mg daily
Norgestrel	0.15 mg daily
Micronized progesterone	100–300 mg daily

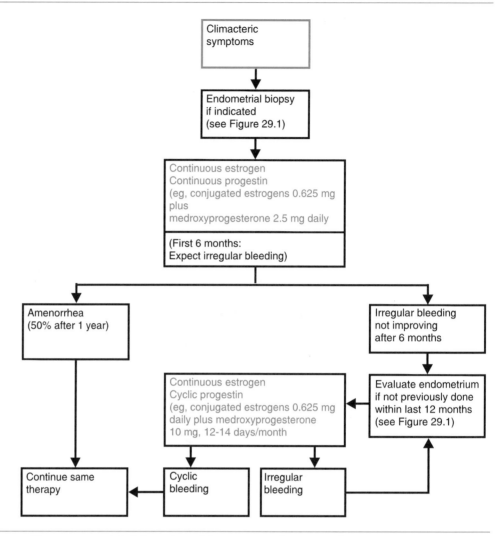

Figure 29.2   Administration of hormone replacement therapy.

effect on the estrogen-induced changes in lipoproteins. Because of a lack of long-term studies of any of these agents, the effects on heart disease and other organ systems are unknown. Until large studies establish a benefit for this type of therapy, androgens should be prescribed with caution. For women who experience decreased sexual responsiveness, appropriate counseling appears to be the most effective therapy.

E is false. Because cyclic progestin therapy may result in symptoms such as breast tenderness, fluid retention, and edema, and psychological symptoms such as anxiety, irritability, or depression, regimens using lower doses of progestins given daily have been developed. Daily progestin therapy (2.5 to 5.0 mg *medroxyprogesterone acetate* or equivalent) protects against endometrial hyperplasia found with cyclic administration at higher doses.
Reference: Pages 999–1001

GYNECOLOGIC ONCOLOGY

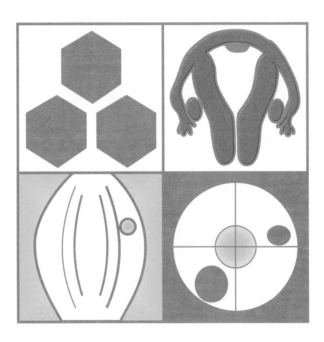

30 General Principles of Cancer Therapy

Robert C. Young
Gillian M. Thomas
Jonathan S. Berek

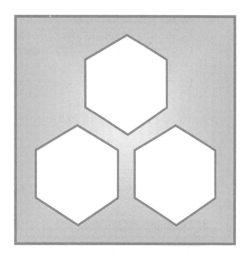

Learning Objectives

1. Be able to provide the scientific and biological rationale upon which cancer chemotherapy is based.

2. Be able to describe the chemotherapeutic agents, their mechanisms of action, toxicities, and spectrum of activity in gynecologic malignancies.

3. Understand the basic principles underlying the use of ionizing radiation in the treatment of malignancy including physics and radiobiology.

4. Be aware of the specific use of radiation therapy and the associated therapeutic ratio in gynecologic malignancies including carcinomas of the cervix, ovary, endometrium, and vulva.

Questions

1. The growth fraction is defined as:

   A. the fraction of growth over a specific interval
   B. the number of tumors that actively grow within a month
   C. the number of cells in the tumor mass that are actively undergoing cell division
   D. the number of tumors that are actively affected by an increase in caloric intake

2. Chemotherapy may not be appropriate in some patients. A situation in which chemotherapy should be omitted is as follows:

   A. the drug causes morbidity
   B. the drug response rate is less than 20%
   C. the doubling time of the tumor is short
   D. the growth fraction of the tumor is high
   E. the malignancy has spread throughout the abdominal cavity

3. The therapeutic index of a drug is defined as the ratio of:

   A. efficacy and toxicity
   B. efficacy over time
   C. toxicity per treatment
   D. cumulative toxicity per patient

4. Methotrexate is a drug which is:

   A. cell cycle specific, proliferation dependent
   B. cell cycle specific, less proliferation dependent
   C. cell cycle nonspecific, proliferation dependent
   D. cell cycle nonspecific, less proliferation dependent

5. A new chemotherapeutic agent is approved for use in the United States. It acts by inhibiting cell division. Which of the following would be *least* likely?

   A. leucopenia
   B. mucosal ulceration
   C. peripheral neuropathy
   D. thrombocytopenia
   E. hair loss

6. The dose intensity of a chemotherapeutic regimen is defined as:

   A. drug (mg)/surface area (M^2)/time (week)
   B. drug (mg)/weight (kg)/time (day)
   C. drug (mg)/height (cm)/time (day)
   D. drug (mg)/time (month)

7. You are asked to care for an elderly (78-year-old) diabetic, hypertensive woman with Stage IIIa epithelial ovarian cancer. She tolerated surgery well and has no residual disease. Which of the following regimens would you select for initial treatment?

   A. no initial therapy
   B. single agent *melphalan*
   C. *cisplatin* and *taxotere*
   D. *cyclophosphamide, hexamethylmelamine, doxorubicin* and *cisplatin*
   E. *carboplatin* and *taxol*

250

8. Conventional external beam radiation therapy is usually given in multiple daily fractions of 180 to 200 cGy per fraction. Why is radiation fractionated over many treatments as opposed to being given in one or two much larger treatments?

   A. A larger number of cancer cells are eradicated with fractionated treatment.
   B. Fractionation allows repair of normal tissues and decreases complications.
   C. Fractionation allows reoxygenation, which improves radiation sensitivity.
   D. A single fraction daily gives the best therapeutic ratio.

9. The rationale for the performance of an operation to define the extent of endometrial cancer before giving postoperative radiation therapy is the:

   A. dose of radiation therapy is much lower
   B. duration of radiation therapy can be shortened
   C. radiation therapy may be used more selectively or omitted
   D. surgery may change the tumor proliferation index and increase hypoxia

10. The inverse square law is defined as the dose of radiation at a given point is:

    A. directly proportional to the square of the dose of radiation
    B. indirectly proportional to the square of the dose of radiation
    C. directly proportional to the square of the distance from the source of the radiation
    D. inversely proportional to the square of the distance from the source of the radiation

11. Radiation therapy for cervical cancer utilizes both external and internal therapy. A useful means of calculating the dose of received radiation is to determine the total dose of radiation at defined points relative to the cervix, specifically "point A" and "point B." Relative to the external cervical os, point A is defined as:

    A. 1 cm lateral and 1 cm superior
    B. 1 cm lateral and 2 cm inferior
    C. 2 cm lateral and 2 cm superior
    D. 3 cm lateral and 3 cm inferior

12. A 42-year-old woman presents with a FIGO Stage IIB carcinoma of the cervix with dimensions of 6 × 4 × 5 cm with infiltration of the right medial parametrium. A retroperitoneal staging laparotomy was performed confirming microscopic involvement of pelvic and para-aoritic nodes at L3 but no intraperitoneal disease. Her radiation therapy should include:

    A. external beam pelvic irradiation
    B. external beam pelvic irradiation plus intracavity irradiation
    C. external beam irradiation to the pelvis and para-aortic nodes plus intracavity irradiation
    D. whole abdominal pelvic irradiation

Answers

1. **C**

   The two major factors that affect the rate at which tumors grow are the growth fraction and cell death. The growth fraction represents the actual number of cells that are actively dividing, and hence, are susceptible to the effects of those chemotherapeutic agents that interfere with cell division. The concept is important because some tumors have a low growth fraction, for example, and are therefore less likely to be affected by the use of some chemotherapeutic drugs.
   Reference: Page 1017

2. B (see Table 30.1)

In a patient whose tumor has a low response rate and no expectation of cure, especially if the patient is in poor general health, it is reasonable to omit chemotherapy. Chemotherapy works best, in general, when the doubling time is short and the growth fraction is high. All chemotherapy has morbidity—it is merely a matter of what kind and how much. In patients with ovarian cancer, diffuse peritoneal carcinomatosis is an appropriate indication for chemotherapy.
Reference: Page 1016

3. A

The therapeutic index of a specific chemotherapeutic agent is the efficacy of the drug relative to the toxicity. For example, if a particular combination of drugs (A) is compared with another combination (B), and A is equally effective as B, but it is more toxic, than the therapeutic index of B is greater than A.
Reference: Page 1018

4. B (see Tables 30.2and 30.3)

The antimetabolite, *methotrexate*, is a cell cycle specific drug because its primary mode of action requires cell division. It is not dependent on the proliferative capacity of the tissue involved.
Reference: Page 1019

5. C

Chemotherapeutic agents that inhibit cell division are cell cycle specific and proliferation dependent and, as such, preferentially effect rapidly proliferating cell populations such as bone marrow, gastrointestinal mucosa, and the epidermis. As a result, one can anticipate toxicity in rapidly proliferating tissues such as the bone marrow (A and D), the gastrointestinal tract (B), and the epidermis (E).
Reference: Page 1019

6. A

The dose intensity is a concept used to compare the amount of one drug given over time to that of another drug, patient, or group of patients. The concept is important because it permits such comparisons, but also because it helps to determine whether higher dose intensities correlate with higher response rates. Drugs may be given at a variety of different dose intensities to determine if the higher doses (typically associated with more side effects) produce a higher response rate. It may be appropriate to give higher dose

---

Table 30.1   Issues To Be Considered Before Using Antineoplastic Drugs

---

1. *Natural History of the Particular Malignancy*
   a. Diagnosis of a malignancy made by biopsy
   b. Rate of disease progression
   c. Extent of disease spread

---

2. *Patient's Circumstances and Tolerance*
   a. Age, general health, underlying diseases
   b. Extent of previous treatment
   c. Adequate facilities to evaluate, monitor, and treat potential drug toxicities
   d. The patient's emotional, social, and financial situation

---

3. *Likelihood of Achieving a Beneficial Response*
   a. Cancers in which chemotherapy is curative in some patients, e.g., ovarian germ cell tumors
   b. Cancers in which chemotherapy has demonstrated improvement in survival, e.g., epithelial ovarian cancer
   c. Cancers that respond to treatment but in which improved survival has not been clearly demonstrated, e.g., cervical cancer
   d. Cancers with marginal or no response to chemotherapy, e.g., melanoma

---

Table 30.2 Cell Cycle-Specificity of Chemotherapeutic Agents

Classification	Examples
Cell cycle specific, proliferation dependent	Hydroxyurea, Ara-C
Cell cycle specific, less proliferation dependent	5-FU, methotrexate
Cell cycle nonspecific, proliferation dependent	Cytoxan, actinomycin D, cisplatin
Cell cycle nonspecific, less proliferation dependent	Nitrogen mustard

Ara-C, cytosine arabinoside; 5-FU, 5-fluorouracil.

Table 30.3 Site of Action in the Cell Cycle

Portion of Cell Cycle	Drugs
G_1	Actinomycin D
Early S	Hydroxyurea, Ara-C, 5-FU, methotrexate
Late S	Doxorubicin, daunomycin
G_2	Bleomycin, etoposide, teniposide
M	Vincristine, vinblastine

Ara-C, cytosine arabinoside; 5-FU, 5-fluorouracil.

intensity at the expense of higher toxicity if there is a substantial gain in response. For many drugs, dose intense regimens do not produce significantly higher response rates.
Reference: Page 1020

7. E
Although some rationale could be given for each of the regimens listed, the selection of appropriate chemotherapy is always a balance between the risks and benefits. In an elderly patient, especially one with diabetes and hypertension, the risk and potential injury from neurotoxic or cardiotoxic agents is great. This makes the use of *cisplatin* and *hexamethylmelamine* less attractive. The potential for cardiovascular compromise make *doxorubicin* and *taxotere* less attractive. Finally, the strong evidence of a survival benefit from modern combination chemotherapy make no therapy unacceptable and single agent *melphalan* inadequate.
Reference: Pages 1023–1030

8. B and C
Fractionated radiation therapy eradicates less cells than the same total dose when given in a single treatment (Figure 30.1). Fractionation of radiation allows the repair of normal tissues between treatments and thus decreases complications. It additionally allows for hypoxic tumors to reoxygenate and become more sensitive to radiation.
Reference: Pages 1034–1035

9. C
The rationale for combining surgery and radiation therapy is based on several theoretic assumptions (Table 30.7). The rationale for the performance of surgery prior to radiation therapy in endometrial cancer is so the disease can be staged, the extent of the disease can be documented, and the radiation can be administered selectively. In some patients, the radiation can be eliminated, and in others, the surgery is used to define the extent of disease (e.g., the para-aortic lymph nodes) so that extended-field radiation can be administered.
Reference: Page 1039

10. D
This important "law" of radiation biology underscores the premise of brachytherapy, i.e., the use of radiation implants. The dose at the distance from the radiation source is

determined by the inverse square law. Thus, in cervical cancer, the tumor can be treated with an implant so that the tumor receives high doses while the tissues several centimeters away receive a much lower dose. In this manner, the treatment minimizes the potential damage to the normal surrounding tissues.
Reference: Page 1044

11. C

Point A is defined by convention as 2 cm lateral and superior to the cervical os. It is used to determine the anticipated dose delivered to the parametria. Point B is 3 cm lateral to point A and corresponds to the pelvic sidewall. Therefore, this gives a practical means of calculating the dose at the pelvic sidewall.
Reference: Pages 1047–1048

12. C

A proportion of patients with disease in the para-aortic nodes in addition to known pelvic disease may be cured with extended field irradiation, thus the radiation field should include the involved para-aortic nodes. Additionally, intracavitary irradiation is critical to bring the pelvic radiation doses to a sufficiently high level to eradicate bulky pelvic disease. These include a dose at point A of approximately 8500 cGy, and a dose on the pelvic sidewall of approximately 6000 cGy. Whole abdominal pelvic irradiation for cervical cancer is unlikely to be curative since the doses required to sterilize bulky cervical cancer are in excess of those tolerated by the large volume irradiated when pelvic and whole abdominal irradiation is prescribed, as in ovarian cancer.
Reference: Pages 1046, 1048

31

Uterine Cancer

John R. Lurain

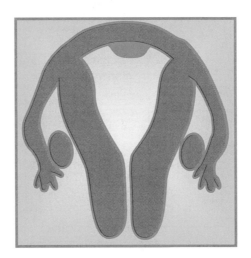

Learning Objectives

1. Understand the epidemiology, risk factors, screening principles, and methods for diagnosis of uterine cancers.

2. Know the different types of endometrial hyperplasias, cancers, and sarcomas, and their natural history.

3. Learn the FIGO surgical staging system for endometrial cancers and be able to identify important prognostic factors.

4. Develop a logical plan for the surgical and postoperative management of endometrial cancers.

Questions
Multiple Choice

1. A 58-year-old, 252-pound, nulliparous woman with diabetes mellitus and a history of irregular menses most of her life until menopause at age 55 is at increased risk for the development of endometrial cancer. The factor which places her at greatest risk is:

   A. Obesity
   B. Nulliparity
   C. Diabetes mellitus
   D. History of irregular menses
   E. Late menopause

2. The recommended follow-up for women with breast cancer receiving tamoxifen therapy is:

   A. Periodic endometrial biopsy
   B. Periodic endovaginal ultrasound
   C. Periodic progesterone challenge test
   D. Endometrial biopsy only for evaluation of abnormal physical examination findings, symptoms (e.g., bleeding), or Pap test results
   E. Prophylactic total abdominal hysterectomy and bilateral salpingo-oophorectomy

3. A 62-year-old woman presents with two days of light vaginal bleeding. She is otherwise asymptomatic and not on hormone replacement therapy. Physical examination is normal except for atrophic cervicovaginal changes. The uterus sounds to 7 centimeters. Aspiration endometrial biopsy yields very little tissue. The pathology report notes mostly mucus and blood with a few fragments of atrophic endometrium. The most likely cause of postmenopausal bleeding in this patient is:

   A. Atrophic vagina
   B. Endometrial atrophy
   C. Endometrial polyps
   D. Endometrial hyperplasia
   E. Endometrial cancer

4. A 52-year-old perimenopausal woman presents with irregular bleeding. An endometrial biopsy shows complex hyperplasia without cytologic atypia. The most appropriate therapy for this patient would be:

   A. Observation
   B. Hysteroscopy
   C. Estrogen therapy
   D. Progestin therapy
   E. Hysterectomy

5. The histologic type of endometrial cancer with the worst prognosis is:

   A. Endometrioid carcinoma with squamous differentiation
   B. Villoglandular
   C. Secretory
   D. Papillary serous
   E. Mucinous

6. A 69-year-old woman is found to have a moderately differentiated endometrial adenocarcinoma on endometrial biopsy done to evaluate postmenopausal bleeding. Physical examination reveals an enlarged uterus which sounds to 10 centimeters. A chest x-ray is within normal limits. The patient undergoes total abdominal hysterectomy, bilateral

salpingo-oophorectomy, and pelvic and para-aortic lymph node sampling. Abdominal exploration is negative. Surgical pathology demonstrates full-thickness myometrial invasion of a poorly differentiated endometrial adenocarcinoma to the uterine serosa; lymph nodes, adnexa, and peritoneal cytology are negative for malignancy. According to the 1988 International Federation of Gynecology and Obstetrics (FIGO) staging system, the patient's endometroid cancer is classified as:

A. Ib G2
B. Ic G3
C. IIIa G3
D. IIIc G3

7. An 81-year-old woman undergoes exploratory laparotomy, total abdominal hysterectomy, bilateral salpingo-oophorectomy, and pelvic and para-aortic lymph node sampling. She is found to have a 2 centimeter, moderately differentiated endometrioid adenocarcinoma with approximately one-third myometrial invasion, negative lymph nodes, and negative peritoneal cytology. What prognostic factor most significantly increases her risk of recurrence?

A. Age
B. Histologic type
C. Tumor grade
D. Myometrial invasion
E. Tumor size

8. A 68-year-old with grade 3 endometrial adenocarcinoma found on endometrial curettage undergoes exploratory laparotomy with total abdominal hysterectomy and bilateral salpingo-oophorectomy, as well as pelvic and para-aortic lymph node sampling. Histopathologic examination reveals a grade 3 endometrioid adenocarcinoma, 80% myometrial invasion, lymphvascular-space invasion, negative lymph nodes, and negative peritoneal cytology. The most commonly employed postoperative treatment plan for this patient with stage Ic G3 disease is:

A. Careful follow-up
B. Vaginal cuff irradiation
C. Irradiation of the pelvis and upper vagina
D. Whole abdomen irradiation
E. Chemotherapy

9. A 59-year-old undergoes total abdominal hysterectomy, bilateral salpingo-oophorectomy, and pelvic and para-aortic lymph node sampling for an endometrial adenocarcinoma. She is found to have a grade 3 tumor, deep (greater than 1/2) myometrial invasion, and microscopically positive para-aortic and pelvic lymph nodes, but no other evidence of disease including negative peritoneal cytology. She subsequently receives extended field irradiation to the pelvis and para-aortic lymph nodes. Five-year survival for her surgical stage of disease (IIIc G3) is approximately:

A. 75%
B. 65%
C. 45%
D. 20%

10. A 61-year-old woman has recently undergone total abdominal hysterectomy, bilateral salpingo-oophorectomy, and lymph node sampling followed by vaginal cuff irradiation for stage Ib G2 adenocarcinoma of the endometrium. Appropriate posttreatment surveillance should include each of the following **except:**

A. Physical examination every three to four months for two to three years, then every six months

B. Vaginal cytology (Pap test) at each visit

C. Chest x-ray every 6 to 12 months

D. Computed tomography (CT) scans yearly

Matching

11–14. For each of the patients described below, select the uterine sarcoma that is the most likely diagnosis.

A. Malignant mixed müllerian tumor

B. Leiomyosarcoma

C. Leiomyomatosis peritonealis disseminata

D. Low-grade stromal sarcoma

11. A 40-year-old woman undergoes hysterectomy for an enlarged uterus and abnormal uterine bleeding. At surgery, the uterus is filled with soft, gray-white tumors with bulging surfaces associated with worm-like elastic extensions into the pelvic veins.

12. A 54-year-old, postmenopausal African-American woman presents with a rapidly enlarging uterus causing pelvic pain and pressure.

13. A 62-year-old woman with a history of pelvic irradiation for cervical cancer 20 years earlier presents with postmenopausal bleeding, vaginal discharge, and pelvic pain. She is discovered to have a polypoid mass protruding from the endocervical canal.

14. At the time of cesarean section, a 32-year-old is found to have nodules scattered throughout the peritoneal cavity on peritoneal surfaces.

Answers
Multiple Choice

1. A (see Table 31.1)

Most risk factors for the development of endometrial cancer are related to prolonged, unopposed estrogen stimulation of the endometrium. The risk of endometrial cancer is increased 3 times for women who are 21 to 50 pounds overweight, and 10 times for those who are more than 50 pounds overweight (excess estrone as a result of peripheral conversion of adrenally derived androstenedione by aromatization in fat). Nulliparous women have 2 to 3 times the risk of parous women. Infertility and a history of irregular menses, as a result of anovulatory cycles (prolonged exposure to estrogen without sufficient progesterone) increases the risk. Natural menopause occurring after age 52 increases the risk of endometrial cancer 2.4 times compared with women in whom menopause occurred before 49 years of age, probably as a result of prolonged exposure of the uterus to progesterone-deficient menstrual cycles. Diabetes mellitus increases a woman's risk of endometrial cancer by 1.3 to 2.8 times. Other medical conditions such as hypertension and hypothyroidism have been associated with endometrial cancer, but a causal relationship has not been confirmed. Other factors leading to long-term estrogen exposure, such as polycystic ovary syndrome, functioning ovarian tumors, and menopausal estrogen replacement therapy, also are associated with an increased risk of endometrial cancer.

Reference: Page 1058

2. D

It has been noted that the use of the antiestrogen *tamoxifen* for treatment of breast cancer is associated with a two- to threefold increased risk for the development of en-

Table 31.1   Risk Factors for Endometrial Cancer

Characteristic	Relative Risk
Nulliparity	2–3
Late menopause	2.4
Obesity	
21–50 lbs	3
>50 lbs	10
Diabetes mellitus	2.8
Unopposed estrogen therapy	4–8
Tamoxifen	2–3
Atypical endometrial hyperplasia	8–29

dometrial cancer. Although this and many other risk factors for endometrial cancer, such as obesity, nulliparity, diabetes mellitus, and postmenopausal estrogen replacement therapy, have been identified, screening for endometrial cancer should *not* be undertaken because of the lack of an appropriate, cost-effective, and acceptable test that reduces mortality. Routine Pap testing is inadequate and endometrial cytologic assessment is too insensitive and nonspecific to be useful in screening for endometrial cancer, even in a high-risk population. A progesterone challenge test will reveal whether the endometrium has been primed by estrogen, but it will not identify abnormal uterine pathology. Transvaginal ultrasound examination of the uterus and endometrial biopsy are too expensive to be employed as screening tests, and endovaginal ultrasound will yield many false positive results.

Even if an appropriate screening test were available, screening of high-risk individuals could at best detect only 50% of all cases of endometrial cancer. Furthermore, no controlled trials have been carried out to evaluate the effectiveness of screening in endometrial cancer. Fortunately, most patients who have endometrial cancer present with abnormal perimenopausal or postmenopausal uterine bleeding early in the development of the disease, when the tumor is still confined to the uterus. Endometrial biopsy performed in this situation usually results in early diagnosis, timely treatment, and a high cure rate. This obviates the need for prophylactic hysterectomy in high-risk patients. Reference: Pages 1059, 1061

3. B (see Table 31.3)

Abnormal perimenopausal or postmenopausal bleeding should always be taken seriously and should be investigated no matter how minimal or nonpersistent. Causes may be nongenital, genital, extrauterine, or uterine. Nongenital tract sites should be considered based on the history or examination, including testing for blood in the urine and stool. Invasive tumors of the cervix, vagina, and vulva are usually evident on examination, and any tumors discovered should be biopsied. Traumatic bleeding from an *atrophic vagina* may account for up to 15% of all causes of postmenopausal bleeding. This diagnosis can be considered if inspection reveals a thin, friable vaginal wall, but the possibility of a uterine source of bleeding first must be eliminated.

Table 31.3   Causes of Postmenopausal Uterine Bleeding

Cause of Bleeding	Frequency (%)
Endometrial atrophy	60–80
Estrogen replacement therapy	15–25
Endometrial polyps	2–12
Endometrial hyperplasia	5–10
Endometrial cancer	10

Possible uterine causes of peri- or postmenopausal bleeding include endometrial atrophy, endometrial polyps, estrogen replacement therapy, hyperplasia, and carcinoma or sarcoma. Uterine leiomyomas should never be accepted as a cause of postmenopausal bleeding. *Endometrial atrophy* is the most common endometrial finding in women with postmenopausal bleeding, accounting for 60 to 80% of such bleeding. Women with endometrial atrophy usually have been menopausal for about 10 years. Endometrial biopsy often yields insufficient tissue or only blood and mucus, and there is usually no additional bleeding after biopsy. *Endometrial polyps* account for 2 to 12% of postmenopausal bleeding. Polyps are often difficult to identify with office endometrial biopsy or curettage. Hysteroscopy, transvaginal ultrasound, or both may be useful adjuncts in identifying endometrial polyps, which may cause continued or recurrent bleeding. *Estrogen therapy* is an established risk factor for endometrial hyperplasia and cancer and may be responsible for 15 to 25% of all causes of postmenopausal bleeding.

Endometrial biopsy should be performed to assess unscheduled bleeding or annually in women not taking a progestin. *Endometrial hyperplasia* occurs in 5 to 10% of patients with postmenopausal uterine bleeding. Only approximately 10% of patients with postmenopausal bleeding have *endometrial cancer*.
Reference: Page 1062

4. D (see Table 31.2)

Endometrial hyperplasias usually evolve within a background of proliferative endometrium as a result of protracted estrogen stimulation in the absence of progestin influence. Endometrial hyperplasias are important clinically because they may precede or occur simultaneously with endometrial cancer.

The risk of endometrial hyperplasia progressing to carcinoma is related to the presence and severity of cytologic atypia. Progression to carcinoma occurs in 1% of patients with simple hyperplasia, 3% of patients with complex hyperplasia, 8% of patients with atypical simple hyperplasia, and 39% of patients with atypical complex hyperplasia. Observation only, diagnostic hysteroscopy, and estrogen therapy would *not* be appropriate therapy.

Progestin therapy is very effective in reversing endometrial hyperplasia without atypia, but is less effective for endometrial hyperplasia with atypia. For women with endometrial hyperplasia without atypia, ovulation induction, cyclical progestin therapy (e.g., *medroxyprogesterone acetate* 10–20 mg/day for 14 days per month), or continuous progestin therapy (e.g., *megestrol acetate* 20–40 mg daily) all seem to be effective therapies. Continuous progestin therapy with *megestrol acetate* 40 mg daily is probably the most reliable treatment for reversing complex or atypical hyperplasia. Therapy should be continued for 2 to 3 months, and endometrial biopsy should be performed at the completion of therapy to assess response. Periodic endometrial biopsy and/or transvaginal ultrasound is advisable, especially in patients treated for atypical hyperplasia, because of the high recurrence rate. In patients with atypical complex hyperplasia de-

Table 31.2   Classification of Endometrial Hyperplasias

Type of Hyperplasia	Progression to Cancer (%)
Simple (cystic without atypia)	1
Complex (adenomatous without atypia)	3
Atypical	
Simple (cystic with atypia)	8
Complex (adenomatous with atypia)	29

Reproduced with permission from **Kurman RJ, Kaminski PF, Norris HJ.** The behavior of endometrial hyperplasia: a long term study of "untreated" hyperplasia in 170 patients. *Cancer* 1985;56:403–12.

tected in an endometrial biopsy or curettage specimen, approximately 25% will have an associated, usually well-differentiated, endometrial carcinoma if a hysterectomy is performed. Therefore, hysterectomy is advised for patients with complex hyperplasia with significant cytologic atypia, a high mitotic rate, and marked cellular stratification. Reference: Pages 1059–1061

5. D (see Table 31.4)
Endometrioid-type adenocarcinomas account for approximately 80% of endometrial carcinomas. The clinical behavior of these tumors is generally related to their differentiation expressed as grade, which is determined by architectural growth pattern and nuclear features. Approximately 15 to 25% of *endometrioid carcinomas have areas of squamous differentiation*. The behavior of these tumors is largely dependent on the grade of the glandular component. A *villoglandular* configuration is present in approximately 2% of endometrioid carcinomas. These are always well-differentiated lesions that behave like the regular endometrioid carcinomas and should be distinguished from papillary serous carcinomas. *Secretory carcinoma* is a rare variant of endometrioid carcinoma that accounts for about 1% of cases. It occurs mostly in early postmenopausal women. The tumors are composed of well-differentiated glands with intracytoplasmic vacuoles similar to early secretory endometrium, and therefore, must be distinguished from the very aggressive clear-cell carcinomas, which also have predominantly clear cells. Secretory carcinomas behave as regular well-differentiated endometrioid carcinomas and generally have an excellent prognosis. Approximately 5% of endometrioid carcinomas have a predominant *mucinous* pattern in which more than 50% of the tumor is composed of cells with intracytoplasmic mucin. Most of these tumors have a well-differentiated glandular pattern; their behavior is similar to common endometrioid carcinomas and their prognosis is good. *Uterine papillary serous carcinomas* (UPSC), which resemble serous carcinomas of the ovary and fallopian tube, make up approximately 3 to 4% of endometrial carcinomas. They are all considered high-grade lesions, even when mixed with other histologic patterns. Serous carcinomas are often associated with lymph-vascular space and deep myometrial invasion; however, even when these tumors appear to be confined to the endometrium or endometrial polyps, they behave more aggressively than endometrioid carcinomas. They also have a propensity to spread intra-abdominally, simulating the behavior of ovarian carcinoma.
Reference: Pages 1063–1067

Table 31.4   Classification of Endometrial Carcinomas

Endometrioid adenocarcinoma
Usual type
Variants
Villoglandular/papillary
Secretory
With squamous differentiation
Mucinous carcinoma
Papillary serous carcinoma
Clear cell carcinoma
Squamous carcinoma
Undifferentiated carcinoma
Mixed carcinoma

6. C

Clinical staging of endometrial carcinoma according to FIGO 1971 should be performed only in patients who are deemed unsuitable candidates for surgery either because of their poor medical condition or the spread of their disease. This patient has clinical stage Ib G2 disease based on her preoperative assessment. In 1988, FIGO adopted a surgical staging system (see Appendix) because of the poor correlation between the preoperative evaluation and clinical staging with the surgical and pathologic findings. Most patients with endometrial cancer should now undergo surgical staging. At a minimum, the surgical procedure should include sampling of peritoneal fluid for cytologic evaluation, exploration of the abdomen and pelvis with biopsy or excision of any extrauterine lesions suggestive of metastatic cancer, extrafascial hysterectomy, and bilateral salpingo-oophorectomy. The uterine specimen should be opened in the operating room and the tumor size, depth of myometrial involvement, and cervical extension should be assessed. Any suspicious pelvic and para-aortic lymph nodes should be removed for pathologic examination. Additionally, clinically negative retroperitoneal lymph nodes should be sampled in all patients with poorly differentiated tumors, deep myometrial invasion, isthmus-cervix extension, tumor size greater than 2 centimeters, or extrauterine disease.

This patient has a poorly differentiated (G3) tumor invading the uterine serosa, and her disease is, therefore, staged as FIGO IIIa G3. Other criteria for stage IIIa disease are positive peritoneal cytology or adnexal spread. Stage Ic connotes deep myometrial invasion without cervical or extrauterine disease. Metastases to pelvic or para-aortic lymph nodes or both indicates Stage IIIc disease.
Reference: Page 1069

7. A (see Tables 31.11 and 31.12; Figure 31.5)

Although the stage of disease is the most significant variable affecting survival, a number of individual prognostic factors for disease recurrence or survival have been identified, including patient age, tumor histopathology and grade, depth of myometrial in-

---

Table 31.11   Surgical-Pathologic Findings in Clinical Stage I Endometrial Cancer

Surgical-Pathologic Finding	*Percentage*
Histology	
Adenocarcinoma	80
Adenosquamous	16
Other (papillary serous, clear cell)	4
Grade	
1	29
2	46
3	25
Nyometrial invasion	
None	14
Inner one-third	45
Middle one-third	19
Outer one-third	22
Lymph-vascular space invasion	15
Isthmic tumor	16
Adnexal involvement	5
Positive peritoneal cytology	12
Pelvic lymph node metastasis	9
Aortic lymph node metastasis	6
Other extrauterine metastasis	6

Modified from **Creasman WT, Morrow CP, Bundy BN, Homesley HD, Graham JE, Heller PB.** Surgical pathologic spread patterns of endometrial cancer. *Cancer* 1987;60:2035–41.

Table 31.12 Prognostic Variables in Endometrial Carcinoma

Age	Lymph node metastasis
Histologic type	Intraperitoneal tumor
Histologic grade	Tumor size
Myometrial invasion	Peritoneal cytology
Lymph-vascular space invasion	Hormone receptor status
Isthmus-cervix extension	DNA ploidy/proliferative index
Adnexal involvement	oncogene amplification/expression

Figure 31.5. The risk of pelvic lymph node metastasis with grade and depth of myometrial penetration in clinical Stage I endometrial cancer. Adjuvant pelvic irradiation is recommended for the high-risk group but not for the low-risk group. (Reproduced with permission from **DiSaia PJ, Creasman WT.** Management of endometrial adenocarcinoma, stage I with surgical staging followed by tailored adjuvant radiation therapy. *Clin Obstet Gynecol* 1986;13:751.)

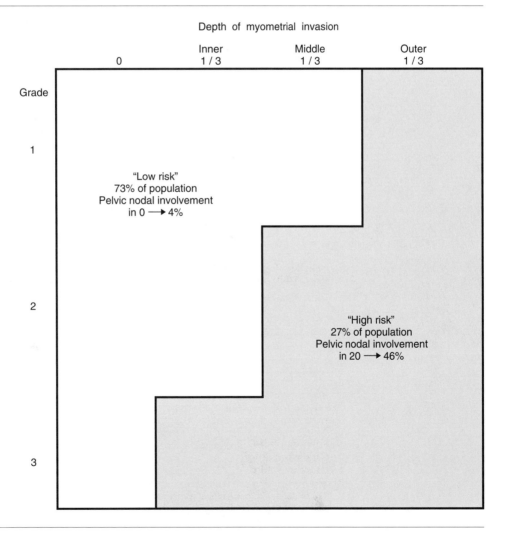

vasion, and surgical- pathologic evidence of extrauterine disease spread. Other factors such as tumor size, peritoneal cytology, hormone receptor status, flow cytometry, and oncogene perturbations have also been implicated as having prognostic importance.

In general, older women with endometrial cancer have a poorer prognosis than younger women. This is related in part to a higher incidence of grade tumor or unfavorable histologic subtypes in older patients, but increasing patient age has also been found to be independently associated with disease recurrence. Nonendometrioid histologic subtypes, such as papillary serous and clear cell, carry an increased risk of recurrence and distant spread. Increasing tumor grade is associated with deep myometrial invasion, cervical extension, lymph node metastasis, and both local recurrence and distant metastasis. Because access to the lymphatic system increases as cancer invades into the outer one-half of the myometrium, increasing depth of invasion has been associated with increasing likelihood of extrauterine spread and recurrence. Tumor size greater than 2 centimeters is also a significant prognostic factor for lymph node metastasis and survival in patients with endometrioid cancer.
Reference: Pages 1073–1077

Table 31.8   Indications for Selective Pelvic and Para-aortic Lymph Node Dissection in Endometrial Cancer

Tumor histology clear cell, serous, squamous, or grade 3 endometrioid

Myometrial invasion $\geq \frac{1}{2}$

Isthmus-cervix extension

Tumor size >2 cm

Extrauterine disease

Table 31.9   Relationship of Grade to Lymph Node Metastasis in Clinical Stage I Endometrial Carcinoma

Grade	No.	Pelvic Nodes		Aortic Nodes	
		No.	Percentage	No.	Percentage
1	180	5	3	3	2
2	288	25	9	14	5
3	153	28	18	17	11

Reproduced with permission from **Creasman WT, Morrow CP, Bundy BN, Homesley HD, Graham JE, Heller PB.** Surgical pathologic spread patterns of endometrial cancer. *Cancer* 1987;60:2035–41.

Table 31.10   Relationship of Myometrial Invasion to Lymph Node Metastasis in Clinical Stage I Endometrial Carcinoma

Myometrial Invasion	No.	Pelvic Nodes		Aortic Nodes	
		No.	Percentage	No.	Percentage
None	87	1	1	1	1
Inner one-third	279	15	5	8	3
Middle one-third	116	7	6	1	1
Outer one-third	139	35	25	24	17

Reproduced with permission from **Creasman WT, Morrow CP, Bundy BN, Homesley HD, Graham JE, Heller PB.** Surgical pathologic spread patterns of endometrial cancer. *Cancer* 1987;60:2035–41.

8. C (see Tables 31.8, 31.9, and 31.10)

Postoperative therapy should be based on prognostic factors determined by surgical-pathologic staging. Patients with grade 1 and 2 lesions without myometrial invasion have an excellent prognosis and require no postoperative therapy. The incidence of vaginal recurrence in patients with tumors apparently confined to the uterus can be reduced from as high as 15% to as low as 1 to 2% by the administration of vaginal vault irradiation. Patients most likely to benefit from vaginal irradiation are those who have surgical stage I grade 1 and 2 tumors with superficial (less than 1/2) myometrial invasion, or grade 3 tumors with no invasion, and some patients with stage IIa disease who otherwise meet the aforementioned criteria. Postoperative external pelvic irradiation decreases the risk of recurrence in the pelvis and may also improve survival in certain high-risk groups. Patients found to benefit most from adjuvant postoperative whole pelvis irradiation are those with cervical involvement, pelvic lymph node metastases, pelvic disease outside the uterus (adnexa, parametria), and especially patients with clinical stage I disease who are at significant risk of nodal metastasis (grade 3 tumors with any degree of myoinvasion; grade 1 and 2 tumors with more than one-half myoinvasion; large (greater then 2 centimeters) grade 2 tumors with superficial myoinvasion; and any grade tumor with lymph-vascular space invasion). Whole abdominal radiation therapy is usually reserved for patients with stage III and IV endometrial cancer. It may also be considered for patients who have papillary serous or mixed müllerian tumors, which have a propensity for upper abdominal recurrence. There is no apparent benefit to the use of adjuvant chemotherapy in combination with or in place of radiation therapy in patients at high risk for recurrence or metastasis.
Reference: Pages 1081–1085

9. C (see Figures 31.6 and 31.7; Table 31.14)

Patients with histologically proven para-aortic lymph node metastases who have no other evidence of disease spread outside the pelvis should be treated with extended field irradiation to the entire pelvis, common iliac lymph nodes, and para-aortic lymph nodes. This type of postoperative radiotherapy appears to improve survival, with reported 5-year survival rates ranging from 42 to 59% depending on tumor grade and degree of lymph node involvement.

Survival in surgical stage I disease ranges from more than 95% for stages Ia G1 and Ib GI, to about 90% for stages Ia G2, Ib G2, and Ic G1, to less than 75% for stage Ic G3. Five-year survival is approximately 75% for surgical stage II, 65% for surgical stage IIIa, and 20% for surgical stage IV disease. Overall 5-year survival in endometrial cancer is about 73%.
Reference: Pages 1083, 1091

10. D

History and physical examination remain the most effective methods of follow-up in patients treated for endometrial cancer. Patients should be examined every 3 to 4 months during the first 2 to 3 years and every six months thereafter. Approximately one-half of patients discovered to have recurrent cancer will be asymptomatic, and 75 to 80% of recurrences will be detected initially on physical examination. Particular attention should be given to peripheral lymph nodes, the abdomen, and the pelvis.

Vaginal cytology should be performed at each visit. Although very few asymptomatic recurrences are detected by vaginal cytology, these early recurrences are often amenable to successful therapy. Chest x-ray every 6 to 12 months is an important method of posttreatment surveillance. Almost one-half of all asymptomatic recurrences are detected by chest x-ray. Other radiologic studies, such as intravenous pyelography and CT scans, are not indicated for routine follow-up of asymptomatic patients.
Reference: Page 1091

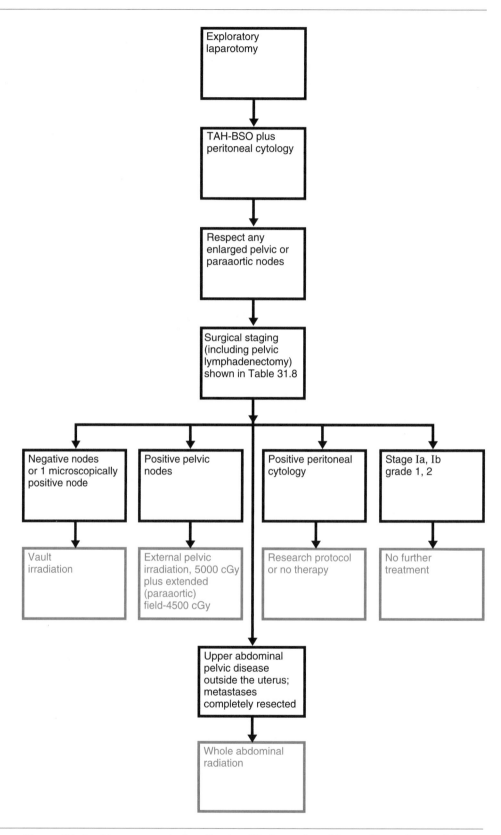

Figure 31.6   Management of patients with Stage I and Stage IIa endometrial carcinoma.

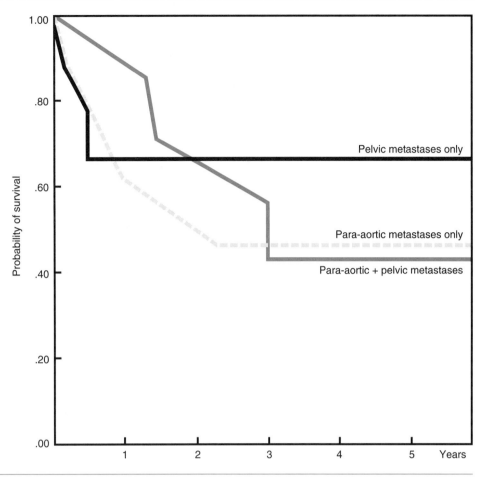

Figure 31.7 Survival of patients with endometrial cancer after extended-field irradiation for surgically confirmed para-aortic lymph node metastasis. (Reproduced with permission from **Potish RA, Twiggs LB, Adcock LL, Savage JE, Levitt SH, Prem KA.** Para-aortic lymph node radiotherapy in cancer of the uterine corpus. *Obstet Gynecol* 1985;65:251.)

Matching

11. D (see Tables 31.18 and 31.19)

12. B

13. A

14. C

Uterine sarcomas are relatively rare tumors of mesodermal origin constituting 2 to 6% of uterine malignancies. The three most common histologic variants of uterine sarcoma are endometrial stromal sarcoma, leiomyosarcoma, and malignant mixed müllerian tumors.

Endometrial stromal tumors occur primarily in perimenopausal women between 45 and 50 years of age. The most frequent symptom is abnormal uterine bleeding. Pelvic examination usually reveals uterine enlargement, sometimes associated with rubbery parametrial induration. At surgery, an enlarged uterus filled with soft, gray-white to yellow necrotic and hemorrhagic tumors with bulging surfaces associated with wormlike extensions into pelvic veins suggests the diagnosis.

Table 31.14   Postoperative Management of Endometrial Carcinoma Based on Surgical-Pathologic Findings and Stage

Surgical-Pathology Findings	Stage	Postoperative Treatment
Low Risk		
G1, G2, no myoinvasion	Ia G1, G2	None
No cervix/isthmus invasion		
Negative peritoneal cytology		
No lymph-vascular space invasion		
No evidence of metastasis		
Intermediate Risk		
G1, G2 less than one-half myoinvasion	Ib G1, G2	Vaginal cuff irradiation
G3, no myoinvasion	Ia G3	
G3, less than one-half myoinvasion	Ib G3	Pelvic vs. vaginal cuff irradiation
G1, G2 isthmus/cervix extension	IIa G1, G2	
G1, G2, G3, more than one-half myoinvasion	Ic G1, G2, G3	Pelvic irradiation plus vaginal cuff boost
G3 isthmus/cervix extension	IIa G3	
G1, G2, G3, cervix invasion	IIb G1, G2, G3 LVSI	
Positive peritoneal cytology	IIIa (+ cytology)	Progestin/^{32}P
High Risk		
Adnexal/serosal/parametrial spread	IIIa G1, G2, G3	Pelvic and vaginal irradiation
Vaginal metastasis	IIIb G1, G2, G3	(extended field radiation therapy if + aortic/common iliac lymph nodes)
Lymph node metastasis	IIIc G1, G2, G3	
Bladder/rectal invasion	IVa	Pelvic and vaginal irradiation
Intraperitoneal spread	IV	Whole abdomen irradiation Systemic chemotherapy

Table 31.18   Classification of uterine Sarcomas

Type	Homologous	Heterologous
Pure	Leiomyosarcoma	Rhabdomyosarcoma
	Stromal sarcoma	Chondrosarcoma
	(i) endolymphatic stromal myosis	Osteosarcoma
	(ii) Endometrial stromal sarcoma	Liposarcoma
Mixed	Carcinosarcoma	Mixed mesodermal sarcoma

Reproduced with permission from **Hacker NF, Moore JG.** *Essentials of Obstetrics and Gynecology.* Philadelphia: WB Saunders, 1986:472.

Table 31.19   AFIP Classification of Endometrial Stromal Tumors

Tumor	Malignant Potential	Cytologic Atypia	Mitoses/10 HPF
Stromal nodule	None	Mild–Moderate (pushing margins)	Less than 10; usually 1–3
Low-grade stromal sarcoma	Low to intermediate	Mild–Moderate (infiltrating margins)	Less than 10; usually 1–3
Stromal sarcoma	High	Moderate–Marked	10 or more

Reproduced with permission from **Zaloubek CJ, Norris HC.** Mesenchymal tumors of the uterus. In: Fengolio C, Wolff M, eds. *Progress in Surgical Pathology.* Vol. 3. New York: Mason Publishing, 1981:1–35.
AFIP, Armed Forces Institute of Pathology.

Low grade stromal sarcoma or endolymphatic stromal myosis is distinguished from the true endometrial stromal sarcoma microscopically by a mitotic rate of less than 10 mitotic figures per 10 high-power fields (10 mf/10 hpf) as well as clinically by a more protracted course characterized by late recurrences, hormone responsiveness, and prolonged survival.

Leiomyosarcomas occur in somewhat younger women (median age 43 to 53 years). There is a higher incidence and a poorer prognosis in African Americans. Presenting symptoms are related to the presence of an enlarged uterus, including pelvic pain and pressure. The diagnosis should be expected if rapid uterine enlargement occurs, especially in a postmenopausal woman. Gross presentation of the tumor at the time of surgery is an important prognostic indicator. Microscopically, the number of mitoses in the tumor seems to be the most reliable indicator of malignant behavior, with tumors having greater than 10 mf/10 hpf being frankly malignant with a poor prognosis. Other histologic indicators of poor prognosis are marked anaplasia, necrosis, and blood vessel invasion.

Leiomyomatosis peritonealis disseminata is a rare clinical entity characterized by benign smooth muscle nodules scattered throughout the peritoneal cavity on peritoneal surfaces. This condition probably arises as a result of metaplasia of subperitoneal mesenchymal stem cells to smooth muscle, fibroblasts, myofibroblasts, and decidual cells under the influence of estrogen and progesterone. Most reported cases have occurred in 30- to 40-year-old women who are or have recently been pregnant or who have a long history of oral contraceptive use. Intriguing features of the disease are its grossly malignant appearance, benign histology, and favorable clinical outcome.

Malignant mixed müllerian tumors are composed histologically of a mixture of sarcoma and carcinoma. Almost all of these tumors occur after menopause, at a median age of 62 years. There is a higher incidence in African-American women. These tumors are often found in association with other medical conditions, such as obesity, diabetes mellitus, and hypertension, as well as a history of previous pelvic irradiation. The most frequent presenting symptom is postmenopausal bleeding. On physical examination, uterine enlargement is present in 50 to 95% of patients, and a polypoid mass may be seen within or protruding from the endocervical canal in up to 50% of patients. Unfortunately, disease has clinically already extended outside the uterus in 40 to 60% of patients at the time of diagnosis, indicating the highly malignant nature of this lesion and contributing to an overall five-year survival of approximately 20 to 30%.
Reference: Pages 1092–1098

32 Cervical and Vaginal Cancer

Anne P. Shapter
Jonathan S. Berek

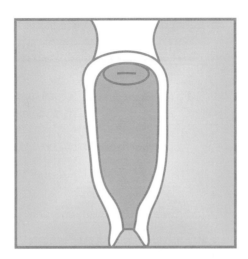

Learning Objectives

1. Be able to identify the histologic characteristics of cervical cancer.

2. Understand the role of colposcopy in the evaluation of cervical lesions.

3. Know the FIGO staging of cervical cancer.

4. Be able to articulate the different treatment modalities for cervical cancer, as well as the advantages and disadvantages of each.

5. Know how to diagnose vaginal cancer.

6. Know the FIGO staging of vaginal cancer.

7. Be able to articulate the different treatment modalities for vaginal cancer, as well as the advantages and disadvantages of each.

Questions

1. Which of the following studies is *not* permitted by FIGO in the determination of stage in patients with cervical cancer?

   A. Intravenous pyelogram (IVP)
   B. Barium enema (BE)
   C. Chest radiograph (CXR)
   D. Computerized axial tomography (CT)
   E. Cervical conization

2. Which of the following types of hysterectomy is a hysterectomy in which the uterine artery is ligated at its origin and in which there is complete removal of the uterosacral and cardinal ligaments are completely removed?

   A. Extrafascial or type I hysterectomy
   B. Modified radical or type II hysterectomy
   C. Radical or type III hysterectomy
   D. Extended radical or type IV hysterectomy
   E. Partial exenteration or type V hysterectomy

3. Which of the following factors has *not* been clearly shown to influence survival after radical hysterectomy and pelvic lymphadenectomy?

   A. The status of the lymph nodes
   B. Tumor size
   C. Involvement of paracervical tissues
   D. Depth of invasion
   E. The presence or absence of lymph vascular space invasion (LVSI)

4. Which of the following treatment modalities is most appropriate in the management of a 30-year-old female diagnosed with a stage Ia2 squamous cell carcinoma of the cervix?

   A. Cervical conization
   B. Type I hysterectomy
   C. Type II hysterectomy without pelvic lymph node dissection
   D. Type II hysterectomy with pelvic lymph node dissection
   E. Radiation therapy

5. Which of the following statistics regarding the treatment of stage Ib cervical cancer is false?

   A. The five-year survival is comparable with primary radical surgery versus primary radiation therapy.
   B. There is a significantly higher urologic fistula rate with radical surgery compared to radiation therapy.
   C. The surgical mortality from radical surgery is approximately the same as that for intracavitary radiation therapy.
   D. Chronic bladder atony occurs in approximately 3% of patients after radical surgery.
   E. Radiation fibrosis of bowel and bladder occurs in 6 to 8% of patients.

6. In the staging of a patient with vaginal carcinoma, extension to the subvaginal tissues is consistent with which of the following stages?

   A. Stage I
   B. Stage II
   C. Stage III
   D. Stage IVa
   E. Stage IVb

7. Which of the following correctly reflects the histologic subtypes of vaginal cancer from most frequent to least frequent?

   A. Squamous cell, adenocarcinoma, melanoma, sarcoma
   B. Squamous cell, melanoma, adenocarcinoma, sarcoma
   C. Adenocarcinoma, squamous cell, melanoma, sarcoma
   D. Adenocarcinoma, squamous cell, sarcoma, melanoma
   E. Squamous cell, sarcoma, melanoma, adenocarcinoma

8. A tumor involving the lower one-third of the vagina and extending to the vulva should be staged as follows:

   A. Stage II vaginal cancer
   B. Stage III vaginal cancer
   C. Stage IVa vaginal cancer
   D. Stage IVb vaginal cancer
   E. At least stage III vulvar carcinoma (T3 lesion)

9. All of the following statements regarding vaginal carcinoma are true **except:**

   A. Approximately 30% of patients with vaginal carcinoma have a history of cervical cancer treated within the five previous years.
   B. Any vaginal cancer diagnosed at least five years after a cervical cancer diagnosis should be considered a new primary.
   C. The most common site of vaginal carcinoma is the upper one-third of the vagina on the anterior wall.
   D. The majority of patients are diagnosed in stages II through IV rather than stage I.
   E. The most common mode of spread is by direct extension.

10. Which of the following statements regarding cervical cancer in pregnancy is false?

   A. Diagnosis is often delayed during pregnancy because bleeding may be attributed to obstetric causes.
   B. If absolutely indicated, cervical conization in pregnancy should be performed in the second trimester.
   C. Patients with more than 5 millimeters of invasion should undergo immediate surgical intervention without consideration of the gestational age.
   D. In advanced stages of disease, radiation therapy should be undertaken, and in the first trimester, spontaneous abortion should be anticipated before the delivery of 4000 cGy.
   E. The diagnosis of cervical cancer in the postpartum period has been associated with more advanced disease and, therefore, decreased survival.

11. A 24-year-woman undergoes a cervical conization after a colposcopically directed biopsy reveals a carcinoma *in situ,* and rules out a microinvasive carcinoma. The cone shows 2 millimeters invasion of a well-differentiated squamous carcinoma. There is no lymph-vascular involvement and the margins are free of disease. She wants to preserve her fertility. The best therapeutic option is:

   A. Observation
   B. Hysterectomy
   C. Repeat conization
   D. Modified radical hysterectomy
   E. Radical hysterectomy

12. A 32-year-old woman has a 5-centimeter cervical lesion. The biopsy shows a poorly differentiated squamous cell carcinoma of the cervix. On clinical assessment, the tumor extends into the right parametrium. The most appropriate therapy is:

A. Pelvic radiation therapy
B. Radical hysterectomy and lymphadenectomy
C. Pelvic radiation therapy followed by chemotherapy
D. Pelvic radiation therapy followed by radical hysterectomy
E. Radical hysterectomy followed by pelvic radiation therapy

13. A 48-year-old woman had undergone pelvic radiation therapy for a stage IIb cervical cancer two years ago, and now presents with vaginal bleeding. The vaginal examination reveals a 3-centimeter central pelvic mass at the vaginal apex. The biopsy is consistent with a recurrent squamous carcinoma. Metastatic evaluation shows no clinical evidence that the disease has spread. The most effective subsequent therapy is:

A. Chemotherapy
B. Radiation therapy
C. Pelvic exenteration
D. Radiation plus chemotherapy
E. Radical hysterectomy and radiation

Answers

1. D

Cervical cancer and vaginal cancer are the two gynecologic malignancies which are currently staged clinically rather than surgically. Once a patient has been assigned to a particular stage, the stage should not be changed. The stage distribution in cervical cancer is as follows: stage I, 38%; stage II, 32%; stage III, 26%; and stage IV, 4%. CT scan, lymphangiography, ultrasonography, magnetic resonance imaging (MRI), radionucleotide scanning, and laparoscopy may all be used in planning treatment but are not allowed by FIGO in the determination of stage. These studies are not universally available throughout the world and, therefore, it is not practical to use them for staging since cervical cancer is the most common gynecologic malignancy worldwide. All of the other diagnostic modalities listed are permissable by FIGO for staging in this malignancy. In addition, physical examination, biopsy, cystoscopy, and proctoscopy are also permitted (see Table 32.2 in Appendix).
Reference: Page 1121

2. C (see Figure 32.8)

The radical hysterectomy (type III hysterectomy) described by Meigs in 1944 includes removal of as much of the uterosacral and cardinal ligaments as possible as well as removal of the upper one-third of the vagina. It also includes ligation of the uterine artery at its origin. Pelvic lymphadenectomy is performed. The type II hysterectomy as described by Wertheim is less extensive and involves removal of the medial one-half of the uterosacral and cardinal ligaments as well as ligation of the uterine artery as it traverses the ureter rather than at its origin. In a type IV hysterectomy, the periureteral tissue, superior vesicle artery, and up to three-fourths of the vagina are removed. The type V hysterectomy or partial exenteration is rarely performed today because of the more widespread availability of radiation therapy.
Reference: Page 1128

3. E (see Figure 32.9)

The status of the lymph nodes has been shown to impact survival in multiple studies. The five-year survival in stage Ib1 cervical cancer is 85 to 90% when the lymph nodes are negative but decreases significantly in the presence of positive nodes. When greater than three positive pelvic nodes are present, the recurrence rate is 68% in contrast to 30

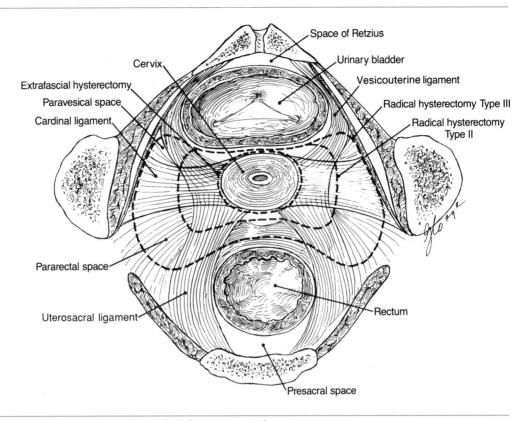

Figure 32.8   The pelvic ligaments and spaces.

Figure 32.9   Radical hysterectomy. Uterine artery is ligated, ureter is dissected, and sites for division of the vesicouterine and uterosacral ligaments are shown.

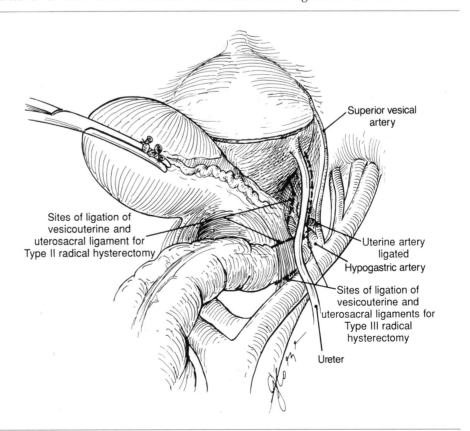

to 50% when less than three nodes are involved. Lesion size has been shown to be an independent predictor of survival with survival rates of approximately 90% with lesions less than 2 centimeters, in contrast to 60% for lesions greater than 2 centimeters. The depth of invasion also influences survival with survival rates significantly decreasing when the depth of invasion is greater than 1 centimeter. The five-year survival is approximately 95% with negative parametrium versus 69% with positive parametrium. The significance of LVSI is somewhat more controversial and LVSI may be more a predictor of lymph node metastasis rather than an independent predictor of survival. Future studies are needed to settle this controversy.
Reference: Pages 1126–1128

4. D (see Tables 32.3 and 32.4)

In a young patient with a stage Ia1 squamous cell cancer of the cervix with no evidence of lymph-vascular space invasion, conization may be adequate treatment provided that margins are negative. The incidence of pelvic lymph node metastases in this setting is less than 1%. If the patient does not desire fertility, she may be treated with type I hysterectomy. If LVSI is present, consideration should be given to performing a type II hysterectomy. In the setting of a stage Ia2 lesion, the incidence of pelvic lymph node metastases is nearly 4% and, therefore, pelvic lymph node dissection is required. A type II hysterectomy is most appropriate. If the patient has a stage Ib lesion (either Ib1 or Ib2), a type III hysterectomy with pelvic lymphadenectomy is appropriate with consideration of para-aortic lymph node evaluation. Surgery is preferrable to radiation therapy in young patients with early-stage disease.
Reference: Pages 1121–1123

5. B (see Table 32.5)

The overall five-year survival is approximately 85% for patients with stage Ib/IIa cervical cancer when treated with either radical surgery or radiation therapy. The choice of treatment is individualized with surgery generally selected for relatively young patients in good health. The urologic fistula rate is approximately 1 to 2% after radical

---

Table 32.3 Incidence of Pelvic and Para-aortic Nodal Metastasis by Stage

Stage	n	% Positive Pelvic Nodes	% Positive Para-aortic Nodes
Ia1 (≤3 mm)	179[†]	0.5	0
Ia2 (>3–5 mm)	84[†]	4.8	<1
Ib	1926[††]	15.9	2.2
IIa	110[§]	24.5	11
IIb	324[§]	31.4	19
III	125[§]	44.8	30
IVa	23[§]	55	40

[†]References 14, 15, 41, 42.
[††]References 4, 23, 28, 29, 31, 33, 35, 50.
[§]References 3, 4, 23, 33, 47, 50.

Table 32.4 Surgical management of Early Invasive Cancer of the Cervix

Stage Ia1	≤3 mm invasion	
	No lymph-vascular space invasion	Conization Type I hysterectomy
	With lymph-vascular space invasion	Type I or II hysterectomy with (?) pelvic lymph node dissection
Stage Ia2	>3–5 mm invasion	Type II hysterectomy with pelvic lymphadenectomy
Stage Ib	>5 mm invasion	Type III hysterectomy with pelvic lymphadenectomy

Table 32.5   Comparison of Surgery Versus Radiation for Stage Ib/IIa Cancer of the Cervix

	Surgery	*Radiation*
Survival	85%	85%
Serious complications	Urologic fistulas 1–2%	Intestinal and urinary strictures and fistulas 1.4–5.3%
Vagina	Initially shortened, but may lengthen with regular intercourse	Fibrosis and possible stenosis particularly in postmenopausal patients
Ovaries	Can be conserved	Destroyed
Chronic effects	Bladder atony in 3%	Radiation fibrosis of bowel and bladder in 6–8%
Applicability	Best candidates are younger than 65 years of age, <200 lb, and in good health	All patients are potential candidates
Surgical mortality	1%	1% (from pulmonary embolism during intracavitary therapy)

surgery and is less than 5% overall after radiation therapy and is therefore not significantly higher with radical surgery. Surgical mortality is approximately 1% with both radical surgery and intracavitary implants and is most commonly related to pulmonary embolism. The most common chronic complication after radical hysterectomy is bladder hypotonia or atony and occurs in approximately 3% of patients.
Reference: Page 1131

6. B

Like cervical cancer, vaginal cancer is clinically staged (see Table 32.6 in Appendix). Cancer of the vagina most often spreads via direct extension and involvement of pelvic lymph nodes may occur in advanced stages of disease. Stage II disease indicates involvement of the subvaginal tissues in the absence of spread to the sidewall of the pelvis. Approximately 75% of patients present in stage II through IV, indicating delay in diagnosis. There is no FIGO category for microinvasive cancer of the vagina as is seen with cervical cancer.
Reference: Pages 1142–1143

7. A

Squamous cell carcinoma is the most common histologic subtype occurring in 80% of vaginal cancers. Like cervical cancer, vaginal carcinoma may have a similar link to the human papilloma virus (HPV). In some cases, invasive vaginal carcinoma may progress from vaginal intraepithelial neoplasia (VAIN) but the true incidence of this progression is not known. VAIN is not felt to have as great a malignant potential as CIN. Approximately 30% of patients with vaginal cancer have a history of cervical cancer treated within the previous five years. Any new vaginal carcinoma diagnosed at least five years after a diagnosis of cervical cancer should be considered a new primary.

Adenocarcinoma of the vagina is the second most common histologic subtype and comprises approximately 9% of all primary vaginal carcinomas. Adenocarcinomas may arise in Wolffian rest elements, periurethral glands, and foci of endometriosis and; in women exposed to DES, adenocarcinomas may arise in vaginal adenosis. Metastatic adenocarcinoma of the vagina may originate from the colon, endometrium, ovary, pancreas, or stomach; in fact, metastatic vaginal adenocarcinoma is more common than primary vaginal adenocarcinoma.

The next most common subtype is melanoma, which is extremely rare. Most of the lesions are deeply invasive at the time of diagnosis and are quite lethal. Vaginal sarcomas are also quite rare and are usually fibrosarcomas or leiomyosarcomas.
Reference: Pages 1141–1146

8. E

The FIGO staging system of gynecologic malignancies mandates that a tumor involving both the vagina and cervix be designated as a cancer of the cervix. Similarly, a tumor involving both the vagina and vulva should be classified as a vulvar cancer. Cancer of the vulva is staged surgically but, at a minimum, a vulvar cancer that extends into the vagina is considered a T3 lesion and is therefore at least a stage III vulvar carcinoma. It may fall into the category of stage IV depending on the status of the nodes on final pathology. If there is no cervical or vulvar involvement of the vaginal cancer, it should then be considered a vaginal carcinoma and should be staged by the FIGO staging system for vaginal cancer (see Table 32.6 in Appendix).
Reference: Page 1141

9. C

The diagnosis of vaginal cancer is usually made after abnormal cytology mandates the pursuit of such a diagnosis. It may also be diagnosed after visualization and biopsy of a gross lesion. The most common site for vaginal cancer is the upper one-third of the vagina on the *posterior* wall. These tumors may be missed when they are in early stages because they may be obscured by the speculum blades at the time of pelvic examination. Colposcopy should be undertaken with abnormal cytology or in the setting of persistent unexplained vaginal bleeding. Unfortunately, a minority of patients are diagnosed in stage I (75% present with stages II through IV), indicating delays in diagnosis. Cancer of the vagina spreads most frequently by direct extension. Metastases to the pelvic and para-aortic lymph nodes may occur in advanced or late disease as does hematogenous spread to lungs, liver, or bone. Lesions in the lower one-third of the vagina may metastasize to the inguinal femoral lymph nodes in addition to the sites described previously.
Reference: Pages 1141–1146

10. C

Cervical cancer is estimated to complicate 1 in 2200 pregnancies. The key to approaching this cancer during pregnancy is individualization with consideration for both mother and fetus. A diagnostic conization may be necessary if there is a high suspicion for malignancy and the diagnosis cannot be made with colpsocopy and biopsy. If required, conization should be performed in the second trimester as the abortion rate may be as high as 33% in the first trimester. If a patient is diagnosed with stage Ib cervical cancer in pregnancy (greater than 5 millimeters of invasion), the timing of treatment depends upon the gestational age and wishes of the patient. If the cancer is diagnosed in the third trimester, fetal pulmonary maturity can be assessed via amniocentesis and therapy undertaken with pulmonary maturity. Treatment should probably not be delayed greater than four weeks and, in the third trimester, consists of cesarean section, radical hysterectomy, and pelvic lymphadenectomy. Conversely, when a patient is diagnosed early in pregnancy, treatment should also not be delayed more than four weeks and radical hysterectomy is generally accomplished without hysterotomy with the fetus *in situ*. When carcinoma of the cervix is diagnosed in the middle of pregnancy, decisions regarding timing of treatment are less clear and again individualization with regard for the wishes of the patient is a most important consideration.
Reference: Pages 1135–1136

11. A

Cervical conization has now become standard treatment for microinvasive carcinoma of the cervix when the patient wishes to preserve fertility. In lesions invasive to less than 3 millimeters without lymph-vascular invasion, the risk of lymph node metastasis is essentially nil.
Reference: Pages 1112–1113, 1122–1123

12. A

The standard treatment for a stage IIb cervical cancer is pelvic radiation therapy. Surgery is contraindicated in such patients. The addition of concurrent or sequential chemotherapy does not clearly improve the outcome.
Reference: Pages 1131–1132

13. C

Pelvic exenteration is used for potentially curable patients whose disease appears confined to the central pelvis. The patient is explored to look for any metastatic disease, and if none is found, then the exenteration is performed. The uterus, cervix, ovaries, tubes, vagina, bladder and if necessary, and, if necessary, the rectosigmoid colon are extirpated.
Reference: Pages 1138–1141

33 Ovarian Cancer

Robert E. Bristow
Jonathan S. Berek

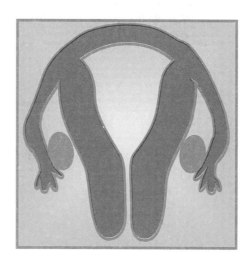

Learning Objectives

1. Understand the principles and surgical techniques involved in staging of epithelial ovarian cancer.

2. Understand the appropriate surgical therapy and indications for surgical staging of germ-cell and sex cord-stromal ovarian malignancies.

3. Understand the genetic transmission of and ovarian cancer risk associated with site-specific familial ovarian cancer, breast-ovarian familial cancer syndrome, and Lynch II syndrome.

4. Know the chemotherapeutic agents used in first-line treatment of epithelial, germ-cell, and sex cord-stromal ovarian cancer and their associated toxicities.

5. Know the clinical factors influencing the prognosis of advanced epithelial ovarian cancer.

6. Be able to identify, based on clinical factors, those patients with recurrent ovarian cancer who are most likely to benefit from secondary cytoreductive surgery.

Questions

1. Which of the following is *not* part of the diagnostic criteria for an ovarian tumor of low malignant potential?

   A. Epithelial proliferation with papillary formation and pseudostratification
   B. Disease confined to one or both ovaries
   C. Nuclear atypia and increased mitotic activity
   D. Abscence of true stromal invasion

2. What is the rate of bilaterality of malignant mucinous carcinomas?

   A. 1 to 2%
   B. 8 to 10%
   C. 20%
   D. 33%

3. What percentage of ovarian neoplasms in postmenopausal women are malignant?

   A. 7%
   B. 20%
   C. 30%
   D. 50%

4. Preoperative testing for a postmenopausal woman with a pelvic mass and suspected ovarian cancer should include all of the following **except:**

   A. Hematologic and biochemical assessment
   B. Chest X-ray
   C. Electrocardiogram
   D. Magnetic resonance imaging of the abdomen and pelvis

5. Which of the following are independent prognostic variables for ovarian cancer?

   A. Stage of disease
   B. Volume of ascites
   C. Extent of residual disease after primary surgery
   D. All of the above

6. Complete surgical staging of those with apparent stage I or II disease will result in the upstaging of what percentage of patients?

   A. 5%
   B. 15%
   C. 30%
   D. 50%

7. The benefits of primary cytoreductive surgery include:

   A. Prolonged progression-free survival
   B. Improved patient comfort
   C. Theoretical enhancement of chemotherapy through cellular kinetic effects
   D. All of the above

8. First-line chemotherapy of choice for advanced epithelial ovarian cancer is:

   A. *Cisplatin, paclitaxel*
   B. *Cyclophosphamide, hexamethylmine, doxorubicin, cisplatin* (CHAP)
   C. *Melphalan*
   D. *Cisplatin, cyclophosphamide*

9. A second-look operation is performed after a prescribed course of chemotherapy to determine the response to therapy on a patient who has:

   A. No clinical evidence of disease
   B. A palpable tumor mass but a negative CA125
   C. No palpable tumor mass but an elevated CA125
   D. A palpable tumor mass and an elevated CA125

10. During the first two decades of life, germ-cell tumors account for what percentage of ovarian malignancies?

    A. 10%
    B. 33%
    C. 66%
    D. None of the above

11. Of germ cell malignancies, bilateral ovarian involvement occurs in 10 to 15% of:

    A. Dysgerminoma
    B. Endodermal sinus tumor
    C. Immature teratoma
    D. Choriocarcinoma

12. Appropriate management of a premenopausal woman with a dysgerminoma apparently confined to one ovary is:

    A. Unilateral salpingo-oophorectomy, ipsilateral pelvic lymph node dissection, and staging
    B. Bilateral salpingo-oophorectomy, bilateral pelvic lymph node dissection, and staging
    C. Karyotype
    D. A and C
    E. B and C

13. Preferred treatment for advanced stage, incompletely resected dysgerminoma is:

    A. three to four cycles of *bleomycin/etoposide/cisplatin* (BEP)
    B. six cycles of *cisplatin/paclitaxel*
    C. three cycles of BEP plus three cycles of *vincristine/actinomycin-D/cyclophosphamide* (VAC)
    D. four cycles of *vinblastine/bleomycin/cisplatin* (VBP)

14. Prognosis of immature teratoma is correlated with the:

    A. Amount of undifferentiated neural tissue
    B. Degree of glandular differentiation
    C. Presence of mature teratoma
    D. Presence of sexual pseudoprecosity

15. A 58-year-old woman undergoes an exploratory laparotomy for an irregularly shaped pelvic tumor. An invasive malignant ovarian cancer is found and she undergoes a total abdominal hysterectomy, bilateral salpingo-oophorectomy, omentectomy, and tumor reductive surgery. All of the macroscopic disease is removed, i.e., she has an "optimally" resected tumor. The diagnosis is a stage IIIb serous adenocarcinoma of the ovary. Based on the current data, of the following chemotherapeutic regimen, which one should be used for this patient:

    A. *Cisplatin, paclitaxel*
    B. *Carboplatin, cisplatin*
    C. *Carboplatin, doxorubicin*
    D. *Cisplatin, cyclophosphamide*

16. A 17-year-old undergoes an exploratory laparotomy for a complex 12-centimeter pelvic tumor. The pathology shows a grade 3 immature teratoma. The staging laparotomy confirms that the disease is a stage Ia tumor. Of the following chemotherapeutic regimens, which one should be administered to this patient:

A. *Cisplatin*
B. *Cisplatin, etoposide*
C. *Cisplatin, etoposide, bleomycin*
D. *Cisplatin, etoposide, bleomycin, methotrexate*

Answers

1. B (see Table 33.1)
Borderline tumors of the ovary, or tumors of low malignant potential, can be unilateral or bilateral. The histologic diagnosis depends on specific criteria, including the presence of papillary formations and pseudostratification. Nuclear atypia is usually seen, as is increased mitotic activity. Lesions lack, however, true stromal invasion, and thus they represent noninvasive, albeit highly proliferative, lesions.
Reference: Pages 1155–1161

2. B
The rate of bilaterality varies depending on the histologic type of the tumor and, importantly, on the stage of the tumor. For apparent low-stage tumors, the rate of bilateral serous tumors is about 5%, whereas for mucinous it is 8 to 10%.
Reference: Pages 1159–1160

Table 33.1	Epithelial Ovarian Tumors	
	Histologic Type	**Cellular Type**
I.	**Serous** A. Benign B. Borderline C. Malignant	Endosalpingeal
II.	**Mucinous** A. Benign B. Borderline C. Malignant	Endocervical
III.	**Endometrioid** A. Benign B. Borderline C. Malignant	Endometrial
IV.	**Clear-Cell "Mesonephroid"** A. Benign B. Borderline C. Malignant	Müllerian
V.	**Brenner** A. Benign B. Borderline ("proliferating") C. Malignant	Transitional
VI.	**Mixed epithelial** A. Benign B. Borderline C. Malignant	Mixed
VII.	**Undifferentiated**	Anaplastic
VIII.	**Unclassified**	Mesothelioma, etc.

Adapted with permission from **Seroy SF, Scully RE, Sobin LH.** *International Histological Classification of Tumours no. 9. Histological Typing of Ovarian Tumors.* Geneva: World Health Organization, 1973.

3. C (see Figure 33.6)

More than 80% of epithelial ovarian cancers are found in postmenopausal women. The peak incidence is 62 years. About 30% of ovarian neoplasms found in postmenopausal women are malignant, compared with only 7% in premenopausal women.
Reference: Page 1163–1164

4. D

The preoperative evaluation of a postmenopausal woman with an adnexal mass should be kept to a minimum. With a few exceptions, these patients warrant surgical exploration, and thus, the tests will add little to the preoperative assessment in the vast majority of women.

Expensive scanning and testing should be kept to a minimum, particularly if there is no clinical suspicion that the pelvic tumor is anything other than an adnexal lesion. The yield on CT scans and MRI scans is low.
Reference: Pages 1166–1167

5. D

These features are each independent variables that have an impact on prognosis. The stage of the disease is highly prognostic, however, within the advanced stage group, the extent of ascites, and the maximum size of the residual disease after cytoreductive surgery correlates with survival. Those patients with stage III disease who have microscopic or small macroscopic (less then 5-millimeter largest tumor diameter) disease have a much longer median survival than those patients whose disease is larger.
Reference: Pages 1168–1171, 1177–1178

Figure 33.6 Ovarian Cancer Incidence: Distribution by age. (Reproduced with permission from *J Natl Cancer Inst* 1995;87(17):1280.

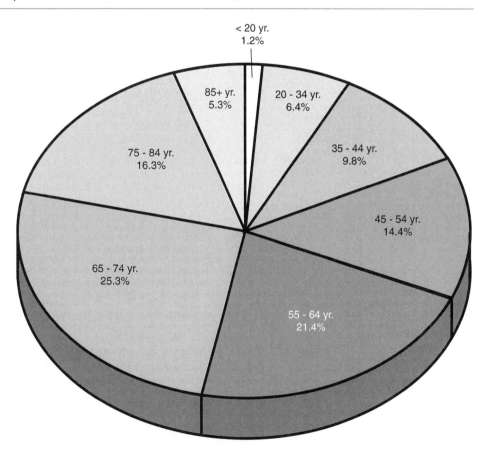

6. C (see Table 33.2 in Appendix)

A comprehensive surgical staging should be performed in patients with epithelial ovarian cancer, i.e., a staging laparotomy, including the aspiration of any free peritoneal fluid, obtaining multiple peritoneal washings, peritoneal biopsies, and the performance of a pelvic and para-aortic lymphadenectomy, and an omentectomy. In doing so, about 30% of patients whose disease appears to be confined to the pelvis (apparent stages I and II) will in fact have microscopic evidence of tumor metastasis. About one-fifth will have positive lymph node metastasis.

Reference: Pages 1169–1171

7. D (see Figure 33.10)

The role of "debulking" surgery or cytoreductive surgery in advanced stage epithelial ovarian cancer is to facilitate the response to subsequent chemotherapy and to survival. There are substantial retrospective and limited prospective data that demonstrate a longer median survival in patients whose disease has been resected so that they have minimal residual or "optimal" residual disease at the initiation of or within a few cycles of chemotherapy.

Reference: Pages 1174–1181

Table 33.2   FIGO Staging for Primary Carcinoma of the Ovary

Stage I		Growth limited to the ovaries.
	Stage Ia	Growth limited to one ovary; no ascites containing malignant cells. No tumor on the external surface; capsule intact.
	Stage Ib	Growth limited to both ovaries; no ascites containing malignant cells. No tumor on the external surfaces; capsules intact.
	Stage Ic*	Tumor either stage Ia or Ib but with tumor on the surface of one or both ovaries; or with capsule ruptured; or with ascites present containing malignant cells or with positive peritoneal washings.
Stage II		Growth involving one or both ovaries with pelvic extension.
	Stage IIa	Extension and/or metastases to the uterus and/or tubes.
	Stage IIb	Extension to other pelvic tissues.
	Stage IIc*	Tumor either stage IIa or IIb but with tumor on the surface of one or both ovaries; or with capsule(s) ruptured; or with ascites present containing malignant cells or with positive peritoneal washings.
Stage III		Tumor involving one or both ovaries with peritoneal implants outside the pelvis and/or positive retroperitoneal or inguinal nodes. Superficial liver metastasis equals stage III. Tumor is limited to the true pelvis, but with histologically proven malignant extension to small bowel or omentum.
	Stage IIIa	Tumor grossly limited to the true pelvis with negative nodes but with histologically confirmed microscopic seeding of abdominal peritoneal surfaces.
	Stage IIIb	Tumor of one or both ovaries with histologically confirmed implants of abdominal peritoneal surfaces, none exceeding 2 cm in diameter. Nodes negative.
	Stage IIIc	Abdominal implants >2 cm in diameter and/or positive retroperitoneal or inguinal nodes.
Stage IV		Growth involving one or both ovaries with distant metastasis. If pleural effusion is present, there must be positive cytologic test results to allot a case to stage IV. Parenchymal liver metastasis equals stage IV.

These categories are based on findings at clinical examination and/or surgical exploration. The histologic characteristics are to be considered in the staging, as are results of cytologic testing as far as effusions are concerned. It is desirable that a biopsy be performed on suspicious areas outside the pelvis.

*In order to evaluate the impact on prognosis of the different criteria for allotting cases to stage Ic or IIc, it would be of value to know if rupture of the capsule was 1) spontaneous or 2) caused by the surgeon and if the source of malignant cells detected was 1) peritoneal washings or 2) ascites.

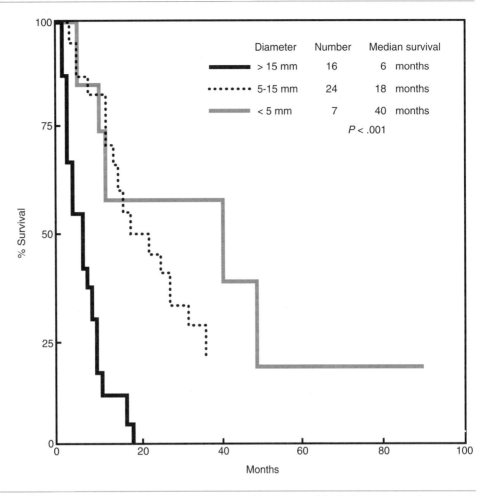

Figure 33.10 Survival versus diameter of largest residual disease. (Redrawn with permission from **Hacker NF, Berek JS, Lagasse LD, et al.** *Obstet Gynecol* 1983; 61:413).

8. A

Based on two large prospective trials, the combination of *cisplatin* plus *paclitaxel* (*Taxol*) is considered the treatment of choice for stages III and IV epithelial ovarian cancer. These trials compared this treatment to the former standard regimen of *cisplatin* and *cyclophosphamide*, and the survival of the patients who received the *paclitaxel*-containing treatment was longer. Current studies are comparing *carboplatin* and *paclitaxel* versus *cisplatin* and *paclitaxel*. The use of these agents in low-stage disease is also being tested.
Reference: Page 1185

9. A

A second-look operation is defined as one performed in a patient who has no clinical evidence of disease after the completion of a planned course of chemotherapy. Such a patient would have a normal CA125, a normal physical examination, and no radiologic evidence of disease. The value of a second-look operation in terms of the prolongation of survival is controversial. Second-look is no longer considered mandatory, but it is used selectively for young patients, and those who are on experimental treatment protocols.
Reference: Pages 1187–1189

10. C (see Table 33.4)

Germ-cell tumors account for about two-thirds of all malignancies in the first two decades of life. Epithelial and stromal tumors are less common. Germ-cell tumors are rare after the third decade of life.

Reference: Page 1193

11. A (see Figure 33.14)

Dysgerminomas are frequently bilateral, whereas the immature teratomas are only rarely bilateral. Endodermal sinus tumors and choriocarcinomas are unilateral lesions. The significance of this issue relates to the need to look for and remove, if necessary, tumors from both ovaries.

Reference: Pages 1195–1208

12. D

The surgical management of a unilateral dysgerminoma is the removal of the involved ovary and the performance of a staging laparotomy. These lesions occur in young women for whom the preservation of fertility is important. Because about 5% of dysgerminomas occur in women with dysgenetic ovaries, a karyotype should be performed as well.

Reference: Pages 1195–1197

13. A (see Figure 33.17)

The use of combination chemotherapy for women with germ-cell tumors is now well established as effective. In addition, this approach permits the preservation of fertility in most of these women as this treatment is given in lieu of radiation therapy that would render the ovary without function.

The combination of *bleomycin*, *etoposide*, and *cisplatin* (BEP) is the most extensively tested for the treatment of germ-cell tumors of the ovary and testes. Three or four cycles appear to be sufficient to produce excellent results and high cure rates.

Reference: Pages 1197–1201

Table 33.4   Histologic Typing of Ovarian Germ Cell Tumors

1. Dysgerminoma

2. Teratoma
   A. Immature
   B. Mature
      1) Solid
      2) Cystic
         a. Dermoid cyst (mature cystic teratoma)
         b. Dermoid cyst with malignant transformation
   C. Monodermal and highly specialized
      1) Struma ovarii
      2) Carcinoid
      3) Struma ovarii and carcinoid
      4) Others

3. Endodermal sinus tumor

4. Embryonal carcinoma

5. Polyembryoma

6. Choriocarcinoma

7. Mixed forms

Reproduced with permission from **Seroy SF, Scully RE, Robin IH.** *Histological Typing of Ovarian Tumors: International Histological Classification of Tumors, No. 9.* Geneva: World Health Organization, 1973.

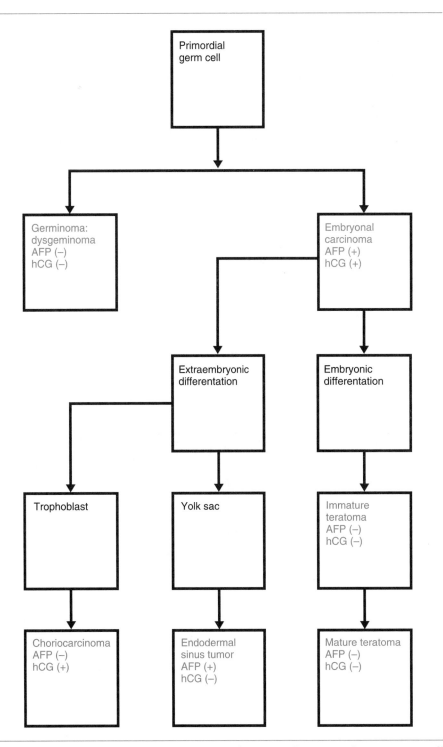

Figure 33.14   Relationship between types of pure malignant patients. Germ cell tumors and their secreted marker substances. (Reproduced with permission from **Berek JS, Hacker NF.** *Practical Gynecologic Oncology.* 2nd ed. Baltimore: Williams & Wilkins, 1994:379.)

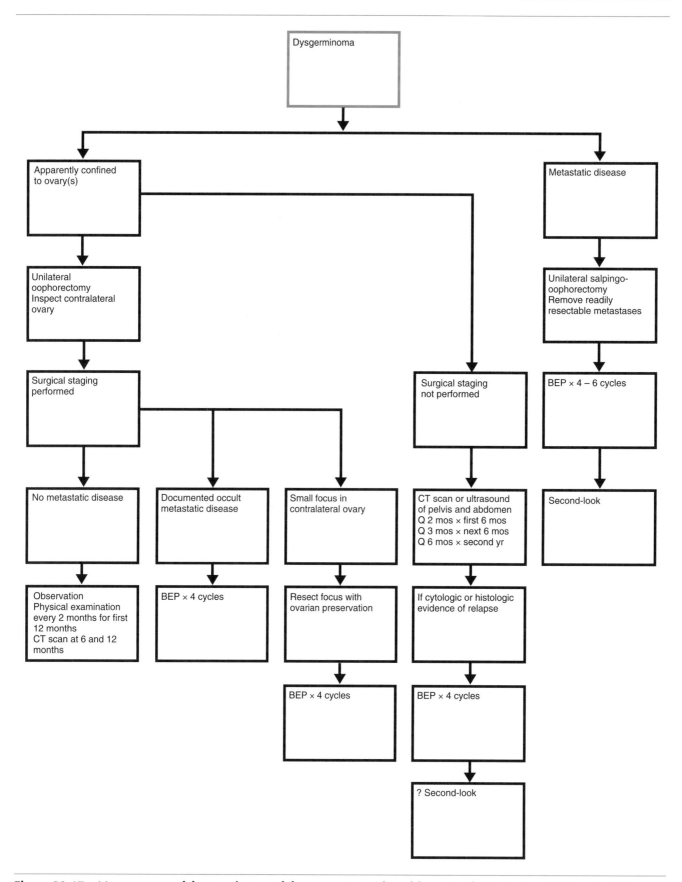

Figure 33.17   Management of dysgerminoma of the ovary. Reproduced from **Berek JS, Hacker NF.** *Practical Gyneco-logic Oncology.* 2nd ed. Baltimore: Williams & Wilkins. 1994:383.

14. A

Most patients who present with a diagnosis of immature teratomas have stage I tumors. Within that group the most important prognostic feature is the extent of immaturity of the elements, i.e., the grade. The elements that correlate best with prognosis are the differentiation of the neural tissues.

Reference: Pages 1201–1202

15. A

As noted above, in question 8, the treatment of choice in these patients is *cisplatin* and *paclitaxel*.

Reference: Page 1185

16. C

As noted above, in question 13, the BEP regimen is the preferred technique.

Reference: Pages 1197–1201

34 Vulvar Cancer

Lee-may Chen

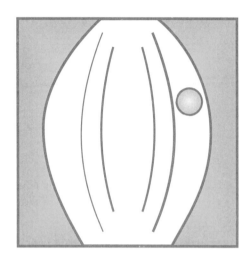

Learning Objectives

1. Know the incidence of patients developing invasive vulvar cancer.

2. Understand the histopathology and routes of disease spread, focusing on the implications of lesion size and depth of invasion to lymph node metastasis, which in turn prognosticates patient outcome.

3. Be able to classify patients by the FIGO surgical staging system.

4. Understand the rationale for individualization of treatment for all patients.

5. Understand the role of conservative surgery, including vulvar conservation, selection of cases for groin dissection, use of separate groin incisions, and elimination of routine pelvic lymphadenectomy.

6. Recognize the role of preoperative radiation to obviate the need for exenteration in patients with advanced disease.

7. Recognize the role of postoperative radiation to decrease the incidence of local groin recurrence in patients with multiple postive groin nodes.

8. Recognize differences in staging and managing patients with vulvar melanoma, as well as treatment of other vulvar malignancies such as Bartholin gland carcinoma, basal cell carcinoma, and vulvar sarcomas.

293

Questions

1. Vulvar cancer accounts for 4% of gynecologic malignancies; over 90% of these are squamous cell carcinomas. Which of the following factors have been associated with invasive vulvar cancer?

   A. Invasive cervical cancer
   B. Chronic granulomatous disease
   C. Syphilis
   D. All of the above

2. Depth of invasion is measured from the most superficial basement membrane to the deepest tumor. Stage Ia, or microinvasive carcinoma, is characterized by lesion size of less than or equal to 2 centimeters, and depth of invasion of:

   A. <1 mm
   B. <2 mm
   C. <5 mm
   D. <7 mm

3. Vulvar cancer may spread by direct extension, lymphatic embolization, or hematogenous spread. Which of the following statements regarding lymphatic metastasis is *false*?

   A. Cloquet's node is the most cephalad of the femoral node group.
   B. Lymphatic drainage of the vulva proceeds from femoral to inguinal to pelvic nodes.
   C. The overall incidence of lymph node metastasis is about 30%.
   D. The incidence of pelvic node metastasis is about 9%.

For Questions 4 and 5:

The TNM classification was adopted by FIGO in 1969. Surgical staging was introduced in 1988 and revised in 1995. Classify the following patients by stage.

4. A 56-year-old woman is found to have a 2-centimeter lesion at the fourchette, impinging on the anal sphincter. No lymph nodes are palpable.

   A. Stage I—$T_1N_0M_0$
   B. Stage II—$T_2N_0M_0$
   C. Stage III—$T_3N_0M_0$
   D. Stage IV—$T_4N_0M_0$

5. A 70-year-old woman presents with a 3-centimeter periclitoral lesion. Both groins have suspicious lymph nodes that are each 1 centimeter in size.

   A. Stage III—$T_3N_0M_0$
   B. Stage III—$T_3N_1M_0$
   C. Stage IV—$T_2N_2M_0$
   D. Stage IV—$T_3N_2M_0$

6. Which of the following lesions would be most appropriately treated by radical local excision alone?

   A. A 2 cm periclitoral lesion with < 1 mm invasion
   B. A 2 cm right labium minus lesion with < 1 mm invasion
   C. A 1 cm right labium minus lesion with < 1 mm invasion in a background of VIN 3
   D. A 1 cm right labium majus lesion with > 1 mm invasion

7. A 67-year-old woman notes a pruritic 3-centimeter mass on the left labium majus. Radical vulvectomy and bilateral groin lympadenectomy reveal two superficial lymph nodes to be involved with microscopic disease on the left. Margins of 1 centimeter are achieved on the primary lesion. The next step in this patient's management should involve:

A. Regular exams and Pap smears every three months
B. Radiation to the site of the primary vulvar lesion
C. Radiation to the pelvis and bilateral groins
D. Bilateral pelvic lymph node dissection

8. A 72-year-old woman has a T_3 lesion involving the lower urethra. Which of the following treatments will provide cure with the least potential for morbidity?

A. Anterior pelvic exenteration
B. Radical vulvectomy by en bloc/butterfly incision
C. Radical vulvectomy by separate vulva and groin incisions
D. Preoperative radiation therapy followed by limited vulvar resection

9. The most common late postoperative complication of inguinal-femoral lymphadenectomy is:

A. Recurrent lymphangitis/cellulitis
B. Chronic leg edema
C. Femoral hernia
D. Femoral nerve injury

10. Prognosis and recurrence of vulvar carcinoma both correlate best with:

A. Size of primary tumor
B. Response of tumor to chemotherapy
C. Number of lymph nodes positive for microscopic disease
D. Preoperative radiation therapy

11. Malignant melanoma is the second most common vulvar malignancy. Differences between vulvar melanoma and squamous cell carcinoma include:

A. Prognosis is related to depth of invasion.
B. Lesions with less than 1 mm of invasion can be treated with radical local excision alone.
C. Pelvic node metastases rarely occur in the absence of groin node metastasis.
D. None of the above

12. Bartholin gland carcinoma may be underdiagnosed if Honan's criteria are strictly followed. Which of the following is *not* among Honan's criteria?

A. Correct anatomic postition
B. Obliteration of normal glandular architecture
C. Overlying skin is intact
D. Tumor is located deep in the labium majus

Answers

1. D (see Table 34.1)
While no specific etiology for vulvar cancer has been identified, a synchronous cervical lesion—either dysplasia or invasive cancer—has been identified in up to 22% of cases. HPV DNA has been reported in 20 to 60% of patients with invasive vulvar cancer, who tend to be younger with a higher incidence of tobacco use and vulvar intraepithelial neoplasia (VIN). Association with lymphogranuloma venereum and gran-

Table 34.1   Types of Vulvar Cancer

Type	Percent
Squamous	92
Melanoma	2–4
Basal cell	2–3
Bartholin gland	1
(adenocarcinoma, squamous cell, transitional cell, adenoid cystic)	
Metastatic	1
Verrucous	<1
Sarcoma	<1
Appendage (e.g., hidradenocarcinoma)	rare

uloma inguinale has also been noted in patients with vulvar cancer. Although the incidence of syphilis is now lower, 5% of patients with vulvar cancer will have a positive serologic test for syphilis; these patients will more likely be younger and have less differentiated lesions.
Reference: Page 1232

2. A (see Table 34.3)
The incidence of lymph node metastasis is related to the depth of stromal invasion. When depth of invasion is less than 1 millimeter, the incidence of postive nodes is 0%. For depth of invasion 1.1 to 2 mm, 2.1 to 3 mm, 3.1 to 5 mm, and greater than 5 mm, the respective incidences of lymph node metastasis are 7.7%, 8.3%, 26.7%, and 34.2%.
Reference: Page 1233

3. B (see Figure 34.3)
Lymphatics of the vulva drain first to the superficial inguinal or groin nodes, then to the femoral nodes along the femoral vessels, which in turn drain to the pelvic lymph node chain. The superficial groin nodes are, therefore, the sentinel nodes of the vulva. Cloquet's node is the most cephalad of the femoral node group; this is the last node involved before the pelvic lymph nodes.
Reference: Pages 1235–1236

4. C

5. D
In the TNM classification, T_2 lesions are confined to the vulva or perineum and are greater than 2 centimeters in the greatest dimension; T_3 lesions are any tumors involv-

Table 34.3   Nodal Status in T, Squamous Cell Carcinoma of the Vulva Versus Depth of Stromal Invasion

Depth of Invasion	No.	Positive Nodes	Nodes
<1 mm	163	0	0
1.1–2 mm	145	11	7.7
2.1–3 mm	131	11	8.3
3.1–5 mm	101	27	26.7
>5 mm	38	13	34.2
Total	578	62	10.7

Data compiled from Parker, 1975 (40); Magrina, 1979 (53); Iversen, 1981 (4); Wilkinson, 1982 (54); Hoffman, 1983 (52); Hacker, 1984 (5); Boice, 1984 (55); Ross, 1987 (56); Rowley, 1988 (57); Struyk, 1989 (58).

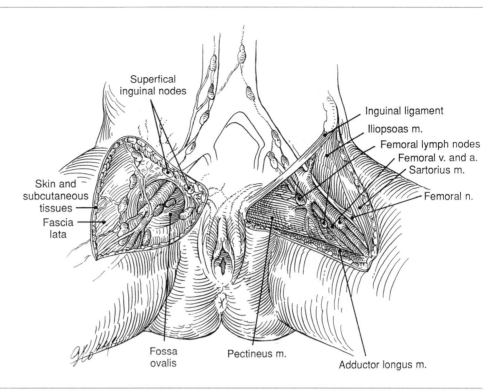

Figure 34.3 Inguinal-femoral lymph nodes.

ing the lower urethra, vagina, or anus. N_0 tumors have no lymph node metastasis; N_1 lesions have unilateral regional lymph node metastasis; and N_2 lesions have bilateral lymph node metastasis.
Reference: Page 1238

6. B

Radical local excision is advocated for T_1 lesions on the lateral or posterior vulva. In achieving a 2 centimeter margin, local recurrence rates are comparable to radical vulvectomy. In periclitoral lesions, alternative treatment with radiation can reduce psychosocial consequences. In cancer arising from a field of VIN, additional superficial local excision beyond radical local excision may be required for the noninvasive component. Regardless of lesion size, all patients with less than 1-millimeter stromal invasion require groin node dissection.
Reference: Pages 1239–1240

7. C

The presence of one positive groin node does not worsen prognosis or survival. With two or more positive nodes, groin irradiation improves survival and provides local control of disease recurrence. There is no data to suggest benefit of pelvic radiation over pelvic lymphadenectomy; however, enlarged pelvic nodes should be removed since radiation will not cure bulky disease. Postoperative radiation to the vulvar primary site may prevent local recurrence in patients with positive or close (less than 5-millimeter) surgical margins.
Reference: Pages 1241, 1243

8. D

To treat primary disease involving the urethra, rectovaginal septum, anus, or rectum, radical vulvectomy alone is insufficient to obtain adequate surgical margins. Morbidity from pelvic exenteration surgery can be avoided by combining preoperative radiation followed by a more limited vulvar resection. If persistent disease is present following preoperative

teletherapy, brachytherapy can potentially reduce tumor volume further to minimize radical surgery. Radiation therapy can be combined with cisplatin, 5-fluorouracil, or mitomycin C to serve as radiation sensitizers.
Reference: Pages 1244–1245

9. B

As many as 69% of patients will have chronic leg edema. Full groin dissection combined with groin irradiation often results in severe leg edema. About 10% of patients will have recurrent lymphangitis or leg cellulitis. Femoral hernia is an uncommon late complication. Femoral nerve injury is noted as an early postoperative complication and resolves slowly over time.
Reference: Page 1244

10. C

The number of positive groin lymph nodes is the most important prognostic variable for survival and recurrent disease. If three or more groin lymph nodes are positive for metastatic disease, a high incidence of disease recurrence and a poor prognosis exist. Patients with N_0 or N_1 lesions are reported to have a 78% two-year survival compared to patients with N_2 or N_3 lesions, who have 52% and 33% two-year survivals, respectively. Local recurrence is more likely if the primary lesion is greater than 4 centimeters in size, although this can be treated by further surgical excision. Tumor ploidy also appears to have prognostic implication for survival.
Reference: Pages 1246–1247

11. D

FIGO staging for squamous cell carcinoma of the vulva cannot be applied to vulvar melanomas; instead, staging is related to depth of invasion as per the Clark, Breslow, and Chung systems. Overall prognosis is poor, but relates to the depth of invasion. In squamous cell carcinoma, prognosis depends on lymph node involvement, but lymph node metastasis depends on depth of invasion. Patients with lesions that have less than 1-millimeter depth of invasion have an excellent prognosis and may be treated with radical local excision alone. Although lesions most commonly are found on the labia minora or clitoris, pelvic node metastasis do not occur if groin lymph nodes are negative for disease.
Reference: Pages 1247–1248

12. B

The best criterion to classify a vulvar tumor as a Bartholin gland carcinoma is the transition of normal and malignant tissue. Some recognizable normal gland should be identifiable to clearly characterize a Bartholin gland carcinoma. The deep location of the gland may result in delay of diagnosis and necessitate extensive dissection, but stage for stage, prognosis is similar.
Reference: Page 1250

35 Gestational Trophoblastic Disease

Ross S. Berkowitz
Donald P. Goldstein

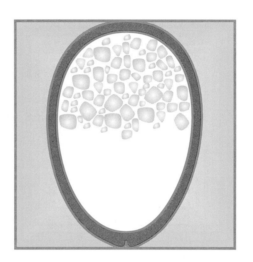

Learning Objectives

1. Understand the histopathologic and cytogenetic differences between complete and partial hydatidiform mole.

2. Understand the natural history of gestational trophoblastic diseases.

3. Understand the principles of management of persistent gestational trophoblastic tumors.

4. Understand later reproductive outcome in patients who are successfully treated for gestational trophoblastic diseases.

Questions

1. What is the most common chromosal pattern in a complete molar pregnancy?

   A. Triploidy
   B. Trisomy 21
   C. 46 XX — All chromosomes are of maternal origin
   D. 46 XY — All chromosomes are of paternal origin
   E. 46 XX — All chromosomes are of paternal origin

2. The most common site of metastasis of a gestational trophoblastic tumor is the:

   A. Vagina
   B. Lung
   C. Liver
   D. Brain
   E. Ovary

3. Of the following features, which one is highly prognostic in patients with stage II and III gestational trophoblastic disease (GTD) ?

   A. Race
   B. Smoking history
   C. The parity of the patient
   D. Socioeconomic status
   E. Interval between the antecedent pregnancy and the occurrence of the GTD

4. Patients with nonmetastatic gestational trophoblastic tumors are most commonly treated with:

   A. Hysterectomy
   B. Pelvic radiation therapy
   C. Primary combination chemotherapy
   D. Single agent chemotherapy with either cisplatin or Taxol
   E. Single agent chemotherapy with either methotrexate or actinomycin-D

5. When a patient has achieved remission with chemotherapy for a gestational trophoblastic tumor, she should be advised that in later pregnancies:

   A. She should expect a higher risk of congenital malformations
   B. She should expect a higher risk of cesarean section
   C. She should expect a higher risk of spontaneous abortion
   D. She should expect a generally normal reproductive outcome
   E. She should expect a greater risk of prematurity

Answers

1. **E (see Figure 35.2)**
   Cytogenetic studies have demonstrated that complete hydatidiform moles usually have a 46 XX karyotype, and the molar chromosomes are entirely of paternal origin. Complete moles appear to usually arise from an ovum that has been fertilized by a haploid sperm, which then duplicates its own chromosomes, and the ovum nucleus may be either absent or inactivated. Although most complete moles have a 46 XX chromosomal pattern, about 10% have a 46 XY karyotpye. The karyotype of the partial mole is 69XXX, 69XYY, or 69XXY (see Figure 35.4).
   Reference: Pages 1262–1264

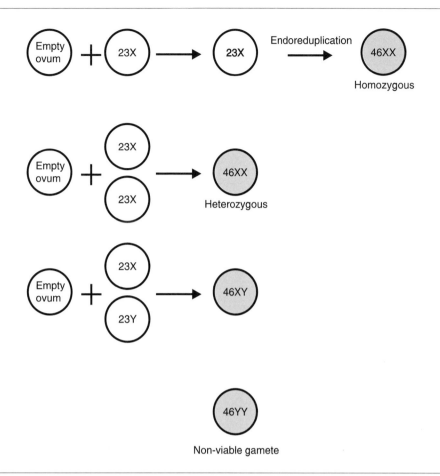

Figure 35.2   The karyotype of complete hydatidiform mole.

2. B
The most common sites of metastases are as follows: lung 80%; vagina 30%; pelvis 20%; liver 10%; brain 10%. At the time of presentation, 80% of the patients with metastatic GTT show lung involvement on chest radiographs. Patients with pulmonary metastases may have chest pain, cough, hemoptysis, dyspnea, or an asymptomatic lesion on chest radiographs. Respiratory symptoms may be acute or chronic, persisting over many months.
Reference: Page 1270

3. E
Stage of the GTD correlates with outcome; however, the majority of women with stages I through III disease, fortunately, are cured. Within stages II and III, there are several prognostic features that correlate with outcome. These have been developed into a scoring system (see Table 35.3). In addition to the interval between antecedent pregnancy and the development of the GTD (the longer the interval, the poorer the prognosis), other risk features include patient age, level of hCG, ABO blood group, size of tumor, size of metastases, and the number of prior chemotherapy regimens.
Reference: Pages 1270–1272

4. E (see Table 35.4 and Figure 35.6)
Single-agent chemotherapy is the preferred treatment in patients with nonmetastatic gestational trophoblastic tumors who desire to retain fertility. Single-agent chemotherapy with either actinomycin-D or methotrexate has achieved comparable and excellent remission rates in both nonmetastatic and low-risk metastatic GTT. Primary single-

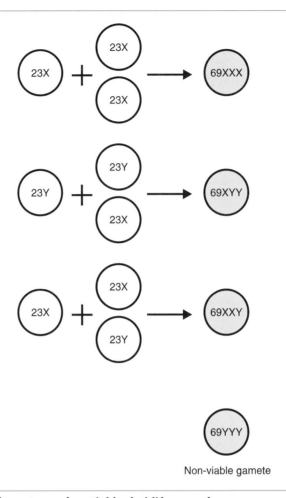

Non-viable gamete

Figure 35.4   The karyotype of partial hydatidiform mole.

Table 35.3   Scoring System Based on Prognostic Factors

	Score			
	0	*1*	*2*	*4*
Age (years)	≤39	>39		
Antecedent pregnancy	Hydatidiform mole	Abortion	Term	
Interval between end of antecedent pregnancy and start of chemotherapy (months)	<4	4–6	7–12	>12
Human chorionic gonadotropin (IU/liter)	<10^3	10^3–10^4	10^4–10^5	>10^5
ABO groups		O or A	B or AB	
Largest tumor, including uterine (cm)	<3	3–5	>5	
Site of metastases		Spleen, kidney	Gastrointestinal tract, liver	Brain
Number of metastases		1–3	4–8	>8
Prior chemotherapy			1 drug	≥2 drugs

The total score for a patient is obtained by adding the individual scores for each prognostic factor. Total score: <4 = low-risk; 5–7 = middle risk; ≥8 = high risk.

Table 35.4   Protocol for Treatment of GTT

Stage I
Initial	Single-agent chemotherapy or hysterectomy with adjunctive chemotherapy
Resistant	Combination chemotherapy
	Hysterectomy with adjunctive chemotherapy
	Local resection
	Pelvic infusion

Stage II and III
Low Risk*
Initial	Single-agent chemotherapy
Resistant	Combination chemotherapy

High Risk*
Initial	Combination chemotherapy
Resistant	Second-line combination chemotherapy

Stage IV
Initial	Combination chemotherapy
Brain	Whole-heat irradiation (3000 cGy)
	Craniotomy to manage complications
Liver	Resection to manage complications
Resistant*	Second-line combination chemotherapy
	Hepatic arterial infusion

*Local resection optional.

agent chemotherapy was administered at the New England Trophoblastic Disease Center to 399 patients with nonmetastatic GTT and 373 (93.5%) attained complete remission. The remaining 26 resistant patients subsequently achieved remission after combination chemotherapy or surgical intervention.
Reference: Pages 1273–1274

5. D

Patients with GTT who are treated successfully with chemotherapy can expect normal reproduction in the future. Patients who were treated with chemotherapy at the New England Trophoblastic Disease Center from 1965 to 1992 had 420 subsequent pregnancies that resulted in 295 term live births (70.2%). First and second trimester spontaneous abortions occured in 65 (15.5%) and 7 (1.6%) pregnancies respectively. Major and minor congenital malformations were detected in only 7 infants (2.2%). Primary cesarean section was performed in 32 (15%) of 214 subsequent term and premature births from 1979 to 1992. It is particularly reassuring that the frequency of congenital anomalies is not increased, although chemotherapeutic agents are known to have teratogenic and mutagenic potential.
Reference: Page 1279

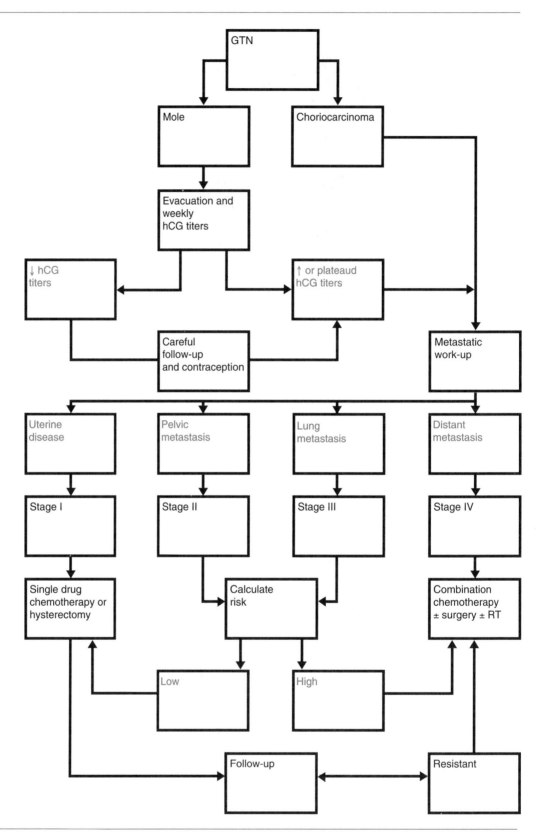

Figure 35.6   Algorithm for the management of persistent gestational trophoblastic tumor. (Reproduced with permission from **Berek JS, Hacker NF,** eds. *Practical Gynecologic Oncology.* 2nd ed. Baltimore: Williams & Wilkins, 1994:473.)

36 Breast Cancer

Armando E. Giuliano

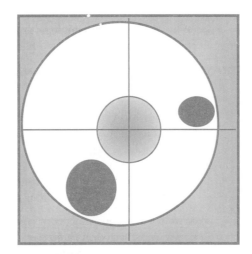

Learning Objectives

1. Know the risk factors for development of breast cancer.

2. Be aware of the methods used to diagnose breast cancer.

3. Be cognizant of the TNM classification for staging breast cancer.

4. Understand the appropriate steps in the preoperative evaluation of breast cancer.

5. Know the treatment options for breast cancer, including the advantages and disadvantages of each.

6. Be aware of the prognosis for different forms of breast cancer.

Questions

1. Significant risk factors for developing breast cancer include which *one* of the following:

    A. Age under 25 years
    B. Mother with bilateral breast cancer diagnosed when premenopausal
    C. Alcoholism
    D. Breast-fed children
    E. Oral contraceptive use

2. Of the following epidemiologic aspects, which is the most significant regarding the relative risk of the development of breast cancer?

    A. Obesity
    B. Patient age
    C. Alcohol consumption
    D. Family history of breast cancer
    E. Personal history of hormone intake

3. Which of the following would be appropriate for an otherwise healthy 60-year-old post-menopausal woman recently diagnosed with a 3-centimeter, estrogen receptor–positive invasive ductal carcinoma with negative axillary lymph nodes and normal blood tests.

    A. Make a diagnosis by mammographic needle localization if palpable
    B. Order a chest x-ray, bone scan, and CT scan of the abdomen
    C. Perform a radical mastectomy if the patient does not wish breast conservation
    D. Perform a lumpectomy with axillary dissection, but no radiation therapy if breast conservation is desired
    E. Label her as stage Iia, $T_2N_0M_0$

4. Compared with women whose breast cancers are detected by palpation, those detected by screening mammography have a lower likelihood of:

    A. *In situ* carcinomas
    B. Axillary lymph node metastases
    C. Estrogen receptor–positive carcinomas
    D. Epidermal growth factor receptor–positive carcinomas

5. A 48-year-old woman is diagnosed with stage II infiltrating ductal carcinoma of the breast. The best results with the lowest morbidity are achieved with which of the following therapy:

    A. Radiation therapy
    B. Modified radical mastectomy
    C. Segmental mastectomy, axillary dissection, and radiation therapy
    D. Modified radical mastectomy, axillary dissection, and chemotherapy

6. Which of the following statements about adjuvant treatment of breast cancer is *false*?

    A. Postmenopausal women with ER-positive, node-negative tumors benefit from tamoxifen.
    B. Tamoxifen gives a decreased incidence of contralateral breast cancer as well as a decreased death rate from heart disease.
    C. Only premenopausal women with ER-negative tumors and no axillary metastasis benefit from chemotherapy if tolerable.
    D. Postmenopausal women with ER-negative tumors and no axillary metastasis benefit from chemotherapy if tolerable.
    E. Adjuvant therapy is not recommended for tumors less than 1 centimeter with negative axillary lymph nodes.

7. A 52-year-old woman undergoes a segmental mastectomy, axillary dissection, and radiation therapy for a stage I, node-negative, estrogen receptor–positive breast cancer. Adjuvant hormonal therapy with tamoxifen is prescribed. The duration of *tamoxifen* therapy that is associated with the longest survival is:

   A. 2 years
   B. 5 years
   C. 10 years
   D. Indefinite

8. Which of the following situations would be inappropriate for mastectomy?

   A. Paget's disease
   B. Inflammatory carcinoma after chemotherapy and radiation
   C. Lobular carcinoma *in situ* for treatment
   D. Intraductal cancer
   E. Ductal cancer during the second trimester

9. Stage for stage, the prognosis for women who are diagnosed with breast cancer during pregnancy compared to women diagnosed with breast cancer who are not pregnant is:

   A. Worse
   B. The same
   C. The same if the pregnancy is aborted
   D. Worse if the pregnancy is the second or greater

Answers

1. **B**
   Women whose mothers or sisters have had bilateral premenopausal breast cancer have at least a 40 to 50% lifetime risk of developing breast cancer. The incidence of breast cancer increases steadily with age. Alcohol consumption may increase the risk of breast cancer, but this relationship is unclear. Lactation does not affect the incidence of breast cancer, and oral contraceptive use does not increase the risk of breast cancer.
   Reference: Pages 1283–1284

2. **B (see Table 36.3)**
   While all of the other variables are significant, the incidence of breast cancer increases as the patient ages, and this is the most significant variable.
   Reference: Pages 1283–1284

Table 36.3   Prognostic Factors in Node-Negative Breast Carcinoma

Factor	Increased Risk of Recurrence
Size	Larger tumors
Histologic grade	High-grade tumors
DNA ploidy	Aneuploid tumors
Labeling index	High index (>3%)
S phase fraction	High fraction (>5%)
Lymphatic/vascular invasion	Present
Cathepsin D	High levels
HER-2/*neu* oncogene expression	High expression
Epidermal growth factor	High levels

Reproduced with permission from **Tierney LM, McPhee SJ, Papadakis MA.** *Current Medical Diagnosis and Treatment.* Lange, 1995.

3. E

Since this patient's tumor is between 2 and 5 centimeters in diameter and she has no evidence of axillary or distant metastasis, she is staged Iia ($T_2N_0M_0$). Diagnosis of a palpable mass can be made by fine needle aspiration, core biopsy, or open biopsy. Needle localization is reserved for nonpalpable mammographically detected lesions. For patients with clinical stage II disease, a bone scan should be obtained, but a CT scan of the liver is not necessary unless symptoms or liver functions suggest liver metastasis. Surgical options include modified radical mastectomy or breast conservation surgery. Modified radical mastectomy has replaced radical mastectomy. Breast conservation surgery includes lumpectomy and axillary node dissection and must be followed by postoperative radiation to decrease local recurrence rates.
Reference: Pages 1285–1293

4. B

Clear evidence suggests that those lesions detected by screening mammography—lesions that are not yet palpable—are less likely to be associated with axillary lymph node metastasis. Because this feature correlates with prognosis, these data explain, in part, the reduction in mortality achieved through the use of screening mammography in the appropriate population.
Reference: Pages 1284–1287

5. C

The survival for patients with this disease is identical for those undergoing a segmental mastectomy, axillary dissection, and postoperative radiation therapy as for those treated with a modified radical mastectomy and an axillary resection. The former approach is less morbid and more cosmetic. Radiation therapy alone or modified mastectomy without axillary dissection would not be sufficient treatments for this disease.
Reference: Pages 1289–1293

6. C

In the NSABP study, both premenopausal and postmenopausal women who had ER-positive tumors with node-negative disease benefited from adjuvant use of tamoxifen. The Early Breast Cancer Trialist's Collaborative Group data demonstrated a decreased incidence of carcinoma of the contralateral breast and a decreased death rate from heart disease. In another NSABP study, the disease-free survival was longer for both pre- and postmenopausal women with ER-negative tumors who underwent adjuvant chemotherapy. When the risk of recurrence is extremely low, as would be expected for tumors less than 1 centimeter with no lymph node metastasis, the reduction in recurrence may not justify the side effects of the drugs.
Reference: Pages 1293–1295

7. B

Data suggest that patients who receive five years of tamoxifen therapy are associated with a longer survival than those patients with ER/PR-positive lesions who do not receive adjuvant therapy. A comparative trial of 5 versus 10 years showed equivalent results.
Reference: Page 1294

8. C

For Paget's disease of the nipple, treatment has always been total mastectomy and lymph node dissection, although radiotherapy with resection of the tumor and nipple areolar complex is being performed. Mastectomy for inflammatory breast cancer may be indicated for patients who remain free of distant metastatic disease after initial chemotherapy and radiation. Lobular carcinoma *in situ* predisposes for an increased risk of developing invasive cancer and, therefore, occasionally a patient may request bilateral *prophylactic* mastectomy. Although modified radical mastectomy has been the standard treatment for intraductal carcinoma, more conservative surgery with or

without radiation can yield good results. Localized disease found during the first or second trimester of pregnancy is probably best treated with definitive surgery and radiation therapy similar to that given nonpregnant women.
Reference: Pages 1296–1297

9. B

Based on all of the available data, it appears that the prognosis for breast cancer is the same for pregnant versus nonpregnant patients when corrected for stage at diagnosis.
Reference: Pages 1297–1298

37 Palliative Care and Pain Management

Jonathan S. Berek

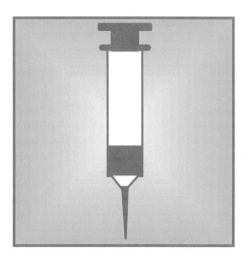

Learning Objectives

1. Be able to articulate the four steps to providing palliative pain management.

2. Understand how to assess and manage lumbosacral plexopathy.

3. Understand how to diagnose and manage psoas muscle spasm.

4. Be able to list other symptoms in need of palliation in terminal cancer patients.

5. Be aware of the principles by which you should treat patients close to death.

Questions

1. In a patient with incurable cancer, the principal tenet of palliative care is that:

   A. life can be prolonged with effective analgesia
   B. investigative therapies can be used to sustain life
   C. patients can live as actively as possible until death
   D. death can be hastened with appropriate medications

2. A 47-year-old woman has cervical cancer metastatic to the pelvic bone. She has been experiencing progressive pain that is no longer responsive to nonsteroidal anti-inflammatory medications. Narcotic medications are chosen. In general opioids should be administered at:

   A. fixed doses and fixed intervals
   B. variable doses and fixed intervals
   C. fixed doses and variable intervals
   D. variable doses and variable intervals

3. A 65-year-old woman with advanced stage ovarian cancer develops diffuse peritoneal carcinomatosis and persistent nausea is a problem. The mechanism for her vomiting is unknown, although she has a fair degree of anxiety associated with her nausea, and has frequent "colicky" abdominal pain. In order to treat her nausea effectively, the most suitable drugs would be:

   A. *prochlorperazine*
   B. *metaclopromide*
   C. *ondansetron*
   D. *cyclizine*

4. A 72-year-old woman has chronic, progressive intestinal obstruction associated with widely metastatic ovarian cancer. The obstruction is considered end stage and all effective chemotherapeutic options have been exhausted. In this patient, the St. Christopher's Hospice approach is recommended. Using this palliative therapy, the use of the following is avoided:

   A. oral nutrition and medications
   B. nasogastric tube and intravenous fluids
   C. rectally administered antiemetics and opioids
   D. subcutaneous antinauseants and intravenous opioids

5. A patient with cervical cancer metastatic to the bone has developed severe hypercalcemia refractory to increasing fluid intake. In this circumstance, the treatment of severe hypercalcemia is best accomplished by using:

   A. *thiazide* and *bicarbonate*
   B. *diazepam* and *phosphate*
   C. *furosemide* and *pamidronate*
   D. *alondrenate* and *corticosteroids*

6. A 56-year-old woman has end-stage ovarian cancer and requests information on the duration of her survival. The most appropriate prognostication should be:

   A. no estimate of survival time
   B. the best estimate of a finite survival time
   C. the best estimate of the shortest survival time
   D. the best estimate of survival time boundaries

Answers

1. C

Palliative care is the active total care of patients whose disease is not responsive to curative treatments. The goal of palliative care is to achieve the best possible quality of life for patients who are dying from their disease, and their families. Control of pain, of other symptoms, and of psychological, social, and spiritual problems is paramount. Many aspects of palliative care are also applicable earlier in the course of the illness, in conjunction with anticancer treatment. In general, palliative care should:

- affirm life and regard dying as a normal process;
- neither hasten nor postpone death;
- provide relief from pain and other distressing symptoms;
- integrate the psychological and spiritual aspects of patient care;
- offer a support system to help patients live as actively as possible until death;
- offer a support system to help the family during the patient's illness and in their bereavement.

Radiotherapy, chemotherapy, and surgery have a place in palliative care if the symptomatic benefits of treatment clearly outweigh the disadvantages. Investigative procedures are kept to a minimum.
Reference: Pages 1303–1304

2. A

It is now widely recognized that opioids should be given regularly at precisely determined doses and at fixed intervals in accordance with the half-life of the drug concerned, rather than haphazardly in response to a severe pain stimulus. The equivalency of various narcotic analgesics to 10 mg of intramuscular morphine are presented in Table 37.1.
Reference: Pages 1307–1309

Table 37.1   Equivalency of Various Narcotic Analgesics to 10 mg of Intramuscular Morphine

Drug	Route*	Dose (mg)	Duration (hr)	Plasma (half-life)	Comments
Morphine	SQ/IM	10	4–6	2–3.5	Also available in a slow-release
	PO	30–60			form and as rectal suppositories
Codeine	SQ/IM	130	4–6	3	Metabolized to morphine
	PO	200			
Oxycodone	SQ/IM	15	3–4	—	Often, 5 mg combined with
	PO	30			ASA and acetaminophen
Levorphanol	IM	2	4–6	12–16	May accumulate and result
	PO	4			in delayed toxities
Hydromorphone	SQ/IM	1.5	4–5	2–3	Available up to 10 mg/ml for
	PO	7.5			injection and as rectal suppositories
Oxymorphone	SQ/IM	1	4–6	2–3	No oral preparation
	PR	10			
Meperidine	SQ/IM	75	2–3	3–4	Toxic metabolite causes CNS
	PO	300			excitation; avoid in renal failure
Methadone	SQ/IM	10	4–6	15–30	May accumulate and result in
	PO	20			delayed toxicities
Fentanyl	IV	0.1	0.5–1	3–12	Transdermal delivery requires
	Patch	0.5	72		days to reach steady state

Reproduced with permission from **Grossman SA.** Is pain undertreated in cancer patients? *Advances Oncol* 1993;9:11.
IM, intramuscular; IV, intravenous; PO, oral; SQ, subcutaneous; ASA, acetylsalicylic acid (aspirin); PR, rectally, CNS, central nervous system.
*Subcutaneous route is preferable to intramuscular in most situations.

Table 37.2   Commonly Used Antinauseant Drugs

Drug	Dose	Comment
Metoclopramide	10–20 mg every 4 hours (oral or subcutaneous)	Avoid if patient has bowel colic
Haloperidol	1–3 mg bid or tid (oral)	Lower doses required than when used as a sedative
Prochlorperazine	5–25 mg bid or tid (oral or rectal)	May be useful if vomiting mechanism is unknown
Meclozine	10–75 mg per day in divided doses (oral)	Antihistamine with doses that produce minimal sedation
Cyclizine	10–75 mg per day in divided doses (oral, rectal, or subcutaneous)	Useful if patient has bowel obstruction
Hyoscine	0.1–0.4 mg every 6–8 hours (subcutaneous)	CNS side effects can occur, particularly drowsiness and confusion
Ondansetron	0.15 mg/kg every 4 hours for 3 doses IV 4–8 mg tid (oral)	Main use is for chemotherapy-related nausea Constipation can be troublesome

See text and manufacturers' information before prescribing; watch for side effects; review frequently; cease ineffective drugs.

3. A (see Table 37.2)

As antinauseants, drugs such as prochlorperazine have some affinity for both muscarinic and histaminic receptors and are moderately useful when the specific etiology of the nausea is somewhat unclear. If vestibular mechanisms are suspected, *cyclizine*, which acts directly on the vestibular center, is appropriate. *Ondansetron* is expensive and typically used in patients receiving chemotherapeutic agents that are strongly emetogenic. *Metoclopramide* should be avoided in patients with bowel colic.
Reference: Pages 1312–1313

4. B

In a patient with end-stage intestinal obstruction associated with cancer, usually associated with peritoneal carcinomatosis, the "totally symptomatic" approach developed at St. Christopher's Hospice may be preferable. In summary, this approach seeks to avoid the unpleasant use of a nasogastric tube and the conventional use of intravenous fluids. It relies on careful mouth care, with as little food or drink as desired. The patient remains mildly dehydrated, but this is beneficial in terms of reducing gastrointestinal secretions and the amount of vomiting.
Reference: Pages 1313–1315

5. C

Hypercalcemia is a recognized complication of metastatic cancer, especially cervical cancer metastatic to the bone. Hypercalcemia can cause unpleasant symptoms in these patients and therefore warrants palliation. The best treatment is the use of a loop diuretic and pamidronate in those patients with skeletal metastases to cause an increase in excretion of calcium and a decrease in production of calcium by osteoclasts.
Reference: Page 1317

6. D

The process of dying is fraught with uncertainty. Predictions of duration of survival are often wrong.
Reference: Pages 1317–1318

Appendix I: Preventive Health Care by Age Groups

Table 8.3 Periodic Evaluation Ages 13–18

Screening	*Evaluation and Counseling*
History	**Sexuality**
Reason for visit	Development
Health status: medical, surgical, family	High-risk behaviors
Dietary/nutritional assessments	Contraceptive options Genetic counseling Prevention of unwanted pregnancy
Physical activity	Sexually transmitted diseases Partner selection Barrier protection
Tobacco, alcohol, other drugs	
Abuse/neglect	**Fitness**
Sexual practices	Hygiene (including dental)
	Dietary/nutritional assessment
Physical	Exercise: discussion of program
Height	
Weight	**Psychosocial evaluation**
Blood pressure	Interpersonal/family relationships
Secondary sexual characteristics (Tanner staging)	Sexual identity
Pelvic examination (yearly when sexually active or by age 18)	Personal goal development
Skin*	Behavioral/learning disorders
	Abuse/neglect
Laboratory tests	**Cardiovascular risk factors**
Pap test (yearly when sexually active or by age 18)	Family history
High-risk groups	Hypertension
Hemoglobin*	Hyperlipidemia
Bacteriuria testing*	Obesity/diabetes mellitus
Sexually transmitted disease testing*	

Table 8.3—continued

Screening	Evaluation and Counseling
Human immunodeficiency virus testing*	**Health-risk behaviors**
Rubella titer*	Injury prevention
Tuberculosis skin test*	Safety belts and helmets
Lipid profile*	Recreational hazards
	Firearms
	Hearing
	Skin exposure to ultraviolet rays
	Suicide: depressive symptoms
	Tobacco, alcohol, other drugs

*In the presence of high-risk factors.
Modified with permission from **ACOG.** *The Obstetrician–Gynecologist and Primary-Preventive Health Care.* Washington, DC: American College of Obstetricians and Gynecologists, 1993:1–22.

Table 8.4   Periodic Evaluation Ages 19–39

Screening	Evaluation and Counseling
History	**Sexuality**
Reason for visit	High-risk behaviors
Health status: medical, surgical, family	Contraceptive options
Dietary/nutritional assessments	Genetic counseling
Physical activity	Prevention of unwanted pregnancy
Tobacco, alcohol, other drugs	Sexually transmitted diseases
Abuse/neglect	Partner selection
Sexual practices	Barrier protection
	Sexual functioning
Physical	
Height	**Fitness**
Weight	Hygiene (including dental)
Blood pressure	Dietary/nutritional assessment
Neck: adenopathy, thyroid	Exercise: discussion of program
Breasts	
Abdomen	**Psychosocial evaluation**
Pelvic examination	Interpersonal/family relationships
Skin*	Domestic violence
	Job satisfaction
	Lifestyle/stress
	Sleep disorders

Table 8.4—*continued*

Screening	*Evaluation and Counseling*
Laboratory tests	
Pap test (physician and patient discretion after three consecutive normal tests)	
Cholesterol (Every 5 years)	**Cardiovascular risk factors**
High-risk groups	Family history
Hemoglobin*	Hypertension
Bacteriuria testing*	Hyperlipidemia
Mammography*	Obesity/diabetes mellitus
Fasting glucose test*	Lifestyle
Sexually transmitted disease testing*	
Human immunodeficiency virus testing*	**Health/risk behaviors**
Genetic testing/counseling*	Injury prevention
Rubella titer*	—Safety belts and helmets
Tuberculosis skin test*	—Occupational hazards
Lipid profile*	—Recreational hazards
Thyroid-stimulating hormone*	—Firearms
	—Hearing
	Breast self-examination
	Skin exposure to ultraviolet rays
	Suicide: depressive symptoms
	Tobacco, alcohol, other drugs

*In the presence of high-risk factors.
Modified with permission from **ACOG.** *The Obstetrician–Gynecologist and Primary-Preventive Health Care.* Washington, DC: American College of Obstetricians and Gynecologists, 1993:1–22.

Table 8.5   Periodic Evaluations Ages 40–64

Screening	*Evaluation and Counseling*
History	**Sexuality**
Reason for visit	High-risk behaviors
Health status: medical, surgical, family	Contraceptive options
Dietary/nutritional assessment	Genetic counseling
Physical activity	Prevention of unwanted pregnancy
Tobacco, alcohol, other drugs	Sexually transmitted disease
Abuse/neglect	Partner selection
Sexual practices	Barrier protection
	Sexual functioning

317

Table 8.5—*continued*

Screening	Evaluation and Counseling
Physical	
Height	**Fitness**
Weight	Hygiene (including dental)
Blood pressure	Dietary/nutritional assessment
Oral cavity	Exercise: discussion of program
Neck: adenopathy, thyroid	
Breasts, axillae	**Psychosocial evaluation**
Abdomen	Family relationships
Pelvic and rectovaginal examination	Domestic violence
Skin*	Job/work satisfaction
	Retirement planning
	Lifestyle/stress
	Sleep disorders
Laboratory tests	
Pap test (physician and patient discretion after three consecutive normal tests)	**Cardiovascular risk factors**
Mammography (Every 1–2 years until age 50, yearly beginning at 50)	Family history
Cholesterol (every 5 years)	Hypertension
Fecal occult blood test	Hyperlipidemia
Sigmoidoscopy (every 3–5 years after age 50)	Obesity/diabetes mellitus
High-risk groups	Life style
Hemoglobin*	
Bacteriuria testing*	**Health/risk behaviors**
Mammography	Hormone replacement therapy
Fasting glucose test*	Injury prevention
Sexually transmitted disease testing*	Safety belts and helmets
Human immunodeficiency virus testing*	Occupational hazards
Tuberculosis skin test*	Recreational hazards
	Sports involvement
Lipid profile*	Firearms
Thyroid-stimulating hormone*	Hearing
Colonoscopy	Breast self-examination
	Skin exposure to ultraviolet rays
	Suicide: depressive symptoms
	Tobacco, alcohol, other drugs

*In the presence of high-risk factors.
Modified with permission from **ACOG.** *The Obstetrician–Gynecologist and Primary-Preventive Health Care.* Washington, DC: American College of Obstetricians and Gynecologists, 1993:1–22.

Table 8.6   Periodic Evaluations Ages 65 Years and Older

Screening	*Evaluation and Counseling*
History	**Sexuality**
Reason for visit	Sexual functioning
Health status: medical, surgical, family	Sexual behaviors
Dietary/nutritional assessment	Sexually transmitted diseases
Physical activity	
Tobacco, alcohol, other drugs, polypharmacy	**Fitness**
Abuse/neglect	Hygiene (general and dental)
Sexual practices	Dietary/nutritional assessment
	Exercise: discussion of program
Physical	
Height	**Psychosocial evaluation**
Weight	Neglect/abuse
Blood pressure	Life style/stress
Oral cavity	Depression/sleep disorders
Neck: adenopathy, thyroid	Family relationships
Breasts, axillae	Job/work/retirement satisfaction
Abdomen	
Pelvic and rectovaginal examination	**Cardiovascular risk factors**
Skin*	Hypertension
	Hypercholesterolemia
	Obesity/diabetes mellitus
Laboratory Tests	Sedentary lifestyle
Pap test (physician and patient discretion after three consecutive normal tests)	
Urinalysis/dipstick	**Health/risk behaviors**
Mammography	Hormone replacement therapy
Cholesterol (every 3–5 years)	Injury prevention
Fecal occult blood test	Safety belts and helmets
Sigmoidoscopy (every 3–5 years)	Occupational hazards
Thyroid-stimulating hormone test (every 3–5 years)	Recreational hazards
High-risk groups	Hearing
Hemoglobin*	Firearms
Fasting glucose test*	Visual acuity/glaucoma
Sexually transmitted disease testing*	Hearing
Human immunodeficiency virus testing*	Breast self-examination
Tuberculosis skin test*	Skin exposure to ultraviolet rays
Lipid profile*	Suicide: depressive symptoms
Colonoscopy*	Tobacco, alcohol, other drugs

*In the presence of high-risk factors.
Modified with permission from **ACOG.** *The Obstetrician–Gynecologist and Primary-Preventive Health Care.* Washington, DC: American College of Obstetricians and Gynecologists, 1993:1–22.

Table 8.7   High-Risk Factors

Bacteriuria Testing

Persons with diabetes mellitus

Colonoscopy

Personal history of:
   Inflammatory bowel disease
   Colonic polyps
Family history of:
   Familiar polyposis
   Colorectal cancer
   Cancer family syndrome

Fasting Glucose Test

Every 3–5 years for persons with family history of diabetes mellitus (one first- or two
   second-degree relatives)
Marked obesity
History of gestational diabetes mellitus

Fluoride Supplement

Persons living in areas with inadequate water fluoridation (< 0.7 parts/million)

Genetic Testing/Counseling

Women of reproductive age who are exposed to teratogens
Women of reproductive age who contemplate pregnancy at 35 years of age or older
Patient, partner, or family member with history of genetic disorder or birth defect
Persons of African-American, Eastern European, Jewish, Mediterranean, or Southeast
   Asian ancestry

Hemoglobin

Caribbean, Latin American, Asian, Mediterranean, or African descent
Menorrhagia

Hepatitis B Vaccine

Intravenous drug users
Current recipients of blood products
Persons in health-related jobs with exposure to blood or blood products
Household and sexual contacts of hepatitis B virus carriers
Prostitutes
Persons with history of multiple sexual partners in the last 6 months

HIV testing

Person seeking treatment for sexually transmitted disease
Past or present intravenous drug use
History of prostitution
Past or present sexual partner HIV +, bisexual, intravenous user
Persons from area of high prevalence HIV infection
History transfusion 1978–1985

Influenza Vaccine

Residents of chronic care facilities
Persons with chronic cardiopulmonary disorders
Persons with metabolic diseases including:
   Diabetes mellitus
   Hemoglobinopathies
   Immunosuppression
   Renal dysfunction

Lipid Profile

Persons with elevated cholesterol level
History of parent or sibling with cholesterol ≥ 240 mg/dl
History of sibling parent, or grandparent with documented premature (younger than 55
years of age) coronary artery disease
Persons with diabetes mellitus
Smoker

Table 8.7—*continued*

Mammography

Women aged 35 years and older with a family history of premenopausally diagnosed breast cancer in a first-degree relative

Pneumococcal Vaccine

Chronic cardiac/pulmonary disease
Sickle cell disease
Nephrotic syndrome
Hodgkin's disease
Asplenia
Diabetes mellitus
Alcoholism
Cirrhosis
Multiple myeloma
Renal disease
Immunosuppression

Rubella Titer/Vaccine

Women of childbearing age lacking evidence of immunity
Immunization (MMR) for all women unable to show proof of immunity

Skin

Recreational or occupation exposure to sunlight
History/family history skin cancer
Precursor lesions (dysplastic nevi, some congenital nevi)

Sexually Transmitted Disease (STD)

Multiple partners/partner with multiple partners
Sexual contacts of persons with culture proven STDs
History repeated episodes STDs
Persons attending STD clinics

Tuberculin (TB) Skin Test

Patients with HIV
Close contacts (household or enclosed environments) of known or suspected persons with TB
Persons with medical risk factors known to increase the risk of disease if infection occurred
Foreign-born persons from countries with high TB prevalence
Medically underserved, low-income populations
Alcoholics and intravenous drug users
Residents of long-term care facilities, jails, mental institutions, nursing homes and facilities, other long-term residential facilities
Health-professional working in high-risk health care facilities

Thyroid-Stimulating Hormone

Individuals with strong family history thyroid disease
Patients with autoimmune disease

Modified with permission from **ACOG.** *The Obstetrician–Gynecologist and Primary-Preventive Health Care.* Washington, DC: American College of Obstetricians and Gynecologists, 1993:1–22.

Table 8.8   Immunizations

Ages 13–18 Years

Periodic
    Tetanus-diphtheria booster (once between ages 14 and 16)
High-Risk Groups
    Measles, mumps, rubella (MMR) (HR7)
    Hepatitis B vaccine (HR 10)
    Fluoride supplement (HR 11)

Ages 19–39 Years

Periodic
    Tetanus-diphtheria booster (every 10 years)
High-Risk Groups
    Measles, mumps, rubella (MMR) (HR7)
    Hepatitis B vaccine (HR 10)
    Influenza vaccine (HR 15)
    Pneumococcal vaccine (HR 16)

Age 40–64 Years

Periodic
    Tetanus-diphtheria booster (every 10 years)
    Influenza vaccine (annually beginning at age 55)
High-Risk Groups
    Mumps, measles, rubella (MMR) (HR7)
    Hepatitis B vaccine (HR 10)
    Influence vaccine (HR 15)
    Pneumococcal vaccine (HR 16)

Ages 65 Years and Older

Periodic
    Tetanus-diphtheria booster (every 10 years)
    Influenza vaccine (annually)
    Pneumococcal vaccine (once)
High-Risk Groups
    Hepatitis B vaccine (HR 10)

Modified with permission from **ACOG.** *The Obstetrician–Gynecologist and Primary-Preventive Health Care.* Washington, DC: American College of Obstetricians and Gynecologists, 1993:1–22.

Appendix II: Primary Care Guidelines

Table 9.5 Selected Medications and Dosage for Control of Essential Hypertension

Medication (Class)	Normal Daily Dosage (mg/day) and Interval	Dispensing Unit (mg)
Angiotensin-converting enzyme (ACE) inhibitors		
Enalapril	5–40 (qd, bid)	2.5, 5, 10, 20
Calcium channel blockers		
Nifedipine sustained release	30–90 (qd)	30, 60, 90
Diltiazem sustained release	120–240 (bid)	60, 90, 120
Alpha blockers		
Terazosin	1–20 (qd)	1, 2, 5, 10
Mixed alpha and beta blockers		
Labetalol	200–800 (bid)	100, 200, 300
Diuretics		
Hydrochlorothiazide	12.5–50 (qd)	25, 50
Triamterene (potassium-sparing)	50–100 (bid)	50, 100
Beta blockers		
Propranolol (lipid soluble)	60–160 (qd)	60, 80, 120, 160
Atenolol (water soluble)	50–100 (qd)	50, 100
Smooth muscle relaxant		
Hydralazine	25–75 (tid, qid)	10, 25, 50, 100

Table 9.6 Schemes for Control of Essential Hypertension

Angiotensin-converting enzyme (ACE) inhibitor

Beta blockers, diuretics, central agents

Calcium channel blockers

Diuretics, beta blockers, central agents

Alpha blockers

Diuretics, beta blockers

Primary Medications are in bold, *Secondary drugs to add in combination with primary are in italics.*
Monotherapy and long-acting agents are recommended for sustained release and compliance. Fixed combinations have an advantage of compliance but are discouraged due to the inability to selectively modify doses.
Reproduced with permission from **Nolan T.** Evaluation and treatment of uncomplicated hypertension. *Clin Obstet Gynecol,* 1995;38:156–65.

Table 9.7   Initial Classification Based on Total Cholesterol and HDL Cholesterol Levels*

Cholesterol Level	Initial Classification
Total Cholesterol	
< 200 mg/dl (5.2 mmol/l)	Desirable blood cholesterol
200–239 mg/dl (5.2–6.2 mmol/l)	Borderline high blood cholesterol
≥ 240 mg/dl (6.2 mmol/l)	High blood cholesterol
HDL Cholesterol	
< 35 mg/dl (0.9 mmol/l)	Low HDL Cholesterol

*HDL, high-density lipoprotein.
Reproduced with permission **Expert Panel on Detection, Evaluation and Treatment of High Blood Cholesterol in Adults.** Summary of the NCEP Adult Treatment Plan II Report. *JAMA* 1993;269:3017.

Table 9.8   Classification of Diabetes Mellitus

Type I:	Insulin-dependent diabetes mellitus (IDDM)
Type II:	Noninsulin-dependent diabetes mellitus (NIDDM) (Subgroups may be classified as obese or nonobese)
Other types of diabetes:	
	Impaired glucose tolerance (IGT) Subgroups—obese or nonobese
	Pancreatic disease Secondary to destruction of islet cells
	Endocrinopathies Cushing's, acromegaly, pheochromocytoma, hyperaldosteronism
	Drug-induced

Table 9.9   Physician Guidelines in the Therapy of Diabetes Mellitus

- Establish diagnosis and classify type of diabetes mellitus (DM).

- If diagnosis of DM is already established, additional oral glucose tolerance tests should not be performed.

- Initiate diabetes education classes to learn blood glucose monitoring and diabetic medications, to learn signs, symptoms, and complications, and to learn how to manage sick days.

- Place patient on American Diabetes Association (ADA) diet with appropriate caloric, sodium, and lipid restrictions.

- Establish cardiac risk factors, kidney function (serum creatinine, 24-hour urine albumin).

- If neuropathy is present, refer to a neurologist.

- Establish extent of fundoscopic lesion (refer to ophthalmologist as needed).

- Check feet and toenails at each visit.

- Use finger stick blood glucose for daily diabetic control and urine check for ketones (but do not use first morning void).

- Follow chronic glycemic control by HgA$_{1c}$ every 2–3 months (every 6 months in elderly) in the office.

- Initial general health evaluation should consist of history and physical examination and the following laboratory tests: Complete blood count (CBC) with differential, chemistry profile, lipid profile, urinalysis, thyroid function tests, and electrocardiogram (base line at 40 years of age or older; repeat yearly).

- Oral hypoglycemic agents (OHA) may be considered if fasting blood glucose (FBG) does not decline or increase, if the patient has had diabetes for less than 10 years, does not have severe hepatic or renal disease, and is not pregnant or allergic to sulfonylurea.

- Fasting blood sugar (FBS) (on diet) $\geq$ 250 mg/dl are not suitable candidates for oral hypoglycemic agents.

- While on oral hypoglycemic agents, check FBS and 2-hour postprandial in the office every 2 months (in conjunction with daily home glucose monitoring).

- If postprandial glucose < 200 mg/dl, omit oral hypoglycemic agents and place on diet alone and follow every 1–2 months.

- If FSG > 200 mg/dl consistently, place patient on insulin.

- If insulin is required, consider sending to an internist, especially if obese.

- If the gynecologist continues to follow patient, the amount of insulin necessary is far less than pregnant patients.

Table 9.10   Patient Guidelines for Treatment of NIDDM

Initiate an American Diabetes Association reducing diet (50% carbohydrate, 30% fat, 20% protein, high fiber) with 3 meals a day.

Maintain ideal body weight or to reduce weight by 5–15% in 3 months if obese.

Modify risk factors (smoking, exercise, fat intake).

Check fasting blood glucose (FBG) by finger stick daily for 2 months.

- If plasma blood sugar declines, no other therapy is needed.

- If FBG does not decline or increases, use of oral hypoglycemic agents may be considered.

Table 9.11   Commonly Used Oral Hypoglycemic Agents

Oral Hypoglycemic Agents	Trade Name	Daily Dose	Duration of Action (Hrs)
Tolbutamide	*Orinase*	750 mg—3.0 g/divided doses	6–12
Tolazamide	*Tolinase*	200–1000 mg/divided doses	12–24
Acetohexamide	*Dymelor*	250–1500 mg/single dose	12–24
Chlorpropamide	*Diabinese*	100–500 mg	up to 60
Glyburide	*Micronase, DiaBeta*	2.5–20 mg variable dose	10–24
Glipizide	*Glucotrol*	2.5–40 mg variable dose	3–8

Appendix III: Contraception

Table 10.1   Current Contraceptive Status and Method: United States, 1982 and 1988

	1988	*1982*
All women	54,009,000	57,900,000
	Percent Distribution	
Total	100.0	100.0
Sterile	29.7	27.2
Surgically sterile	28.3	25.7
Contraceptively sterile	23.6	19.0
Female	16.6	12.9
Male	7.0	6.1
Noncontraceptively sterile	4.7	6.6
Female	4.7	6.3
Male	0.0	0.3
Nonsurgically sterile	1.4	1.5
Pregnant or postpartum	4.8	5.0
Seeking pregnancy	3.8	4.2
Nonuser	25.0	26.9
Never had intercourse	11.5	13.6
No intercourse in last 3 months	6.2	5.9
Intercourse in last 3 months	6.5	7.4
Nonsurgical contraception	36.7	36.7
Pill	18.5	15.6
Intrauterine device	1.2	4.0
Diaphragm	3.5	4.5
Condom	8.8	6.7
Foam	0.6	1.3
Periodic abstinence	1.4	2.2
Withdrawal	1.3	1.1
Douche	0.1	0.1
Other methods	1.2	1.3

From **Mosher WD, Pratt WF.** *Contraceptive Use in the United States, 1973–1988.* Advance Data from Vital and Health Statistics of the National Center for Health Statistics. All races combined. Washington, DC: National Center for Health, 1990:182.

Table 10.2   Percentage of Women Experiencing a Contraceptive Failure During the First Year of Use and the Percentage Continuing Use at the End of the First Year

Method	Women Experiencing Accidental Pregnancy within the First Year of Use (%)		Women Continuing Use at 1 Year (%)
	Typical Use	*Perfect Use*	
Chance	85	85	
Spermicides	21	6	43
Periodic abstinence			67
Calendar		9	
Ovulation method		3	
Symptothermal		2	
Postovulation		1	
Withdrawal	19	4	
Cap			
Parous women	36	26	45
Nulliparous women	18	9	58
Diaphragm	18	6	58
Condom			
Female (Reality)	21	5	56
Male	12	3	63
Pill	3		72
Progestin Only		0.5	
Combined		0.1	
Intrauterine device			
Progesterone T	2.0	1.5	81
Copper T380A	0.8	0.6	78
Levonorgestrel T20	0.1	0.1	81
DepoProvera	0.3	0.3	70
Norplant*	0.3	0.3	85
Female Sterilization	0.4	0.4	100
Male Sterilization	0.15	0.10	100

*Cumulative 5-year pregnancy rate for pliable tubing, divided by 5.
Reproduced with permission from **Hatcher RA, Trussell J, Stewart F, et al.** *Contraceptive Technology.* 16th ed. New York: Irvington Publishers Inc., 1994:113.

Table 10.3 Overview of Contraceptive Methods

Method	Advantages	Disadvantages	Risks	Noncontraceptive Benefits
Coitus interruptus	Available, free	Depends on male control	Pregnancy	?Decreased STD risk
Lactation	Available, free	Unreliable duration of effect	Pregnancy	?Decreased breast cancer
Periodic abstinence	Available, free	Complex methodology; motivation is essential	Pregnancy	None
Condoms	Available, no prescription needed	Motivation is essential; must be used each time; depends on male	Pregnancy	Proven to decrease STDs and cervical cancer
Spermicides	Available, no prescription needed	Must be used each time	Pregnancy	Some decrease in STDs
Diaphragm/ cap	Nonhormonal	Must be used each time; fitting required	Pregnancy, cystitis	Proven to decrease STDs and cervical cancer
IUD T380A	High efficacy for 10 years, unrelated to coitus	Initial cost; skilled inserter; pain and bleeding	Initial mild risk of PID and septic abortion	None
Progestasert	Reasonable efficacy	Initial cost; skilled inserter; replace every year	Initial mild risk of PID, ectopic pregnancy	Reduced dysmenorrhea and menstrual blood loss
Oral contraceptives	High efficacy	Motivation to take daily; cost	Thrombosis; older smokers have increased risk of MI and stroke	Many benefits (see text)
DMPA	High efficacy, convenience	Injection required; bleeding pattern	Probably none	Many (see text)
Implants	High efficacy, convenience	Surgical insertion and removal; initial cost; bleeding pattern	Functional cysts	Unknown
Postcoital hormones	Moderate efficacy	Frequent use disrupts menses; nausea	None	Unknown

STDs, sexually transmitted diseases; IUD, intrauterine device; PID, pelvic inflammatory disease; MI, myocardial infarction; *DMPA, depomedroxyprogesterone acetate.*

Table 10.9 Pregnancies after Tubal Sterilization

	Pregnancies/1000	Sterilizations
Laparoscopy*		
Bipolar coagulation	2.1–4.0	65,971
Endocoagulation	1.1	40,425
Falope ring	0.8–4.0	498,232
Hulka clip	1.8–5.9	5503
Filshie clip	0–2	2317
Minilaparotomy†		
Modified Pomeroy	1.46	2050
Pomeroy	2	6717
Cesarean Section		
Pomeroy	3	1739
Interval laparotomy‡	6	1115

*From **Khandwala SD.** Laparoscopic sterilization: a comparison of current techniques. *J Reprod Med* 1988;33:463–7.
†From **Rimdusit P.** Separate stitches tubal sterilization, a modified Pomeroy's technique. An analysis of the procedure, complaints and failures. *J Med Assoc Thai* 1984;67:602–5.
‡From **Shephard MK.** Female contraceptive sterilization. *Obstet Gynecol Surv* 1974; 29:739–87.

Table 10.11 Death to Case Rates for Legal Abortion Mortality by Weeks of Gestation, United States, 1972–1987

Weeks of Gestation	Deaths	Abortions	Rate*	Relative Risk
≤8	33	8,673,759	0.4	1.0
9–10	39	4,847,321	0.8	2.1
11–12	33	2,360,768	1.4	3.7
13–15	28	962,185	2.9	7.7
16–20	74	794,093	9.3	24.5
≥21	21	175,395	12.0	31.5

*Legal abortion deaths per 100,000 procedures, excludes deaths from ectopic pregnancies or pregnancy with gestation length unknown.
From **Lawson HW, Frye A, Atrash HK, Smith JC, Shulman RB, Ramick M, et al.** Abortion mortality, United States, 1972–1987. *Am J Obstet Gynecol* 1994;171:1365–72.

Table 10.12 Rates for Legal Abortions by Type of Procedure and Weeks of Gestation, United States, 1974–1987*

Procedure	≤8	9–10	11–12	13–15	16–20	≥21
Vacuum curettage†	0.3	0.7	1.1	—	—	—
Dilation and evacuation	—	—	—	2.0	6.5	11.9
Instillation‡	—	—	—	3.8	7.9	10.3
Hysterectomy/ hysterotomy	18.3	30.0	41.2	28.1	103.4	274.3

*Legal induced abortion deaths per 100,000 legal induced abortions.
†Includes all suction and sharp curettage procedures.
‡Includes all instillation methods (saline, prostaglandin).
From **Lawson HW, Frye A, Atrash HK, Smith JC, Shulman HB, Ramick M, et al.** Abortion mortality, United States, 1972–1987. *Am J Obstet Gynecol* 1994;171:1365–72.

330

Appendix IV: Medications for PMS and Psychiatric Conditions

Table 12.2   Scientific Basis of Selected Medications Used to Treat PMS

Treatment	Scientific Basis	Advantages	Disadvantages	Notes
Alprazolam	Several double-blind, placebo-controlled, randomized crossover studies. Results were mixed. Placebo was as effective as alprazolam in some studies.	Oral medication appears to be more effective in alleviating depression and anxiety symptoms than physical symptoms.	Potential for dependence, requires tapering, drowsiness reported by many subjects; long-term effects unknown, safety during pregnancy unknown.	The studies involved highly selective groups of women. There was a high dropout rate in one of the positive studies. In one study that found alprazolam effective, 87% of the women had a history of major depression or an anxiety disorder. Different doses were used in the studies (0.75–2.25 mg); the standard effective dose is unknown.
Fluoxetine (Prozac)	Several double-blind, randomized, placebo-controlled, crossover trials. All found fluoxetine effective.	Well tolerated, single daily oral dose. Significant decrease in psychic and behavioral symptoms.	Long-term effects unknown. Safety during pregnancy unknown. Appears less effective in controlling physical symptoms.	Trials involved very small, highly select groups of women. Duration of treatment did not exceed 3 months. All trials used 20 mg orally daily.
Gonadotropin-releasing hormone agonist	Several small, double-blind, randomized, placebo-controlled, crossover trials. Most patients experienced improvement.	Rapidly reversible, many patients report being virtually symptom-free during therapy.	Produces pseudomenopause, expensive, risk for osteoporosis, hypo-estrogenic symptoms. Usually given for only short periods of time.	An "add-back" regimen of estrogen-progestin in addition to gonadotropin-releasing hormone agonist has been reported. If replicated, it may have potential for an effective, long-term treatment for premenstrual syndrome.
Spironolactone	Several double-blind, randomized, placebo-controlled trials. Mixed results.	May alleviate bloating and improve symptoms related to mood. Oral medication taken once or twice a day. Nonaddictive.	Effectiveness not proven consistently across studies.	Spironolactone is the only diuretic that has shown effectiveness in treating premenstrual syndrome in controlled, randomized trials. Method of action may be antiandrogen properties.
Vitamin B$_6$	Ten randomized double-blind trials. About one-third of the trials reported positive results, one-third reported negative results, and one-third reported ambiguous results.		No conclusive evidence that vitamin B$_6$ is more effective than placebo.	Doses ranged from 50 to 500 mg. Only one study involved more than 40 subjects. The large multicenter trial (N = 204) reported similar results for placebo and vitamin B$_6$.

Reproduced with permission from **The American College of Obstetricians and Gynecologists.** *Committee Opinion.* Washington, DC: ACOG, 1995.

331

Table 12.3   Pharmacology of Antidepressant Medications

Drug	Therapeutic Dosage Range (mg/day)	Average (Range) of Elimination Half-Lives (hours)*	Potentially Fatal Drug Interactions
Tricyclics			
Amitriptyline (Elavil, Endep)	75–300	24 (16–46)	Antiarrhythmics, MAO inhibitors
Clomipramine (Anafranil)	75–300	24 (20–40)	Antiarrhythmics, MAO inhibitors
Desipramine (Norpramin, Pertofrane)	75–300	18 (12–50)	Antiarrhythmics, MAO inhibitors
Doxepin (Adapin, Sinequan)	75–300	17 (10–47)	Antiarrhythmics, MAO inhibitors
Imipramine (Janimine, Tofranil)	75–300	22 (12–34)	Antiarrhythmics, MAO inhibitors
Nortiptyline (Aventyl, Pamelor)	40–200	26 (18–88)	Antiarrhythmics, MAO inhibitors
Protiptyline (Vivactil)	20–60	76 (54–124)	Antiarrhythmics, MAO inhibitors
Trimipramine (Surmontil)	75–300	12 (8–30)	Antiarrhythmics, MAO inhibitors
Heterocyclics			
Amoxapine (Asendin)	100–600	10 (8–14)	MAO inhibitors
Bupropion (Wellbutrin)	225–450	14 (8–24)	MAO inhibitors (possibly)
Maprotiline (Ludiomil)	100–225	43 (27–58)	MAO inhibitors
Trazodone (Desyrel)	150–600	8 (4–14)	—
Selective serotin reuptake inhibitors			
Fluoxetine (Prozac)	10–40	168 (72–360)[†]	MAO inhibitors
Paroxetine (Paxil)	20–50	24 (3–65)	MAO inhibitors[‡]
Sertraline (Zoloft)	50–150	24 (10–30)	MAO inhibitors[‡]
Monoamine oxidase inhibitors (MAO inhibitors)[§]			
Isocarboxazid (Marplan)	30–50	Unknown	For all three MAO inhibitors: vasoconstrictors,[‖] decongestants,[‖] meperidine, and possibly other narcotics
Phenelzine (Nardil)	45–90	2 (1.5–4.0)	
Tranylcypromine (Parnate)	20–60	2 (1.5–3.0)	

*Half-lives are affected by age, sex, race, concurrent medications, and length of drug exposure.
†Includes both fluoxetine and norfluoxetine.
‡By extrapolation from fluoxetine data.
§MAO inhibition lasts longer (7 days) than drug half-life.
‖Including pseudoephedrine, phenylephrine, phenylpropanolamine, epinephrine, norepinephrine, and others.
From **Depression Guideline Panel.** *Depression in Primary Care: Detection, Diagnosis, and Treatment.* Quick Reference Guide for Clinicians, No. 5. AHCPR Publication No. 93-0552. Rockville, MD: U.S. Department of Health and Human Services, Public Health Service, Agency for Health Care Policy and Research, 1993:15.

Table 12.4   Side-Effect Profiles of Antidepressant Medications

| | Side Effect* | | | | | | |
| | Central Nervous System | | | Cardiovascular | | | |
	Anticholinergic†	Drowsiness	Insomnia/ Agitation	Orthostatic Hypotension	Cardiac Arrhythmia	Gastrointestinal Distress	Weight Gain (over 6 kg)
Amitriptyline	4+	4+	0	4+	3+	0	4+
Desipramine	1+	1+	1+	2+	2+	0	1+
Doxepin	3+	4+	0	2+	2+	0	3+
Imipramine	3+	3+	1+	4+	3+	1+	3+
Nortriptyline	1+	1+	0	2+	2+	0	1+
Protriptyline	2+	1+	1+	2+	2+	0	0
Trimipramine	1+	4+	0	2+	2+	0	3+
Amoxapine	2+	2+	2+	2+	3+	0	1+
Maprotiline	2+	4+	0	0	1+	0	2+
Trazodone	0	4+	0	1+	1+	1+	1+
Bupropion	0	0	2+	0	1+	1+	0
Fluoxetine	0	0	2+	0	0	3+	0
Paroxetine	0	0	2+	0	0	3+	0
Sertraline	0	0	2+	0	0	3+	0
Monoamine oxidase inhibitors	1	1+	2+	2+	0	1+	2+

*Numerals indicate the likelihood of side effect occuring ranging from 0 for absent or rare to 4+ for relatively common.
†Dry mouth, blurred vision, urinary hesitancy, constipation.
From **Depression Guideline Panel.** *Depression in Primary Care: Detection, Diagnosis, and Treatment.* Quick Reference Guide for Clinicians, No. 5. AHCPR Publication No. 93-0553. Rockville, MD: U.S. Department of Health and Human Services, Public Health Service, Agency for Health Care Policy and Research, 1993:14.

Table 12.5   Compounds Used for Anxiety

Medication	Trade Name	Rate of Absorption*	Half-Life†	Active Long-Acting Metabolite	Comments
Benzodiazepines					
					Metabolism of benzodiazepines is inhibited by cimetidine, disulfiram, isoniazid, and oral contraceptives. Metabolism of benzodiazepines is enhanced by rifampin.
Alprazolam	Xanax	Intermediate	Intermediate	No	Preferred in elderly patients or patients with poor hepatic functions.
Chlordiazepoxide	Librium, others	Intermediate	Intermediate	Yes	
Clonazepam	Klonopin	Long	Long	No	
Clorazepate	Tranxene, others	Short	Short	Yes	
Diazepam	Valium, others	Short	Long	Yes	Half-life increased three or four times in elderly patients.
Lorazepam	Ativan, others	Intermediate	Intermediate	No	Preferred in elderly patients or patients with poor hepatic function.
Oxazepam	Serax	Long	Intermediate	No	Preferred in elderly patients or patients with poor hepatic function.
Prazepam	Centrax	Long	Short	Yes	
Atypical agent					
Buspirone	BuSpar				Not effective in panic disorder, little sedation, little risk of dependence/tolerance.

*Long ≥ 2 hours; Intermediate = 1–2 hours; Short ≤ 1 hour.
†Long > 20 hours; Intermediate = 6–20 hours; Short < 6 hours.
Adapted from **Gilman AG, Rall TW, Nies AS, Taylor P.** *The Pharmacological Basis of Therapeutics.* 8th ed. New York: McGraw-Hill, 1990.
From **Stotland NL.** Psychiatric and psychosocial issues in primary care for women. In: **Seltzer VL, Pearse WH,** ed. *Women's Primary Health Care: Office Practice and Procedures.* New York: McGraw-Hill, 1995.

Appendix V: Benign Gynecologic Conditions

Table 13.1 **Classification of Benign Conditions of the Vulva, Vagina, and Cervix**

Vulva

Skin conditions
Pigmented lesions
Tumors and cysts
Ulcers
Dystrophies

Vagina

Embryonic origin
    Mesonephric, paramesonephric, and urogenital sinus cysts
    Adenosis (related to diethylstilbestrol)
    Vaginal septa/duplications
Disorders of pelvic support
    Cystocele
    Rectocele
    Urethrocele
Other
    Condyloma
    Urethral diverticuli
    Fibroepithelial polyp
    Vaginal endometriosis

Cervix

Infectious
    Condyloma
    Herpes simplex virus ulceration
    Chlamydial cervicitis
    Other cervicitis
Other
    Endocervical polyps
    Nabothian cysts
    Columnar epithelium eversion

Table 13.2 Benign Ovarian Tumors

Functional

Follicular
Corpus luteum
Theca lutein

Inflammatory

Tubo-ovarian abscess or complex

Neoplastic

Germ cell
  Benign cystic teratoma
  Other and mixed
Epithelial
  Serous cystadenoma
  Mucinous cystadenoma
  Fibroma
  Cystadenofibroma
  Brenner tumor
  Mixed tumor

Other

Endometrioma

Table 13.3 Causes of Bleeding and Pelvic Mass by Approximate Frequency and Age Group

Bleeding

Prepubertal	Adolescent	Reproductive	Perimenopausal	Postmenopausal
Vulvovaginal and external lesions Foreign body Precocious puberty Tumor	Anovulation Pregnancy Exogenous hormone use Coagulopathy	Pregnancy Anovulation Exogenous hormone use Fibroids Cervical and endometrial polyps Thyroid dysfunction	Anovulation Fibroids Cervical and endometrial polyps Thyroid dysfunction	Endometrial lesions, including cancer Exogenous hormone use Atrophic vaginitis Other tumor— vulvar, vaginal, cervical

Pelvic Mass

Infancy	Prepubertal	Adolescent	Reproductive	Perimeno-pausal	Postmeno-pausal
Functional ovarian cyst Germ cell	Germ cell tumor	Functional cyst Pregnancy Dermoid/ other germ cell tumors Obstructing vaginal/uterine anomalies Epithelial ovarian tumors	Functional cyst Pregnancy Uterine fibroids Ovarian epithelial tumors	Fibroids Ovarian epithelial tumors Functional cysts	Ovarian tumor (malignant or benign) Bowel, malignant tumor or inflammatory Metastases

Table 13.4   Causes of Vaginal Bleeding in Prepubertal Girls

Vulvar and external

Vulvitis with excoriation
Trauma (e.g., straddle injury)
Lichen sclerosus
Condylomas
Molluscum contagiosum
Urethral prolapse

Vaginal

Vaginitis
Vaginal foreign body
Trauma (abuse, penetration)
Vaginal tumor

Uterine

Precocious puberty

Ovarian tumor

Exogenous estrogens

Topical
Enteral

Table 13.6   Abnormal Menses—Terminology

Term	Interval	Duration	Amount
Menorrhagia	Regular	Prolonged	Excessive
Metrorrhagia	Irregular	± Prolonged	Normal
Menometrorrhagia	Irregular	Prolonged	Excessive
Hypermenorrhea	Regular	Normal	Excessive
Hypomenorrhea	Regular	Normal or less	Less
Oligomenorrhea	Infrequent and/or irregular	Variable	Scanty

Table 13.7   Etiology of Postmenopausal Bleeding

Factor	Approximate Percentage
Exogenous estrogens	30
Atrophic endometritis/vaginitis	30
Endometrial cancer	15
Endometrial or cervical polyps	10
Endometrial hyperplasia	5
Miscellaneous (e.g., cervical cancer, uterine sarcoma, urethral caruncle, trauma)	10

Reproduced with permission from **Hacker NF, Moore JG.** *Essentials of Obstetrics and Gynecology.* Philadelphia: WB Saunders, 1986:467.

Table 13.8   Conditions Diagnosed as a "Pelvic Mass" in Women of Reproductive Age

---

Full urinary bladder

Urachal cyst

Sharply anteflexed or retroflexed uterus

Pregnancy (with or without concomitant leiomyomas)
   Intrauterine
   Tubal
   Abdominal

Ovarian or adnexal masses
   Functional cysts
   Inflammatory masses
      Tubo-ovarian complex
      Diverticular abscess
      Appendiceal abscess
   Matted bowel and omentum
   Peritoneal cyst
   Stool in sigmoid
   Neoplastic tumors
      Benign
      Malignant

Paraovarian or paratubal cysts

Intraligamentous myomas

Less common conditions that must be excluded:
   Pelvic kidney
   Carcinoma of the colon, rectum, appendix
   Carcinoma of the fallopian tube
   Retroperitoneal tumors (anterior sacral meningocele)
   Uterine sarcoma or other malignant tumors

Table 13.9   Ultrasound Scoring System for Adnexal Masses*

Clear cyst and smooth borders	1
Clear cyst with slightly irregular border; cyst with smooth walls but low-level echoes (i.e., endometrioma)	2
Cyst with low-level echoes with slightly irregular border but no nodularity (i.e., endometrioma); clear cyst in postmenopausal patient	3
Equivocal, nonspecific ultrasound appearance: solid ovarian enlargement or small cyst with irregular borders and internal echoes (hemorrhagic cyst or benign ovarian tumor)	4–6
Multiseptated or irregular cystic mass consistent in appearance with ovarian tumor (7 = less nodularity; 8–9 = more nodularity)	7–9
Pelvic mass as above, with ascites	10

1 = benign; 10 = malignant.
Modified from **Finkler NJ, Benacerraf B, Lavin PT, Wojciechowski C, Knapp RC.** Comparison of CA 125, clinical impression, and ultrasound in the preoperative evaluation of ovarian masses. Reprinted with permission from The American College of Obstetricians and Gynecologists (*Obstet Gynecol 1988;72:659*).

Table 13.10   Subacute and Chronic Recurrent Conditions of the Vulva

Noninfectious	Infectious
Acanthosis nigricans	Cellulitis
Atopic dermatitis	Folliculitis
Behcet's disease	Furuncle/carbuncle
Contact dermatitis	Insect bites (e.g., chiggers, fleas)
Crohn's disease	Necrotizing fasciitis
Diabetic vulvitis*	Pubic lice
Hidradenitis suppurativa*	Scabies
Hyperplastic dystrophy	Tinea
Lichen sclerosus	
Mixed dystrophy	
Paget's disease	
Pseudo folliculitis	
Razor bumps	
Psoriasis	
Seborrheic dermatitis	
Vulvar intraepithelial neoplasia	

*Etiology unknown, often secondarily infected.

Table 13.11   Types of Vulvar Tumors

1. Cystic lesions	3. Anatomic
Bartholin duct cyst	Hernia
Cyst in the canal of Nuck (hydrocele)	Urethral diverticulum
Epithelial inclusion cyst	Varicosities
Skene duct cyst	
	4. Infections
2. Solid Tumors	Abscess—Bartholin, Skene, periclitoral, other
Acrocordon (skin tag)	Condyloma lata
Angiokeratoma	Molluscum contagiosum
Bartholin gland adenoma	Pyogenic granuloma
Cherry angioma	
Fibroma	5. Ectopic
Hemangioma	Endometriosis
Hidradinoma	Ectopic breast tissue
Lipoma	
Granular cell myoblastoma	
Neurofibroma	
Papillomatosis	

Appendix VI: Pelvic Pain

Table 14.2   Nerves Carrying Painful Impulses from the Pelvic Organs

Organ	*Spinal Segments*	*Nerves*
Perineum, vulva, lower vagina	S2–S4	Pudendal, inguinal, genitofemoral, posterofemoral cutaneous
Upper vagina, cervix, lower uterine segment, posterior urethra, bladder trigone, uterosacral and cardinal ligaments, rectosigmoid, lower ureters	S2–S4	Sacral afferents traveling through the pelvic plexus
Uterine fundus, proximal fallopian tubes, broad ligaments, upper bladder, cecum appendix, terminal large bowel	T11–T12, L1	Thoracolumbar splanchnic nerves through uterine and hypogastric plexes
Outer two-thirds of fallopian tubes, upper ureter	T9–T10	Thoracolumbar splanchnic nerves through mesenteric plexus
Ovaries	T9–T10	Thoracolumbar splanchnic nerves traveling with ovarian vessels via renal and aortic plexus and celiac and mesenteric ganglia

Table 14.3 Peripheral Causes of Chronic Pelvic Pain

Gynecologic

Noncyclic

1. Adhesions
2. Endometriosis
3. Salpingo-oophoritis
   a. Acute
   b. Subacute
4. Ovarian remnant syndrome
5. Pelvic congestion syndrome (varicosities)
6. Ovarian neoplasms
7. Pelvic relaxation

Cyclic

1. Primary dysmenorrhea
2. Secondary dysmenorrhea
   a. Imperforate hymen
   b. Transverse vaginal septum
   c. Cervical stenosis
   d. Uterine anomalies (congenital malformation, bicornuate uterus, blind uterine horn)
   e. Intrauterine synechiae (Asherman's syndrome)
   f. Endometrial polyps
   g. Uterine leiomyoma
   h. Adenomyosis
   i. Pelvic congestion syndrome (varicosities)
   j. Endometriosis
3. Atypical cyclic
   a. Endometriosis
   b. Adenomyosis
   c. Ovarian remnant syndrome
   d. Chronic functional cyst formation

Gastrointestinal

1. Irritable bowel syndrome
2. Ulcerative colitis
3. Granulomatous colitis (Crohn's disease)
4. Carcinoma
5. Infectious diarrhea
6. Recurrent partial small bowel obstruction
7. Diverticulitis
8. Hernia
9. Abdominal angina
10. Recurrent appendiceal colic

Genitourinary

1. Recurrent or relapsing cystourethritis
2. Urethral syndrome
3. Interstitial cystitis
4. Ureteral diverticuli or polyps
5. Carcinoma of the bladder
6. Ureteral obstruction
7. Pelvic kidney

Neurologic

1. Nerve entrapment syndrome
2. Neuroma

Table 14.3—*continued*

Musculoskeletal

Low back pain syndrome

1. Congenital anomalies
2. Scoliosis and kyphosis
3. Spondylolysis
4. Spondylolisthesis
5. Spinal injuries
6. Inflammation
7. Tumors
8. Osteoporosis
9. Degenerative changes
10. Coccydynia

Myofascial Syndrome

Systemic

1. Acute intermittent porphyria
2. Abdominal migraine
3. Systemic lupus erythematosis
4. Lymphoma
5. Neurofibromatosis

Appendix VII: Chemotherapy

Table 30.5 Drug Dose Adjustments for Combination Chemotherapy
(Sliding Scale Based on Bone Marrow Toxicity)

If White Blood Count Before Starting the Next Course Is:	*Then Dosage Is:*
>4000/mm^3	100% of all drugs
3999–3000/mm^3	100% of nonmyelotoxic agents and 50% of each myelotoxic agent
2999–2000/mm^3	100% of nonmyelotoxic agents and 25% of each myelotoxic agent
1999–1000/mm^3	50% of nonmyelotoxic agents and 25% of myelotoxic agents
999–0/mm^3	No drug until blood counts recover

If the Platelet Count Before Starting Next Course Is:	*Then Dosage Is:*
>100,000/mm^3	100% of all drugs
50,000–100,000/mm^3	100% of nonmyelotoxic drugs and 50% of myelotoxic drugs
<50,000/mm^3	No drug until blood counts recover

Table 30.6   Chemotherapeutic Drugs Used in Gynecologic Cancers

Drug	Route of Administration	Common Treatment Schedules	Common Toxicities	Diseases Treated
Alkylating agents				
Cyclophosphamide (Cytoxan)	Oral, I.V.	1.5–3.0 mg/kg/day p.o. 10–50 mg/kg I.V. every 1–4 weeks	Myelosuppression, cystitis ± bladder fibrosis, alopecia, hepatitis, amenorrhea, azoospermia	Breast, ovary, soft tissue sarcomas
Melphalan (Alkeran, L-PAM)	Oral	0.2 mg/kg/day × 5 days every 4–6 weeks	Myelosuppression, nausea and vomiting (rare), mucosal ulceration (rare), second malignancies	Ovary, breast
Triethylene thiophosphoramide (TSPA, Thiotepa)	I.V. \ Intracavitary	I.V.: 0.8 mg/kg every 4–6 weeks \ Intracavitary: 45–60 mg	Myelosuppression, nausea and vomiting, headaches, fever (rare)	Ovary, breast; intracavitary for malignant effusions
Iphosphamide (Ifex)	I.V.	1.0 or 1.2 g/m²/day × 5 days With mesna: 200 mg/m² immediately before and 4 and 8 hr after iphosphamide	Myelosuppression, bladder toxicity, CNS dysfunction, renal toxicity	Cervix, ovary
Alkylating-Like Agents				
Cis-dichlorodiamino-platinum (cisplatin)	I.V.	10–20 mg/m²/day × 5 every 3 weeks or 50–75 mg/m² every 1–3 weeks	Nephrotoxicity, tinnitis and and hearing loss, nausea and vomiting, myelosuppression, peripheral neuropathy	Ovarian and germ cell carcinomas, cervical cancer
Carboplatin	I.V.	300–400 mg/m² × 6 every 3–4 weeks	Less neuropathy, ototoxicity, and nephrotoxicity than cisplatin; more hemato-poeitic toxicity, especially thrombocytopenia, than cisplatin	Ovarian and germ cell carcinomas
Decarbazine (DTIC)	I.V.	2–4.5 mg/kg/day × 10 days every 4 weeks	Myelosuppression, nausea and vomiting, flulike syndrome, hepatotoxicity	Uterine sarcomas, soft tissue sarcomas
Antitumor Antibiotics				
Actinomycin D (dactinomycin, Cosmegen)	I.V.	0.3–0.5 mg/m² I.V. × 5 days every 3–4 weeks	Nausea and vomiting, skin necrosis, mucosal ulceration, myelosuppression	Germ cell ovarian tumors, choriocarcinoma, soft tissue sarcoma
Bleomycin (Blenoxane)	I.V., S.C., I.M., I.P.	10–20 units/m² 1–2 times/week to total dose of 400 units; for effusions: 60–120 units	Fever, dermatologic reactions, pulmonary toxicity, anaphylactic reactions	Cervix, germ cell ovarian tumors, malignant effusions
Mitomycin-C (Mutamycin)	I.V.	10–20 mg/m² every 6–8 weeks	Myelosuppression, local vesicant, nausea and vomiting, mucosal ulcerations, nephrotoxicity	Breast, cervix, ovary
...bicin *...ycin)*	I.V.	60–90 mg/m² every 3 weeks or 20–35 mg/m² every day × 3 every 3 weeks	Myelosuppression, alopecia, cardiotoxicity, local vesicant, nausea and vomiting, mucosal ulcerations	Ovary, breast, endometrium

Table 30.6—*continued*

Drug	Route of Administration	Common Treatment Schedules	Common Toxicities	Diseases Treated
Mithramycin (Mithracin)	I.V.	20–50 mg/kg/day every 4–6 weeks; Hypercalcemia: 25 mg/kg every 3–4 days	Nausea and vomiting, hemorrhagic diathesis, hepatotoxicity, renal toxicity, fever, myelosuppression, facial flushing	Hypercalcemia of malignancy
Antimetabolites				
5-Fluorouracil (Fluorouracil, 5-FU)	I.V.	10–15 mg/kg/week	Myelosuppression, nausea and vomiting, anorexia, alopecia	Breast, ovary
Methotrexate (MTX, amethopterin)	P.O., I.V., Intrathecal	Oral: 15–40 mg/day × 5 days; I.V.: 240 mg/m² with leucovorin rescue; Intrathecal: 12–15 mg/m²/week	Mucosal ulceration, myelosuppression, hepatotoxicity, allergic pneumonitis; with intrathecal: meningeal irritation	Choriocarcinoma, breast, ovary
Hydroxyurea (Hydrea)	P.O., I.V.	1–2 gm/m²/daily for 2–6 weeks	Myelosuppression, nausea and vomiting, anorexia	Cervix
Plant Alkaloids				
Vincristine (Oncovin)	I.V.	0.01–0.03 mg/kg/week	Neurotoxicity, alopecia, myelosuppression, cranial nerve palsies, gastrointestinal	Ovarian germ cell, sarcomas, cervical cancer
Vinblastine (Velban)	I.V.	5–6 mg/m² every 1–2 weeks	Myelosuppression, alopecia, nausea and vomiting, neurotoxicity	Ovarian germ cell, choriocarcinoma
Epipodophyllotoxin (Etoposide, VP-16)	I.V.	300–600 mg/m² divided over 3–4 days every 3–4 weeks	Myelosuppression, alopecia, hypotension	Ovarian germ cell, choriocarcinoma
Paclitaxel (Taxol)	I.V.	135–250 mg/m² as a 3- to 24-hour infusion every 3 weeks	Myelosuppression, alopecia, allergic reactions, cardiac arrhythmias	Ovarian cancer, breast cancer
Taxotere	I.V.	50–100 mg/m²	Myelosuppression, alopecia, dermatologic reactions	Ovarian cancer, breast cancer
Miscellaneous Agent				
Hexamethylmelamine, Altretamine (Hexalen)	Oral	120 mg/m²/day × 14 days every 4 weeks	Nausea and vomiting myelosuppression, neurotoxicity, skin rashes	Ovary, breast

I.V., intravenous; S.C., subcutaneous; I.M., intramuscular; I.P., intraperitoneal; CNS, central nervous system, P.O., postoperative.

Table 30.8   Isotopes

Isotope		Half-Life	γ-Ray Energy (MeV)	β-Ray Average Energy at 1 cm	γ-Factor* R/mc/hr
Phosphorus	³²P	14.3 days		0.698	
Technesium	⁹⁹Tc	6.0 hours	0.14	0.014	0.56
Iodine	¹³¹I	8.07 days	Many 0.08–0.72	0.188	2.24
Cesium	¹³⁷Cs	30 years	0.662	0.242	3.2
Iridium	¹⁹²Ir	74 days	Several 0.32–0.61		5.0
Gold	¹⁹⁸Au	2.7 days	Several 0.41–1.1	0.328	2.43
Radium	²²⁶Ra	1620 years	Several 0.19–0.6		8.25

*γ(gamma) factor: Dose rate from a γ-emitting isotope expressed as the exposure rate in roentgens per hour at 1 cm from a point source of 1 mc.

Table 33.3   Chemotherapeutic Regimens for Advanced Ovarian Cancer

	Regimen	Interval
PT	Cisplatin (75–100 mg/M²) Paclitaxel (175–210 mg/M²)	Q 3 weeks
CT	Carboplatin (starting dose, AUC = 5) Paclitaxel (135–175 mg/M²)	Q 3–4 weeks
PC	Cisplatin (75–100 mg/M²) Cyclophosphamide (650–1000 mg/M²)	Q 3 weeks
CC	Carboplatin (AUC = 5–7) Cyclophosphamide (600 mg/M²)	Q 4 weeks
PAC	Cisplatin 50 mg/M² Doxorubicin 50 mg/M² Cyclophosphamide 500 mg/M²	Q 3–4 weeks

AUC, area under the curve.

Table 33.5   Combination Chemotherapy for Germ Cell Tumors of the Ovary

Regimen and Drugs	Dose and Schedule*
BEP	
Bleomycin	15 units/M²/week × 5; then on day 1 of course 4
Etoposide	100 mg/M²/day × 5 days every 3 weeks
Cisplatin	20 mg/M²/day × 5 days, or 100 mg/M²/day × 1 day every 3 weeks
VBP	
Vinblastine	0.15 mg/kg days 1 and 2 every 3 weeks
Bleomycin	15 units/M²/week × 5; then on day 1 of course 4
Cisplatin	100 mg/M² on day 1 every 3 weeks
VAC	
Vincristine	1–1.5 mg/M² on day 1 every 4 weeks
Actinomycin-D	0.5 mg/day × 5 days every 4 weeks
Cyclophosphamide	150 mg/M²/day × 5 days every 4 weeks

·doses given intravenously.

348

Table 33.6   POMB/ACE Chemotherapy for Germ Cell Tumors of the Ovary

POMB

Day 1	*Vincristine* 1 mg/M^2 intravenously; *methotrexate* 300 mg/M^2 as a 12-hr infusion
Day 2	*Bleomycin* 15 mg as a 24-hr infusion: *folinic acid* rescue started at 24 hrs after the start of *methotrexate* in a dose of 15 mg every 12 hrs for 4 doses
Day 3	*Bleomycin* infusion 15 mg by 24-hr infusin
Day 4	*Cisplatin* 120 mg/M^2 as a 12-hr infusion, given together with hydration and 3 g magnesium sulfate supplementation

ACE

Days 1–5	*Etoposide* (VP16-213) 100 mg/M^2, days 1–5
Days 3, 4, 5	*Actinomycin D* 0.5 mg IV, days 3, 4, and 5
Day 5	*Cyclophosphamide* 500 mg/M^2 IV, day 5

OMB

Day 1	*Vincristine* 1 mg/M^2 intravenously; *methotrexate* 300 mg/M^2 as a 12-hr infusion
Day 2	*Bleomycin* 15 mg by 24-hr infusion; *folinic acid* rescue started at 24 hrs after start of *methotrexate* in a dose of 15 mg every 12 hrs for 4 doses
Day 3	*Bleomycin* 15 mg by 24-hr infusion

The sequence of treatment schedules is two courses of POMB followed by ACE. POMB is then alternated with ACE until patients are in biochemical remission as measured by hCG and AFP, PLAP and LDH. The usual number of courses of POMB is three to five. Following biochemical remission, patients alternate ACE with OMB until remission has been maintained for approximately 12 weeks. The interval between courses of treatment is kept to the minimum (usually 9 to 11 days). If delays are caused by myelosuppression after courses of ACE, the first 2 days of etoposide are omitted from subsequent courses of ACE. Reproduced with permission from **Newlands ES, Southall PJ, Paradinas FJ, Holden L.** Management of ovarian germ cell tumours. In: **Williams CJ, Kaikorian JG, Green MR, Ragharan D,** eds. *Textbook of Uncommon Cancer.* New York: John Wiley & Sons, 1988:47.

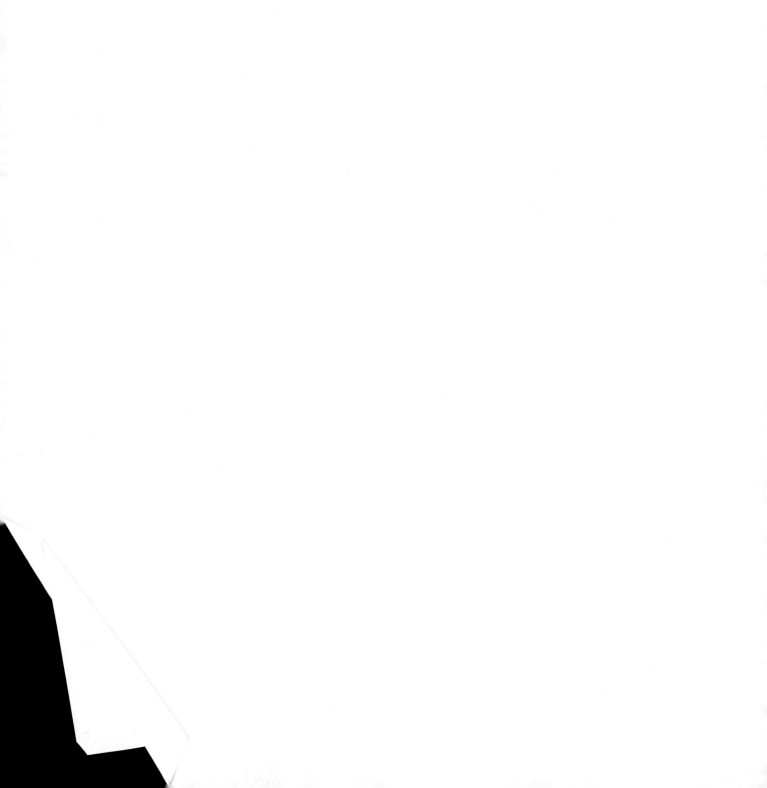

Appendix VIII: Staging of Cancer

Table 31.5   FIGO Definition for Grading of Endometrial Carcinoma

Histopathologic degree of differentiation:

G1: ≤5% nonsquamous or nonmorular growth pattern
G2: 6–50% nonsquamous or nonmorular growth pattern
G3: >50% nonsquamous or nonmorular growth pattern

Notes on pathologic grading:

1. Notable nuclear atypia, inappropriate for the architectural grade, raises the grade of a grade 1 or grade 2 tumor by one grade.
2. In serous adenocarcinoma, clear cell adenocarcinoma and squamous cell carcinoma, nuclear grading takes precedence.
3. Adenocarcinomas with squamous differentiation are graded according to the nuclear grade of the glandular component.

FIGO, International Federation of Gynecology and Obstetrics.

Table 31.6   1988 FIGO Surgical Staging for Endometrial Carcinoma

Stage Ia	**G123**	Tumor limited to endometrium
Ib	**G123**	Invasion to less than one-half of the myometrium
Ic	**G123**	Invasion to more than one-half of the myometrium
Stage IIa	**G123**	Endocervical glandular involvement only
IIb	**G123**	Cervical stromal invasion
Stage IIIa	**G123**	Tumor invades serosa and/or adnexa and/or positive peritoneal cytology
IIIb	**G123**	Vaginal metastases
IIIc	**G123**	Metastases to pelvic and/or para-aortic lymph nodes
Stage IVa	**G123**	Tumor invasion of bladder and/or bowel mucosa
IVb		Distant metastases including intra-abdominal and/or inguinal lymph nodes

FIGO, International Federation of Gynecology and Obstetrics.

Table 32.1   FIGO Staging of Carcinoma of the Cervix Uteri

Preinvasive Carcinoma
Stage 0   Carcinoma *in situ,* intraepithelial carcinoma (cases of Stage 0 should not be included in any therapeutic statistics).

Invasive Carcinoma
Stage I*   Carcinoma strictly confined to the cervix (extension to the corpus should be disregarded).
   Stage Ia   Preclinical carcinomas of the cervix, that is, those diagnosed only by microscopy.
     Stage Ia1   Lesion with ≤3 mm invasion
     Stage Ia2   Lesions detected microscopically that can be measured. The upper limit of the measurement should show a depth of invasion of >3–5 mm taken from the base of the epithelium, either surface or glandular, from which it originates, and a second dimension, the horizontal spread, must not exceed 7 mm. Larger lesions should be staged as Ib.
   Stage Ib   Lesions invasive >5 mm.
     Stage Ib1   Lesion less than or equal to 4 cm.
     Stage Ib2   Lesions larger than 4 cm.

Stage II†   The carcinoma extends beyond the cervix but has not extended onto the wall. The carcinoma involves the vagina, but not the lower one-third.
     Stage IIa   No obvious parametrial involvement.
     Stage IIb   Obvious parametrial involvement.

Stage III‡   The carcinoma has extended onto the pelvic wall. On rectal examination, there is no cancer-free space between the tumor and the pelvic wall. The tumor involves the lower one-third of the vagina. All cases with hydronephrosis or nonfunctioning kidney.
     Stage IIIa   No extension to the pelvic wall.
     Stage IIIb   Extension onto the pelvic wall and/or hydronephrosis or nonfunctioning kidney.

Stage IV§   The carcinoma has extended beyond the true pelvis or has clinically involved the mucosa of the bladder or rectum. A bullous edema, as such, does not permit a case to be allotted to Stage IV.
     Stage IVa   Spread to the growth to adjacent organs.
     Stage IVb   Spread to distant organs.

*The diagnosis of both Stage Ia1 and Ia2 should be based on microscopic examination of removed tissue, preferably a cone, which must include the entire lesion. The depth of invasion should not be more than 5 mm taken from the base of the epithelium, either surface or glandular, from which it originates. The second dimension, the horizontal spread, must not exceed 7 mm. Vascular space involvement, either venous or lymphatic, should not alter the staging but should be specifically recorded as it may affect treatment decisions in the future. Lesions of greater size should be staged as Ib. As a rule, it is impossible to estimate clinically whether a cancer of the cervix has extended to the corpus. Extension to the corpus should therefore be disregarded.
†A patient with a growth fixed to the pelvic wall by a short and indurated, but not nodular, parametrium should be allotted to Stage IIb. At clinical examination, it is impossible to decide whether a smooth, indurated parametrium is truly cancerous or only inflammatory. Therefore, the case should be assigned to Stage III only if the parametrium is nodular to the pelvic wall or the growth itself extends to the pelvic wall.
‡The presence of hydronephrosis or nonfunctioning kidney due to stenosis of the ureter by cancer permits a case to be allotted to Stage III even if, according to other findings, it should be allotted to Stage I or II.
§The presence of the bullous edema, as such, should not permit a case to be allotted to Stage IV. Ridges and furrows into the bladder wall should be interpreted as signs of submucous involvement of the bladder if they remain fixed to the growth at palpation (i.e., examination from the vagina or the rectum during cystoscopy). A cytologic finding of malignant cells in washings from the urinary bladder requires further examination and a biopsy specimen from the wall of the bladder.
FIGO, International Federation of Gynecology and Obstetrics.

Table 32.2   Staging Procedures

Physical examination*	Palpate lymph nodes
	Examine vagina
	Bimanual rectovaginal examination
	(under anesthesia recommended)
Radiologic studies*	Intravenous pyelogram
	Barium enema
	Chest x-ray
	Skeletal x-ray
Procedures*	Biopsy
	Conization
	Hysteroscopy
	Colposcopy
	Endocervical curettage
	Cystoscopy
	Proctoscopy
Optional studies†	Computerized axial tomography
	Lymphangiography
	Ultrasonography
	Magnetic resonance imaging
	Radionucleotide scanning
	Laparoscopy

*Allowed by the International Federation of Gynecology and Obstetrics (FIGO).
†Information that is not allowed by FIGO to change the clinical stage.

Table 32.6   FIGO Staging of Vaginal Cancer

Stage 0	Carcinoma *in situ,* intraepithelia carcinoma.
Stage I	The carcinoma is limited to the vaginal wall.
Stage II	The carcinoma has involved the subvaginal tissue but has not extended to the pelvic wall.
Stage III	The carcinoma has extended to the pelvic wall.
Stage IV	The carcinoma has extended beyond the true pelvis or has involved the mucosa of the bladder or rectum.
Stage IVa	Spread of the growth to adjacent organs.
Stage IVb	Spread to distant organs.

FIGO, International Federation of Gynecology and Obstetrics.

Table 33.2   FIGO Staging for Primary Carcinoma of the Ovary

Stage I		Growth limited to the ovaries.
	Stage Ia	Growth limited to one ovary; no ascites containing malignant cells. No tumor on the external surface; capsule intact.
	Stage Ib	Growth limited to both ovaries; no ascites containing malignant cells. No tumor on the external surfaces; capsules intact.
	*Stage Ic**	Tumor either stage Ia or Ib but with tumor on the surface of one or both ovaries; or with capsule ruptured; or with ascites present containing malignant cells or with positive peritoneal washings.
Stage II		Growth involving one or both ovaries with pelvic extension.
	Stage IIa	Extension and/or metastases to the uterus and/or tubes.
	Stage IIb	Extension to other pelvic tissues.
	*Stage IIc**	Tumor either stage IIa or IIb but with tumor on the surface of one or both ovaries; or with capsule(s) ruptured; or with ascites present containing malignant cells or with positive peritoneal washings.
Stage III		Tumor involving one or both ovaries with peritoneal implants outside the pelvis and/or positive retroperitoneal or inguinal nodes. Superficial liver metastasis equals stage III. Tumor is limited to the true pelvis, but with histologically proven malignant extension to small bowel or omentum.
	Stage IIIa	Tumor grossly limited to the true pelvis with negative nodes but with histologically confirmed microscopic seeding of abdominal peritoneal surfaces.
	Stage IIIb	Tumor of one or both ovaries with histologically confirmed implants of abdominal peritoneal surfaces, none exceeding 2 cm in diameter. Nodes negative.
	Stage IIIc	Abdominal implants >2 cm in diameter and/or positive retroperitoneal or inguinal nodes.
Stage IV		Growth involving one or both ovaries with distant metastasis. If pleural effusion is present, there must be positive cytologic test results to allot a case to stage IV. Parenchymal liver metastasis equals stage IV.

These categories are based on findings at clinical examination and/or surgical exploration. The histologic characteristics are to be considered in the staging, as are results of cytologic testing as far as effusions are concerned. It is desirable that a biopsy be performed on suspicious areas outside the pelvis.

*In order to evaluate the impact on prognosis of the different criteria for allotting cases to stage Ic or IIc, it would be of value to know if rupture of the capsule was 1) spontaneous or 2) caused by the surgeon and if the source of malignant cells detected was 1) peritoneal washings or 2) ascites.

Table 33.8   Surgical Stage of Fallopian Tube Cancer

Stage I   Carcinoma confined to fallopian tube(s)
    Stage Ia   Unilateral disease; no ascites
    Stage Ib   Bilateral disease; no ascites
    Stage Ic   Either *a* or *b* with ascites and/or neoplastic cells in peritoneal
            washings

Stage II   Carcinoma extends beyond fallopian tube(s) but confined to pelvis
    Stage IIa   Extension to uterus and/or ovary
    Stage IIb   Extension to other pelvic organs
    Stage IIc   Either *a* or *b* with ascites and/or neoplastic cells in peritoneal
            washings

Stage III   Carcinoma extends beyond pelvis but confined to abdominal cavity
    Stage IIIa   Tumor microscopic only
    Stage IIIb   Tumor metastasis ≤ 2 cm
    Stage IIIc   Tumor metastasis >2 cm

Stage IV   Carcinoma extends beyond abdominal cavity

Modified with permission from **Podratz KC, Podczaski ES, Gaffey TA, O'Brien PC, Schray MF, Malkasian GD Jr.** Primary carcinoma of the fallopian tube. *Am J Obstet Gynecol* 1986; 154:1319–26.

Table 34.5   Revised FIGO Staging for Vulvar Cancer

1988 FIGO Stage	*TNM*	*Clinical/Pathological Findings*
Stage 0	T_{IS}	Carcinoma *in situ,* intraepithelial carcinoma.
Stage I	$T_1N_0M_0$	Tumor confined to the vulva or perineum, <2 cm in greatest dimension, nodes are negative
Ia		Stromal invasion <1 mm
Ib		Stromal invasion $\geq$1 mm
Stage II	$T_2N_0M_0$	Tumor confined to the vulva and/or perineum, >2 cm in greatest dimension, nodes are negative.
Stage III	$T_3N_0M_0$	Tumor of any size with
	$T_3N_1M_0$	1. Adjacent spread to the lower urethra or the anus
	$T_1N_1M_0$	2. Unilateral regional lymph-node metastasis.
	$T_2N_1M_0$	
Stage IVA	$T_1N_2M_0$	Tumor invades any of the following:
	$T_2N_2M_0$	Upper urethra, bladder mucosa, rectal mucosa, pelvic bone or bilateral regional node metastasis.
	$T_3N_2M_0$	
	T_4 any N M_0	
Stage IVB	Any T, any N M_1	Any distant metastasis including pelvic lymph nodes

TNM Classification

T:	**Primary Tumor**
T_x	Primary tumor cannot be assessed
T_0	No evidence of primary tumor
T_{IS}	Carcinoma *in situ* (preinvasive carcinoma)
T_1	Tumor confined to the vulva and/or perineum 2 cm or less in greatest dimension
T_2	Tumor confined to the vulva and/or perineum more than 2 cm in greatest dimension
T_3	Tumor involves any of the following: lower urethra, vagina, anus
T_4	Tumor involves any of the following: bladder mucosa, rectal mucosa, upper urethra, pelvic bone

N:	**Regional Lymph Nodes**
	Regional lymph nodes are the femoral and inguinal nodes
N_x	Regional lymph nodes cannot be assessed
N_0	No lymph node metastasis
N_1	Unilteral regional lymph node metastasis
N_2	Bilateral regional lymph node metastasis

M:	**Distant Metastasis**
M	Presence of distant metastasis cannot be assessed
M_0	No distant metastasis
M_1	Distant metastasis (pelvic lymph node metastasis is M_1)

Table 34.6   Microstaging of Vulvar Melanomas

	Clark's Levels	Chung	Breslow
I	Intraepithelial	Intraepithelial	<0.76 mm
II	Into papillary dermis	≤1 mm from granular layer	0.76–1.50 mm
III	Filling dermal papillae	1.1–2 mm from granular layer	1.51–2.25 mm
IV	Into reticular dermis	>2 mm from granular layer	2.26–3.0 mm
V	Into subcutaneous fat	Into subcutaneous fat	>3 mm

Table 35.2   Staging of Gestational Trophoblastic Tumors

Stage I	**Disease confined to uterus**
Stage Ia	Disease confined to uterus with no risk factors
Stage Ib	Disease confined to uterus with one risk factor
Stage Ic	Disease confined to uterus with two risk factors
Stage II	**Gestational trophoblastic tumor extending outside uterus but limited to genital structures (adnexa, vagina, broad ligament)**
Stage IIa	Gestational trophoblastic tumor involving genital structures without risk factors
Stage IIb	Gestational trophoblastic tumor extending outside uterus but limited to genital structures with one risk factor
Stage IIc	Gestational trophoblastic tumor extending outside uterus but limited to genital structures with two risk factors
Stage III	**Gestational trophoblastic disease extending to lungs with or without known genital tract involvement**
Stage IIIa	Gestational trophoblastic tumor extending to lungs with or without genital tract involvement and with no risk factors
Stage IIIb	Gestational trophoblastic tumor extending to lungs with or without genital tract involvement and with one risk factor
Stage IIIc	Gestational trophoblastic tumor extending to lungs with or without genital tract involvement and with two risk factors
Stage IV	**All other metastatic sites**
Stage IVa	All other metastatic sites without risk factors
Stage IVb	All other metastatic sites with one risk factor
Stage IVc	All other metastatic sites with two risk factors

Risk factors affecting staging include the following: 1) human chorionic gonadotropin > 100,000 MIU/ml and 2) duration of disease longer than 6 months from termination of antecedent pregnancy.
The following factors should be considered and noted in reporting: 1) prior chemotherapy has been given for known gestational trophoblastic tumor; 2) placental site tumors should be reported separately; 3) histologic verification of disease is not required.

Table 36.1   Tumor–Nodes–Metastasis (TNM) Classification

Primary Tumor (T)

TX	Primary tumor cannot be assessed
TO	No evidence of primary tumor
Tis	Carcinoma *in situ:* intraductal carcinoma, lobular carcinoma *in situ,* or Paget's disease of the nipple with no tumor
T1	Tumor 2 cm or less in greatest dimension
T1a	0.5 cm or less in greatest dimension
T1b	More than 0.5 cm but not more than 1 cm in greatest dimension
T1c	More than 1 cm but not more than 2 cm in greatest dimension
T2	Tumor more than 2 cm but not more than 5 cm in greatest dimension
T3	Tumor more than 5 cm in greatest dimension
T4	Tumor of any size with direct extension to chest wall or skin
T4a	Extension to chest wall
T4b	Edema (including peau d'orange) or ulceration of the skin of breast or satellite skin nodules confined to same breast
T4c	Both T4a and T4b
T4d	Inflammatory carcinoma

Lymph Node (N)

NX	Regional lymph nodes cannot be assessed (e.g., previously removed)
N0	No regional lymph node metastasis
N1	Metastasis to movable ipsilateral axillary lymph node(s)
N2	Metastasis to ipsilateral axillary lymph node(s) fixed to one another or to other structures
N3	Metastasis to ipsilateral internal mammary lymph node(s)

Pathologic Classification (pN)

pNX	Regional lymph nodes cannot be assessed (e.g., previously removed or not removed for pathologic study)
pN0	No regional lymph node metastasis
pN1	Metastasis to movable ipsilateral axillary lymph node(s)
pN1a	Only micrometastasis (none larger than 0.2 cm)
pN1b	Metastasis to lymph nodes, any larger than 0.2 cm
pN1bi	Metastasis in one to three lymph nodes, any more than 0.2 cm and all less than 2 cm in greatest dimension
pN1bii	Metastasis to four or more lymph nodes, any more than 0.2 cm and all less than 2 cm in greatest dimension
pN1biii	Extension of tumor beyond the capsule of a lymph node metastasis less than 2 cm in greatest dimension
pN1biv	Metastasis to a lymph node 2 cm or more in greatest dimension
pN2	Metastasis to ipsilateral axillary lymph nodes that are fixed to one another or to other structures
pN3	Metastasis to ipsilateral internal mammary lymph node(s)

Distant Metastasis (M)

MX	Presence of distant metastasis cannot be assessed
M0	No distant metastasis
M1	Distant metastasis (includes metastasis to ipsilateral supraclavicular lymph node(s))

Reproduced with permission from **Beahrs OH, Henson DE, Hutter RVP, Kennedy BJ.** *American Joint Committee on Cancer: Manual for Staging of Cancer.* 4th ed. Philadelphia: JB Lippincott, 1992:153.

Table 36.2   Staging of Breast Carcinoma

| Stage | <TNM Classification* | | |
	Tumor	Node	Metastasis
Stage 0	Tis	N0	M0
Stage I	T1	N0	M0
Stage IIA	T0	N1†	M0
	T1	N1*	M0
	T2	N0	M0
Stage IIB	T2	N1	M0
	T3	N0	M0
Stage IIIA	T0	N2	M0
	T1	N2	M0
	T2	N2	M0
	T3	N1	M0
	T3	N2	M0
Stage IIIB	T4	Any N	M0
	Any T	N3	M0
Stage IV	Any T	Any N	M1

*See Table 36.1.
†*Note:* The prognosis of patients with N1a is similar to that of patients with pN0.
Reproduced with permission from **Beahrs OH, Henson DE, Hutter RVP, Kennedy BJ.** *American Joint Committee on Cancer: Manual for Staging of Cancer.* 4th ed. Philadelphia: JB Lippincott, 1992:152.

Appendix IX: Reference Values

Measure	SI	Conventional (C)	Conversion Factor (CF) $C \times CF = SI$
Acetoacetate, plasma	<100 μmol/l	<1.0 mg/dl	97.95
Adrenal steroids, plasma			
Aldosterone, supine, saline suppression	<220 pmol/l	<8 ng/dl	27.74
Cortisol			
8:00 AM	220–660 nmol/l	8–24 μg/dl	27.59
4:00 PM	50–410 nmol/l	2–15 μg/dl	27.59
Overnight dexamethasone suppression	<140 nmol/l	<5 μg/dl	27.59
Dehydroepiandrosterone (DHEA)	0.6–70 nmol/l	0.2–20 μg/l	3.467
Dehydroepiandrosterone sulfate (DHEAS)	5.4–9.2 μmol/l	820–3380 ng/ml	0.002714
11-Deoxycortisol (compound S)	<60 nmol/l	<2 μg/dl	28.86
17α-Hydroxyprogesterone, women	1–13 nmol/l	0.3–4.2 μg/l	3.026
Adrenal steroids, urinary excretion			
Aldosterone	15–70 nmol/d	5–26 μg/d	2.774
Cortisol, free	30–300 nmol/d	10–100 μg/d	2.759
17-Hydroxycorticosteroids	5.5–28 μmol/d	2–10 mg/d	2.759
17-Ketosteroids, women	14–52 μmol/d	4–15 mg/d	3.467
Ammonia (as NH_3), venous whole blood	6–45 μmol/l	10–80 μg/dl	0.5872
Angiotensin II, plasma, 8 AM	10–30 ng/l	10–30 pg/ml	1.0
Arginine vasopressin (AVP), plasma, random fluid intake	2.3–7.4 pmol/l	2.5–8 ng/l	0.92
Bicarbonate, serum	18–23 mmol/l	18–23 meq/l	1.0
Calciferols (see vitamin D)			
Calcitonin, serum	<50 ng/l	<50 pg/ml	1.0
Calcium			
Ionized serum	1–1.5 mmol/l	4–4.6 mg/dl	0.2495
Total serum	2.2–2.6 mmol/l	9–10.5 mg/dl	0.2495
β-Carotene, serum	0.9–4.6 μmol/l	50–250 μg/dl	0.01863
Catecholamines, plasma			
Epinephrine, basal supine	170–520 pmol/l	30–95 pg/ml	5.458
Norepinephrine, basal supine	0.3–2.8 nmol/l	15–475 pg/ml	0.005911
Catecholamines, urinary			
Epinephrine	<275 nmol/d	<50 μg/d	5.458
Normetanephrine	0–11 μmol/d	0–2.0 mg/d	5.458
Total catecholamines (as norepinephrine)	<675 nmol/d	<120 μg/d	5.911
Vanillylmandelic acid (VMA)	<35 μmol/d	<68 mg/d	5.046
Chloride, serum	98–106 mmol/l	98–106 meq/l	1.0
Cholesterol, plasma			
Total cholesterol			
Desirable	<5.20 mmol/l	<200 mg/dl	0.02586
Borderline high	5.2–6.18 mmol/l	200–239 mg/dl	0.02586
High	≥6.21 mmol/l	≥240 mg/dl	0.02586
High-density lipoprotein (HDL) cholesterol			
Desirable	≥1.29 mmol/l	≥50 mg/dl	0.02586
Borderline high	0.9–1.27 mmol/l	36–49 mg/dl	0.02586
High	≤0.91 mmol/l	≤35 mg/dl	0.02586
Low-density lipoprotein (LDL) cholesterol			
Desirable	<3.36 mmol/l	<130 mg/dl	0.02586
Borderline high	3.39–4.11 mmol/l	131–159 mg/dl	0.02586
High	≥4.14 mmol/l	≥160 mg/dl	0.02586
Corticotropin (ACTH), plasma	4–22 pmol/l	20–100 pg/ml	0.2202
C peptide, plasma	0.5–2 μg/l	0.5–2 ng/ml	1.0
Creatinine, serum	<133 μmol/l	<1.5 mg/dl	88.40
Fatty acids, nonesterified or free (FFA), plasma	<0.7 mmol/l	<18 mg/dl	0.03906
Gastrin, serum	<120 ng/l	<120 pg/ml	1.0
Glucagon, plasma	50–100 ng/l	50–100 pg/ml	1.0
Glucose, plasma			
Overnight fast, normal	4.2–6.4 mmol/l	75–115 mg/dl	0.05551
Overnight fast, diabetes mellitus	7.8 mmol/l	>140 mg/dl	0.05551
72-hour fast, normal women	>2.2 mmol/l	>40 mg/dl	0.05551
Glucose tolerance test, 2-hour postprandial plasma glucose			
Normal	<7.8 mmol/l	<140 mg/dl	0.05551
Imparied glucose tolerance	7.8–11.1 mmol/l	140–200 mg/dl	0.05551
Diabetes mellitus	>11.1 mmol/l	>200 mg/dl	0.05551

Measure	SI	Conventional (C)	Conversion Factor (CF) C × CF = SI
Gonadal steroids, plasma			
Androstenedione, women	3.5–7.0 nmol/l	1–2 ng/ml	3.492
Estradiol, women			
Basal	70–220 pmol/l	20–60 pg/ml	3.671
Ovulatory surge	>740 pmol/l	>200 pg/ml	3.671
Dihydrotestosterone, women	0.17–1.0 nmol/l	0.05–3 ng/ml	3.467
Progesterone, women			
Luteal phase	6–64 nmol/l	2–20 ng/ml	3.180
Follicular phase	<6 nmol/l	<2 ng/ml	3.180
Testosterone			
Women	<3.5 nmol/l	<1 ng/ml	3.467
Prepubertal boys and girls	0.2–0.7 nmol/l	0.05–0.2 ng/ml	3.467
Gonadotropins, plasma			
Women, basal			
Follicle-stimulating hormone	5–20 IU/l	5–20 mIU/ml	1.0
Luteinizing hormone	5–25 IU/l	5–25 mIU/ml	1.0
Women, ovulatory peak			
Follicle-stimulating hormone	12–30 IU/l	12–30 mIU/ml	1.0
Luteinizing hormone	25–100 IU/l	25–100 mIU/ml	1.0
Prepubertal boys and girls			
Follicle-stimulating hormone	<5 IU/l	<5 mIU/ml	1.0
Luteinizing hormone	<5 IU/l	<5 mIU/ml	1.0
Growth hormone, plasma			
After 100 g glucose orally	<5 µg/l	<5 ng/ml	1.0
After insulin-induced hypoglycemia	>9 µg/l	>9 ng/ml	1.0
Human chorionic gonadotropin, beta subunit, plasma; nonpregnant women	<3 IU/l	<3 mIU/ml	1.0
β-Hydroxybutyrate, plasma	<300 nmol/l	<3.0 mg/dl	96.05
Insulin, plasma			
Fasting	35–145 pmol/l	5–20 µU/ml	7.175
During hypoglycemia (plasma glucose <2.8 nmol/l [<50 mg/dl])	<35 pmol/l	<5 µU/ml	7.175
Insulin-like growth factor I (IGF I, somatomedin-C), women	0.45–2.2 kU/l	0.45–2.2 U/ml	1.0
Lactate, plasma	0.56–2.2 mmol/l	5–20 mg/dl	0.111
Magnesium, serum	0.8–1.20 mmol/l	1.8–3.0 mg/dl	0.4114
Osmolality, plasma	285–295 mmol/kg	285–295 mosm/kg	1.0
Oxytocin, plasma			
Random	1–4 pmol/l	1.25–5 ng/l	0.80
Ovulatory peak in women	408 pmol/l	5–10 ng/l	0.80
Parathyroid hormone, serum (intact PTH using immunoradiometric assay [IRMA])	10–65 ng/l	10–65 pg/ml	1.0
Phosphorus, inorganic, serum	1–1.5 mmol/l	3.0–4.5 mg/dl	0.3229
Potassium, serum	3.5–5.0 mmol/l	3.5–5.0 meq/l	1.0
Prolactin, serum	2–15 µg/l	2–15 ng/ml	1.0
Pyruvate, blood	39–102 µmol/l	0.3–0.9 mg/dl	0.01129
Renin activity, plasma, normal-sodium diet			
Supine	3.2 ± 1 µg/l/h	3.2 ± 1.1 ng/ml/h	1.0
Standing	9.3 ± 4.3 µg/l/h	9.3 ± 4.3 ng/ml/h	1.0
Sodium, serum	136–145 mmol/l	136–145 meq/l	1.0
Thyroid function tests			
Radioactive iodine uptake, 24 hours	0.05–0.30	5–30%	—
Reverse triiodothyronine (rT_3), serum	0.15–0.61 nmol/l	10–4 ng/dl	0.01536
Thyrotropin (TSH), highly sensitive assay, serum	0.6–4.6 mU/l	0.6–4.6 µU/ml	1.0
Thyroxine (T_4), serum	51–42 nmol/l	4–11 µg/dl	12.87
Thyroxine-binding globulin, serum (as thyroxine)	150–360 nmol/l	12–28 µg/ml	12.87
Triiodothyronine (T_3), serum	1.2–3.4 nmol/l	75–220 ng/dl	0.01536
Triiodothyronine resin uptake, serum	0.25–0.35	25–35%	—
Triglycerides, plasma (as Triolein)	<1.80 mmol/l	<160 mg/dl	0.01129
Uric acid, serum	120–420 µmol/l	2–7 mg/dl	59.48
Vitamin D (as vitamin D_3, cholecalciferol), plasma			
1,25-Dihydroxycholecalciferol (1,25($OH)_2$D)	36–144 pmol/l	15–60 pg/ml	2.400
25-Hydroxycholecalciferol (25-OHD)	20–100 nmol/l	8–40 ng/ml	2.496

Modified with permission from **Wilson JD, Foster DW.** *Williams Textbook of Endocrinology,* 8th ed. Philadelphia: WB Saunders, 1991.

Index